Outcome-Based Massage

Outcome-Based Massage

Carla-Krystin Andrade, PhD, PT

Assistant Clinical Professor
University of California-San Francisco/San Francisco State University Graduate Program
   in Physical Therapy
Department of Physical Therapy and Rehabilitation Sciences, School of Medicine,
   University of California San Francisco
San Francisco, California
Physical Therapist (on call)
Pacifica Nursing and Rehabilitation Center
Pacifica, California

Paul Clifford, BSc, MT

Professor, Massage Therapy Program
Sir Sandford Fleming College
Peterborough, Ontario, Canada
Private practice: Peterborough, Ontario, Canada

Photographs by **Marc Boulay**

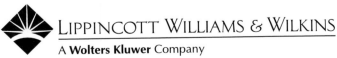

LIPPINCOTT WILLIAMS & WILKINS
A **Wolters Kluwer** Company
Philadelphia · Baltimore · New York · London
Buenos Aires · Hong Kong · Sydney · Tokyo

Editor: John Butler
Managing Editor: Ulita Lushnycky
Marketing Manager: Debby Hartman
Production Editor: Lisa JC Franko

351 West Camden Street
Baltimore, Maryland 21201-2436 USA

530 Walnut Street
Philadelphia, Pennsylvania 19106-3621 USA

Printed in the United States of America

Library of Congress Cataloging-in-Publication Data

Andrade, Carla-Krystin
   Outcome-based massage / Carla-Krystin Andrade, Paul Clifford
      p. cm.
   ISBN 0-7817-1743-4
    1. Massage. 2. Massage—Decision making. I. Andrade, Carla-Krystin, 1962. II. Title.
   RA780.5 .C575 2000
   615.8'22—dc21
                                                  00-050677

To purchase additional copies of this book call our customer service department at **(800) 638-3030** or fax orders to **(301) 824-7390.** International customers should call **(301) 714-2324.**

Visit Lippincott Williams & Wilkins on the Internet: http://www.lww.com. Lippincott Williams & Wilkins customer service representatives are available from 8:30 am to 6:00 pm, EST, Monday through Friday, for telephone access.

01 02
1 2 3 4 5 6 7 8 9 10

Life is short, the art long, opportunity fleeting,
experience treacherous, judgment difficult.

HIPPOCRATES, APHORISMS I.I.

TO
Dr. Ernest James Clifford, MB (1891–1981)
Dr. John Frank Kramer, PhD, PT

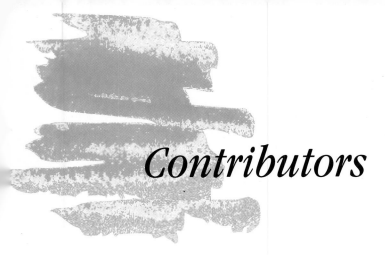

Contributors

Paula Tanksley, BA, MPT
Private practice: Tanksley Physical Therapy
Oakland, California
(Soft-tissue examination techniques and
    complementary techniques)

Stephen Goring, BSc, MA, MT
Private practice
Toronto, Ontario, Canada
(Client's emotional response to massage treatment)

Teresa Randall, MPT
Staff Physical Therapist
Alameda County Medical Center—Fairmont Campus
Oakland, California
(Strategies to enhance client adherence)

List of Reviewers

The authors wish to extend their sincerest thanks to the following individuals who reviewed portions of the manuscript and provided constructive feedback during critical stages of the development of this text. Their thought-provoking comments prompted much discussion and helped us refine the final content.

Lippincott Williams & Wilkins Reviewers

Carol J. Bancroft, PT
Coordinator, Physical Therapist
  Assistant Program
Delaware Technical and
  Community College
Wilmington, Delaware

James Creelman, PT, MS, OCS, MTC
Assistant Professor
Idaho State University
Pocatello, Idaho

James W. Farris, PhD
Assistant Professor
Arkansas State University
State University, Arkansas

Marie L. Koch, MS, PT
Assistant Professor & Director of
  Clinical Education
Quinnipiac College
Hamden, Connecticut

Kathy Mercuris, PT, MGS
Associate Professor
Des Moines University
Des Moines, Iowa

E. Anne Rura, MEd, PT
Instructor
Howard University
Washington, District of Columbia

Ellen Ward, PT, MHS
Academic Coordinator/Assistant Professor
Arizona School of Health Sciences
Phoenix, Arizona

Kriota Willburg, BA, LMT
Chair
Western Massage Department
Swedish Institute
New York, New York

Donna Ziarkowski-Herb, MEd, PT, CHT
Gersinger Medical Center
Danville, Pennsylvania

Clinician Reviewers

Bridget Bouyssounouse, BS, PT
Senior Physical Therapist
Kaiser Permanente: Santa Clara Occupational
    Health Center
Santa Clara, California

Sandi Chan, BS, PT
Senior Physical Therapist
Kaiser Permanente: Santa Clara Occupational
    Health Center
Santa Clara, California

Tara Detwiler, Certified Advanced Rolfer
Private practice
Toronto, Ontario, Canada

Alexandra N. Fallot, BA, MPT
Physical Therapist
Pacifica Nursing and Rehabilitation Center
Pacifica, California

Meghan Gordineer, MPT
Physical Therapy Coordinator
Kaiser Permanente: Santa Clara Occupational
    Health Center
Santa Clara, California

Stephen Goring, BSc, MA, MT
Private practice
Toronto, Ontario, Canada

Betty Ann Harris, BSc, MT
Mobile Massage
Peterborough, Ontario, Canada
Director, Chair of Research and Clinical Issues
    Committee
Ontario Massage Therapist Association

Shawn Jarman, MPT
Senior Physical Therapist
Kaiser Permanente: Santa Clara Occupational
    Health Center
Santa Clara, California

Lee Kalpin, MT
Park Avenue Massage Therapy
Holland Landing, Ontario, Canada
Peer Assessor, College of Massage Therapist of Ontario

Liz Lester, MT
Mulock Chiropractic
Newmarket, Ontario, Canada

Wendy Moore, BA, MSc, MD, FRCP(C)
St. Joseph's Health Centre
Toronto, Ontario, Canada

Gaye Raymond, BS, MS, PT
Director of Rehabilitation
Pacifica Nursing and Rehabilitation Center
Pacifica, California

Kenneth Resznyak, MT
West End Massage Therapy
Toronto, Ontario, Canada

**Jarek Szymczak, MT, Certified Lymph Drainage
    Therapist (Uodder, Germany)**
Manual Lymph Drainage Practitioner
Private practice
Toronto, Ontario, Canada

Paula Tanksley, BA, MPT
Private practice: Tanksley Physical Therapy
Oakland, California

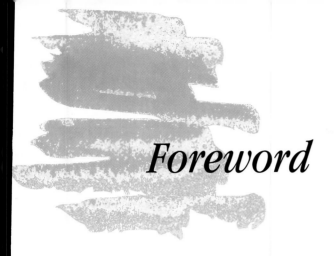

Foreword

I am delighted to write this Foreword for *Outcome-Based Massage* written by Carla-Krystin Andrade, PhD, PT, and Paul Clifford, BSc, MT. Dr. Andrade, Mr. Clifford, and their editor, Margaret Biblis, along with experienced clinicians and clinical specialists, need to be commended on the rigorous outcome-based content that serves as the foundation for this book. This is the first text I have reviewed on the subject of massage that meets the criteria to promote scientific investigation and evidence-based practice. This book is not only appropriate as a text for an entry-level academic program, but it is also an excellent review and guide for the practicing clinician.

Dr. Andrade and Mr. Clifford provide an excellent conceptual framework for clinicians to understand the different types of massage. They outline the theories about outcome-based assessment, as well as the various disablement models that need to be considered when applying massage techniques. While providing a structured framework to evaluate outcomes, they also review the concepts of touch and logically categorize the various techniques that have been developed within the framework of massage.

The authors carefully lay the foundation for the client examination needed to provide the basis for treating with massage techniques. The authors highlight the differences in the clinical examination for treatment with massage as distinguished from the standard clinical examination. In this process, the relevant impairments receptive to remediation by massage are outlined.

In addition to comprehensive descriptions of massage techniques and their variations, each chapter on techniques ends with a specific clinical example that takes the reader through the process from diagnosis to discharge, including measurement, treatment planning, and treatment outcomes. In their discussions of treatment planning, the authors make it very clear that massage is one aspect of the client's total treatment. Furthermore, they emphasize that providers must be sensitive to the broad, as well as the specific, issues that challenge recovery, regardless of the impairment.

Massage is no longer the most common treatment in rehabilitation. Unfortunately, within the current health care environment, many clinicians have moved away from "hands-on" treatment as a regular part of their intervention strategy. In some cases, this is driven by the lack of the provider's time with the client, reimbursement issues, the passive nature of the technique, or the perceived lack of research evidence supporting the specific physiological effects of the different massage techniques. However, we know that touching a person in a safe environment can have measurable benefits. For these reasons, *Outcome-Based Massage* is timely. In this book, the principles of scientific inquiry are meticulously integrated into the technical and humanistic aspects of care. This link between science and practice is not only strong at the beginning of the book, but is emphasized throughout every chapter.

I commend Dr. Andrade, Mr. Clifford, and their team for preparing a rigorous academic text on massage. This is long overdue. I feel confident that clinicians, faculty, students, and even some patients will find this an excellent reference textbook for learning.

Nancy N. Byl, PhD, PT, FAPTA
Professor and Interim Chair
Department of Physical Therapy and Rehabilitation
*   Science School of Medicine, University of*
*   California San Francisco*
University of California San Francisco/San Francisco
*   State University Graduate Program in Physical*
*   Therapy*
San Francisco, California

Acknowledgments

We are indebted to Margaret Biblis for sharing our vision for this book and for her dedication to making this project a reality. We thank Peg Waltner, Ulita Lushnycky, Amy Amico, and all the staff at Lippincott Williams & Wilkins who shepherded our manuscript through the various stages of production. We are grateful for the assistance of Marc Boulay, our photographer, for his expertise and endurance during demanding photography sessions, and for the fine photographs that contribute so much to this book. We extend our sincere thanks to the clinicians and client models who worked with patience and discipline in circumstances as unlike a practice setting as can be imagined: Christopher Alger, Tricia Bachman, Joanne Baker, Dan Boon, Paul Bucciero, Brian Burgess, Melissa Cole, D!ONNE (Francis), Lee Kalpin, Rahima Kassam, Michael Kitney, Amy Knapp, Frank Marincola, Colin Outram, Shahnaz Sadrudin, Jarek Szymczak, and Jane Wellwood. We appreciate the support of the administration of the Canadian College of Massage and Hydrotherapy who donated the space for the photography sessions. We recognize that, in many ways, this book reflects the contribution of the numerous clinicians who have educated us with their hands, hearts, and minds and the countless students and clients who unwittingly goaded us into creating this book, and we thank them wholeheartedly. On a personal note, we are deeply grateful to all the members of our families who have supported us in countless ways with unfailing grace and generosity throughout our careers and during the course of a grueling five-year project.

Paul also wishes to thank his dear friends Anne-Shirley Clough, Stephen Goring, Kerry Garvey, Patrick McNamara, Marion Moore, Wendy Moore, Dave Moulton, Rita O'Connor, Ruth Roberts, Shelley Smith, and Mike Sweeney for being such unapologetically unique individuals and for keeping in touch and enduring this obsession; his friends and guides at St. Andrew's United, Affirm United Sunday Evening Meditation, and the Dharma Centre of Canada for bringing him back to what matters; and Carla-Krystin for persevering with this project when she had really good reasons to drop it on two occasions.

Carla-Krystin also wishes to thank John Kramer, her mentor in physical therapy, for unselfishly providing professional guidance, assistance, and all-round good advice since 1987; her son Alan for being an endless source of joy and for reintroducing her to the wonders of everyday life; her husband Len for his support; and Paul for being a true friend and for sustaining this project while she endured "the pregnancy from hell" and experienced the joys and travails of new motherhood.

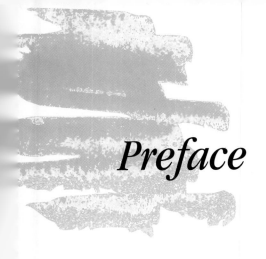

Preface

Although in North America massage is currently characterized as a part of "alternative" or "complementary" medicine, throughout much of medical history and elsewhere in the world, massage has been regarded as an important component of mainstream health care. Indeed, many of the greatest and most rigorous proponents of the clinical use of massage techniques—from Hippocrates to Mezger, Kellogg, Mennell, Cyriax, and most recently Travell and Simons—have been physicians. Recently, the health care community has shown a renewed interest in the clinical use of massage techniques and in research on the clinical outcomes that can be achieved with massage techniques. This change has created a need for an approach to education in massage that is consistent with the outcome-based focus of current health care practices.

We believe that there is a place for the appropriate use of massage techniques within the clinical practice of a number of diverse health care professions whose scopes of practice incorporate manual techniques, such as physical therapy, occupational therapy, physiatry, nursing, massage therapy, chiropractic, and athletic training. Furthermore, we observe that the use of massage techniques to achieve specific outcomes of clinical care most often demands highly developed cognitive and psychomotor skills, not merely a mechanical laying on of hands. Consequently, *Outcome-Based Massage* is a detailed exposition of the clinical decision-making and psychomotor skills that we believe are required for health care professionals to use massage techniques effectively to achieve specified outcomes related to the promotion of wellness and the remediation of the impairments, functional limitations, and disability associated with clinical conditions.

The goal of *Outcome-Based Massage* is to provide both a conceptual framework and a concrete methodology for using massage techniques to achieve specified clinical outcomes. This book is intended to be used by health care professionals whose scope of practice permits them to perform manual techniques. We have deliberately included material at a range of different levels so that this text can be useful to students, to novice clinicians, and to advanced clinicians who wish to use an outcome-based approach in their clinical practice.

Outcome-Based Massage will guide you through the steps of a four-phase clinical decision-making model that comprises the evaluative phase, the treatment planning phase, the treatment phase, and the discharge phase. Through this process, you will learn how to identify relevant impairments through the client examination, select appropriate massage techniques for treating these impairments and achieving relevant functional outcomes, plan interventions that integrate massage techniques with other appropriate techniques, apply massage techniques using correct manual technique, and progress treatment regimens from the initial intervention to discharge.

Part 1 of *Outcome-Based Massage,* titled Client Examination and Treatment Planning, is concerned with, the initial stages of clinical decision making that form the foundation of clinical care. Chapter 1 outlines the role of conceptual frameworks in clinical practice and presents the conceptual frameworks that provide the foundation for outcome-based massage: the current disablement models, Donabedian's framework of the components of clinical care, and the authors' framework of Intelligent Touch. This chapter also introduces a classification system for massage techniques that is based on the tissue layers that are treated and the outcomes that can be achieved with a technique, rather than the customary division between "traditional" and "modern" techniques. Chapter 2 provides the details of the four-phase clinical decision-making process, along with a clinical case that illustrates the application of this process to clinical care. This decision-making model outlines the steps that the clinician uses to formulate a clinical hypothesis about the client's clinical condition, select tests and measures for the client examination, summarize and analyze clinical findings, confirm or refute the clinical hypothesis, identify appropriate impairment-level and functional outcomes of care, select treatment techniques that can be used to achieve the identified outcomes, develop a plan of care, use the findings from client reexaminations to refine and progress interventions, plan for discharge, and discharge the client. It also addresses the interpersonal aspects of the process of clinical care, such as the client–clinician interaction and the client's emotional response to treatment, as well as the technical aspects of providing care. In addition, this chapter introduces 23 categories of musculoskeletal, neurological, cardiopulmonary, and psychoneuroimmunological impairment-level outcomes of care that can be achieved using massage techniques. Chapter 3 identifies the unique aspects of the client examination for massage and provides an overview of palpatory and nonpalpatory approaches to assessing impairments, functional limitations, disability, and quality-of-life issues that are relevant to the use of massage techniques.

Treatment and Discharge is the second part of *Outcome-Based Massage,* which has a greater emphasis on psychomotor skills, in addition to discussing the clinical decision-making skills used to refine and progress treatment regimens. Chapter 4 describes the methods by which the clinician completes the psychological, physical, and material preparation for treatment, as well as the techniques for positioning and draping the client for treatment. Chapters 5 through 10 introduce categories of related massage techniques: Superficial Reflex Techniques, Superficial Fluid Techniques, Neuromuscular Techniques, Connective Tissue Techniques, Passive Movement Techniques, and Percussive Techniques. These chapters detail the cognitive and psychomotor skills required to apply the 17 types of massage techniques presented within a therapeutic treatment. These chapters also include discussions of the descriptive components, outcomes of care, indications, contraindications, cautions, complementary techniques, and posttreatment care associated with each technique. In each chapter, a clinical example is used to demonstrate how to use the client's impairments and functional limitations to guide the selection of massage and other techniques for a plan of care. Finally, Chapter 11 describes the principles and process that clinicians can use

to design massage sequences and to progress treatment regimens that incorporate massage techniques from the initial intervention to discharge.

A combination of diverse backgrounds is required to do justice to the different, yet complementary, components—clinical decision-making and psychomotor skills—that are presented in *Outcome-Based Massage.* Paul, a registered Massage Therapist, brought to this text his expertise in massage and treatment planning that he developed through his extensive manual training and his background practicing massage in varied clinical settings. He created the approach to Intelligent Touch and teaching the psychomotor skills of massage through his experience in classroom and clinical teaching of massage theory and technique, orthopedic assessment, treatment planning, and remedial exercise. Paul conceptualized the classification of massage techniques used in *Outcome-Based Massage* based on his comprehensive training in classical massage, Rolfing®, and Trager®, and on his studies on other massage-related techniques. Carla-Krystin's areas of specialization, in addition to being a licensed Physical Therapist, were critical thinking, clinical decision-making, and outcome measurement. She developed the approach to using conceptual frameworks and outcomes to guide treatment planning and clinical practice presented in *Outcome-Based Massage* through her doctoral studies in measurement and program evaluation theory; her years as a clinical researcher; and her experience teaching courses in conceptual frameworks, clinical decision making, foundations of evaluation and diagnosis, program evaluation, and quality assurance and research methodologies for physical therapists, occupational therapists, nurses, and physicians. In addition, she used her background in teaching clinical skills to physical therapy and massage therapy students and novice clinicians to provide a clinical context for the conceptual material. Together we contributed our years of clinical experience and our passionate belief in a problem-solving approach to the provision of exemplary clinical care and the central role of massage techniques in health care. We trust that our approach does justice to the lineage of fine authors of works on massage techniques and physical medicine and rehabilitation to whom we are in debt, and that contributes to the ongoing restoration of an ancient discipline to a more honored place among the healing arts.

Carla-Krystin Andrade
Paul Clifford
April 2000

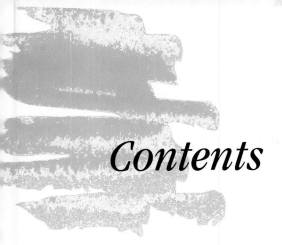

Contents

Outcome-Based Massage

I

Client Examination and Treatment Planning

*T*o use massage aright, we must consider it entirely as a means to an end, the end being the restoration of function. Every movement performed should have this end in view; and the masseur should be able to show, in reasoned detail, what effect it is hoped will result from each movement of the hand or finger, and what part this effect is expected to play in the restoration of function.

Dr. James B. Mennell. Massage: Its Principles and Practice. 2ND Ed. Philadelphia, PA: Blakistons; 1920:4.

The chapters in this section provide the conceptual foundation for outcome-based massage and cover the first two phases of the clinical decision-making process: the Evaluative Phase and the Treatment Planning Phase. Chapter 1 outlines the role of conceptual frameworks in clinical practice and presents the conceptual frameworks that provide the foundation for outcome-based massage: the disablement model, Donabedian's framework of the components of clinical care, and the authors' framework of Intelligent Touch. This chapter also introduces a classification system for massage techniques that is based on the tissue layers that are treated and the outcomes of care that can be achieved with a technique. Chapter 2 details the steps in the 4-phase clinical decision-making process that guide the approach to outcome-based massage used throughout the text: Evaluative Phase, Treatment Planning Phase, Treatment Phase, and Discharge Phase. In addition, this chapter introduces 23 categories of impairment-level outcomes of care that can be achieved using massage techniques. Chapter 3 identifies the unique aspects of the client examination for massage and provides an overview of palpatory and nonpalpatory approaches to assessing impairments, functional limitations, disability, and quality-of-life issues that are relevant to the use of massage techniques.

Section Objectives

After studying this section, the reader will be able to:

1. Outline the clinician's skills that are essential for the practice of Intelligent Touch.
2. Define the terms disease, pathophysiology, impairment, functional limitation, disability, and quality of life.
3. Identify the components of the structure, process, and outcomes of clinical care.
4. Distinguish between the technical and interpersonal aspects of the process of clinical care.
5. Describe the four phases of the clinical decision-making process for outcome-based massage: Evaluative Phase, Treatment Planning Phase, Treatment Phase, and Discharge Phase.
6. Describe how to formulate and select tests and measures to confirm a clinical hypothesis about a client's clinical condition.
7. List the steps in synthesizing clinical findings and creating a clinical problem list.

8. List impairments that can be treated and the impairment-level outcomes that can be achieved with massage techniques.

9. Formulate impairment-level and functional outcomes of care that are relevant to the use of massage techniques.

10. Outline how to select massage and other appropriate techniques required to remediate impairments and achieve identified functional outcomes of care and integrate these into a plan of care.

11. Identify the process by which the findings from the client re-examinations are used to modify, refine, and progress interventions.

12. Describe how to identify the client's discharge needs, plan for discharge, and discharge a client.

13. Identify the ethical issues involved in clinical care.

14. Discuss the client's possible emotional response to treatment and strategies for handling this response appropriately.

15. Outline strategies that can be used to enhance the client's adherence to the plan of care.

16. Describe the unique elements of a client examination for massage.

17. Discuss how to perform palpation.

18. Identify the impairments that can be assessed using palpation.

19. Describe a variety of nonpalpatory approaches to assessing the impairments that are relevant to massage.

1

Conceptual Frameworks for Outcome-Based Massage

Conceptual frameworks provide clinicians with a means of making sense of their clinical observations, and conceptual models enable them to communicate these frameworks. The models of disablement,[1] Donabedian's conceptual framework of the Components of Clinical Care,[2] the conceptual framework of Intelligent Touch, and the approach to classification of massage techniques presented in this text can be used to guide outcome-based massage and to clarify the concept of functional outcomes that are currently central to clinical care.

Outcome-Based Massage

Traditionally, the practice of massage has involved the application of general or regional sequences of massage strokes as a means of achieving specific therapeutic effects in the treatment of clinical conditions.[3] Outcome-based massage builds on that foundation to provide clinicians from a variety of health care disciplines with a strategy for integrating the use of massage techniques into their clinical practice. Outcome-based massage has several defining features that are outlined in Box 1-1.

First, this approach is based on clearly articulated conceptual frameworks of clinical care and the practice of massage that are described in this chapter. It proposes a system of classifying massage techniques on the basis of the tissue layers that they treat and the outcomes they achieve. Outcome-based massage also involves the use of a systematic clinical decision-making process and a defined process for integrating massage techniques into clinical interventions.

Theories, Conceptual Frameworks, and Conceptual Models

THEORIES

Clinicians are familiar with numerous theories: organized sets of facts that explain the relationships between a group of phenomena that have been observed.[4] Theories are not to be confused with conceptual frameworks because these two entities are developed at different points in the process of theory development and testing. A set of facts or insights is first organized into a conceptual framework, or a set of empirical generaliza-

tions. This conceptual framework is tested and refined until it becomes a theory and can be used to explain relationships between phenomena. In daily clinical practice, clinicians use theories to understand their clinical observations and to predict what will occur in a given situation. Furthermore, they can use research to test the validity of the predictions that are made using a particular theory. For example, motor learning theory describes the phases in which motor learning occurs and defines the relationship between sensory and somatic

> **Box 1-1**
> **Defining Features of Outcome-Based Massage**
>
> - Based on disablement models—focuses on functional limitations and disability
> - Guided by the concept of Intelligent Touch
> - Considers the structure, process, and outcomes of care
> - Classifies massage techniques on the basis of the tissue layer they treat and the outcomes they achieve
> - Adopts a client-centered approach to practice
> - Uses a systematic clinical decision-making process
> - Integrates massage techniques into interventions

receptors, the central and peripheral nervous systems, and the musculoskeletal system in the production of movement. Clinicians use this theory to predict how their clients will respond to motor reeducation and to plan clinical interventions. In addition, research on motor learning systematically examines the proposed mechanisms and predicted outcomes for this theory and determines whether they are supported by evidence.

CONCEPTUAL FRAMEWORKS

A conceptual framework, on the other hand, cannot be used to predict behaviors. Instead it provides a means of organizing and integrating observations about a specific set of behaviors that one observes in a particular setting.[4] Clinicians can draw upon several theories, their clinical observations, and their knowledge of the context in which they practice to suggest interactions between the behaviors they observe.[5] Without such an organizing framework, it would be difficult for clinicians to make

sense of the countless observations they make about clients during the course of daily clinical practice, such as their clients' presenting symptoms and response to treatment regimens. Most clinicians have their own personal conceptual frameworks about the treatment process that evolve during the course of their clinical practice. They formulate these conceptual frameworks as they observe and analyze what occurs with their clients.

Take, for example, a clinician who observes that her clients with chronic pain have better adherence with their self-care programs and report better pain management when she involves them in planning clinical goals and home programs. She may use psychological theories about factors that increase adherence and biopsychosocial theories about relationships between autonomy and pain to propose that involving clients in treatment planning can result in a sense of increased autonomy and control that, in turn, affects their perception of pain and their adherence to self-care. While she can use her personal conceptual framework in an informal manner, this framework can also be formalized and used to guide professional clinical practice and to form the basis of theories and research. Conceptual frameworks can be represented and communicated using conceptual models.[5]

CONCEPTUAL MODELS

A conceptual model in health care, according to Earp and Ennett,[5] is a diagram that shows the proposed causal linkages among a set of concepts that the individual believes to be related to a particular health problem. Using boxes or text to represent the factors and arrows to show the direction of causality, these diagrams illustrate relationships between behaviors or other observed phenomena. The conceptual model in Figure 1-1 could represent the clinician's conceptual framework in the example outlined above.

Conceptual Models of Disablement

A recent need to redefine concepts of disability, handicap, and functional limitation has prompted the development of several conceptual frameworks to show the relationships between components of the disablement process and the role of rehabilitation. The International Classification of Impairments, Disabilities, and Handicaps (ICIDH) and the Nagi functional limitations model have been the starting point for several recent models of

disablement.[6,7] One such model is the National Center for Medical Rehabilitation Research (NCMRR)[1] conceptual model of disablement. These conceptual models exist to assist clinicians in understanding the components of the disablement process and how functional limitations and disability occur. Clinicians can also use these models to determine where in the disablement process they can most effectively intervene.

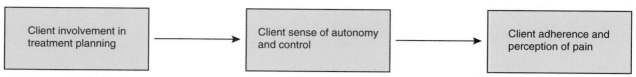

Figure 1-1. Conceptual model of client participation in treatment planning and adherence and perceptions of pain.

The modified Nagi model (Fig. 1-2) and the NCMRR model (Fig. 1-3) define four basic components of the process of disablement. Box 1-2 presents a clinical example of a data entry clerk with carpal tunnel syndrome, which illustrates the disablement process suggested by these models.

The pathophysiology occurs at the cellular level. It is the disease, syndrome, or lesion that interferes with the body's normal processes or structures. In the case of carpal tunnel syndrome, the pathophysiology involves the inflammation of the flexor retinaculum across the carpal tunnel and the wrist and finger flexor tendons in that region. This inflammation results in pressure on the median nerve as it passes through the carpal tunnel. An impairment, loss, or abnormality of the affected individual's physiological, anatomical, cognitive, or emotional structure or function occurs as a result of the initial or subsequent pathophysiology. In the clinical example, the pressure on the median nerve leads to the primary impairments of pain, paresthesia, weakness, and atrophy of the thenar muscles and lumbricals. These primary impairments can contribute to the development of secondary impairments, such as decreased joint range of motion at the wrist, adhesions and tightness of the flexor retinaculum, and weakness of wrist and hand muscles secondary to disuse. Physical and psychological impairments lead to a functional limitation: a restriction of the individual's ability to perform actions or activities within the range considered normal for the organ or organ system. As a consequence of the primary and secondary impairments outlined, this client is unable to perform work-related activities, leisure activities, and activities of daily living with hand and wrist joint range of motion and strength that are within normal limits. When an individual is unable to perform his or her socially defined tasks, activities, or roles to the expected level, this is considered a disability. The client in the clinical example is unable to perform his socially defined roles as a data entry clerk and a member of a racquetball club.

The NCMRR model contributes a fifth component to the disablement process, societal limitations.[1] Societal limitations are those limitations to an individual's level of function that can be attributed to physical or attitudinal barriers in society. In this clinical example, the societal limitation of reduced health insurance restricts the amount of rehabilitation that the data entry clerk can obtain, thereby limiting the level of function that he may be able to achieve.

Finally, health-related quality of life is a dimension that can be superimposed on the basic components of the disablement model. Health-related quality of life as defined by Jette[8] is the objective and subjective dimensions of an individual's ability to function in, and derive satisfaction from, a variety of social roles in the presence of impaired health status. Health-related quality of life encompasses, therefore, both functional limitations and disability (Fig. 1-4). For example, the functional limitations and disability experienced by the data entry clerk may lead him to perceive that he has a decreased quality of life or decreased ability to function in and enjoy his social roles as a data entry clerk and a member of a racquetball club.

Prior to the emphasis on conceptual models of disablement and functional limitations, clinicians focused on measuring and treating the client's presenting impairments. The models of disablement have provided a new perspective from which to view clinical care. This perspective broadens the clinician's approach to examination, evaluation, and treatment to encompass the client's functional limitations and disability, as well as his or her presenting impairments.[1,6,7] In addition, there is also greater acknowledgment of the impact of society as a whole on a client's potential level of function. For example, a clinician who used an impairment-oriented approach in the treatment of the client outlined in the aforementioned example would address the client's physical impairments in the clinical treatment planning. By contrast, a clinician who was treating the patient by using a functional limitations approach based on the models of disablement would also assess the client's functional and societal limitations and address these in treatment planning as appropriate. The differences in these two approaches are illustrated in Table 1-1.

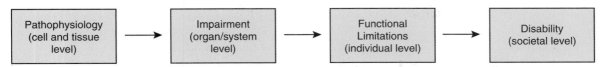

Figure 1-2. Modified Nagi model of disablement. Reprinted with adaptations from Pope A, and Tarlov A (Ed), Disability in America: Toward a national agenda for prevention, 1991: p 9 with the permission of the National Academy Press.

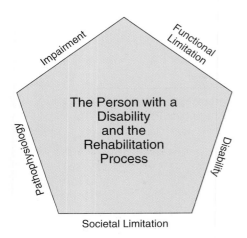

Figure 1-3. National Center for Medical Rehabilitation Research's model of components of the disablement process. Reprinted from the Research Plan for the National Center for Medical Rehabilitation Research. National Institute of Child Health and Human Development. Public Health Service NIH Publication No. 93-3509. Bethesda; MD: National Institutes of Health, US Department of Health and Human Services, 1993.

Box 1-2
Clinical Example of Disablement Model

Client profile	Thirty-year-old male employed as a data entry clerk has long-standing carpal tunnel syndrome on the right side as a result of long periods of keyboarding
Pathophysiology	Inflammation of the flexor retinaculum across the carpal tunnel and the wrist and finger flexor tendons in that region; this inflammation results in pressure on the median nerve as it passes through the carpal tunnel
Impairments	Pain, edema, paresthesia, decreased wrist and finger range of motion, and weakness and atrophy of thenar muscles and lumbricals, adhesions and tightness of the flexor retinaculum, secondary weakness of wrist muscles
Functional limitations	Inability to perform customary job-related activities, especially typing, filing, and writing Inability to perform leisure activity of playing racquetball Inability to perform activities of daily living, especially grooming and household tasks that involve lifting Fear of experiencing pain during functional activity Currently wears a wrist splint
Disability	Inability to carry out social roles as a data entry clerk and a member of a racquetball club
Societal limitation	Limited health insurance to cover the cost of treatment for carpal tunnel syndrome

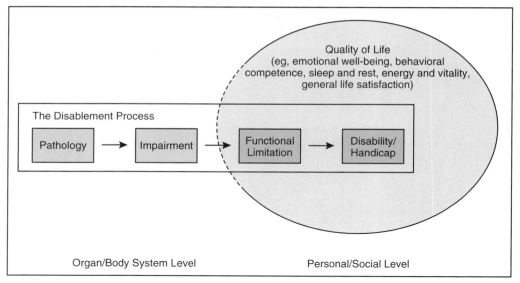

Figure 1-4. Conceptual Model of Quality of Life. Reprinted from Jette AM. Using health-related quality of life measures in physical therapy outcomes research. Phys Ther, 1993;73:531 with the permission of the American Physical Therapy Association.

Table 1-1
Comparison of Impairment-Oriented and Functional Limitations Approaches

Impairment-Oriented Approach	*Functional Limitations Approach*
Impairments · Pain · Edema · Paresthesia · Decreased joint range of motion of wrist and fingers · Decreased strength of hand and wrist muscles · Adhesions and tightness of the flexor retinaculum	1. Impairments 　· Pain 　· Edema 　· Paresthesia 　· Decreased joint range of motion of wrist and fingers 　· Decreased strength of hand and wrist muscles 　· Adhesions and tightness of the flexor retinaculum 2. Functional limitations 　· Duration of typing activities performed 　· Duration of writing activities performed 　· Duration of filing activities performed 　· Weight of objects client is able to lift as a reflection of ability to perform household tasks requiring lifting 　· Duration of grooming activities performed 　· Fear of exacerbating pain limits initiation of functional activity 3. Disability 　· Inability to perform job of data entry clerk 　· Inability to perform social role as a member of a racquetball club 4. Societal limitation 　· Limited health insurance 5. Quality of life 　· Perceived decreased ability to function in and enjoy his social roles of data entry clerk and member of a racquetball club

Table 1-2
Examples of the Components of Clinical Care

Structure	*Process*	*Outcome*
Human resources · Organization of staff · Number and distribution of staff · Qualifications and training of staff	**Technical aspects** · Utilization patterns · Appropriateness of referrals · Completeness of diagnosis · Appropriateness of examinations and evaluations performed by clinicians · Adequacy of interventions selected and provided by clinicians · Relevance of treatment goals set by clinicians · Patterns of treatment by clinicians	**Effectiveness of care** · Effect of care on client's physical impairments · Effect of care on client's psychological impairments · Effect of care on client's functional limitations · Effect of care on client's quality of life · Client's satisfaction with care provided · Cost-effectiveness of care
Physical and financial resources · Size of facility · Geographical location of facility · Organization of facility · Equipment available · Formal financing · Informal financing	**Interpersonal aspects** *Client* · Client's physical and psychological characteristics · Client's expectations of treatment · Level of client participation in care *Clinician* · Clinician's interpersonal skills · Clinician's skill as an educator · Client-clinician interaction · Client-clinician communication · Level of client adherence to plan of care	**Efficiency of care**

Donabedian's Framework of the Components of Clinical Care

In addition to the model of disablement, there are conceptual models of clinical care, such as Donabedian's model,[2] that focus on the components of clinical care. Although clinical outcomes have generated much excitement, outcomes are but one of the three components defined by Donabedian's conceptual framework of the components of clinical care. The other two—equally important—components are the structure and process of clinical care. As Table 1-2 shows, in addition to the outcomes that are achieved by the plan of care, numerous elements of the structure and process of care are integral to the clinical care that a client receives.

STRUCTURE OF CARE

In Donabedian's conceptual framework, the structure of care refers to the human, physical, and financial re-

sources available for the delivery of care. This includes the staffing complement, the clinical environment, and the organization's financing. Often, despite the clinician's best intentions, the structure in which care is provided has an impact on the clinician's approach to treatment. For example, a busy outpatient setting with a capitated reimbursement structure, 20-minute treatment sessions, and a high proportion of aides assisting with treatment delivery presents different constraints and facilitators to treatment than those that the clinician would encounter in a rehabilitation center with 60-minute treatment sessions, few adjunct personnel, and a noncapitated reimbursement structure. A clinician treating clients with industrial injuries in the outpatient setting is less likely to have time for extensive use of hands-on massage techniques and will have a greater component of education in self-care than the clinician treating clients with neurological conditions in the rehabilitation setting. For this reason, clinicians need to be aware of the context in which they treat their clients, even though this will not be an explicit component of treatment planning.

PROCESS OF CARE

The process of care, according to Donabedian, is the manner in which care is delivered—how the activities between the clinician and the client take place. This encompasses the interpersonal aspects of the client-clinician interaction and the technical aspects of how the clinician provides care. The importance of the process of care cannot be emphasized enough. Examining the process by which care is delivered not only provides clinicians with information that they can use to improve their interventions, but it also enables them to determine if they can improve the outcomes they achieve by changing the process by which they deliver care.

TECHNICAL ASPECTS OF CARE DELIVERY
The technical aspects of the process of care that are most relevant to the practicing clinician relate to the appropriateness and adequacy of the examination performed, the clinician's evaluation of the client's presenting problems, the treatment plan outlined, and the interventions selected and provided by the clinician. As the chapter "Clinical Decision-Making Process" outlines, examination, evaluation, treatment planning, and intervention are interdependent processes. A clinician's failure to adequately evaluate the salient impairments related to the client's medical condition will lead to a treatment regimen that does not address these impairments effectively. In turn, this will limit the likelihood that the functional limitations resulting from these impairments will be ameliorated. In the case of the client with carpal tunnel syndrome, had the clinician evaluated only strength, pain, and paresthesia, the treatment regimen provided would not address the adhesions and tightening of the client's flexor retinaculum that could be limiting his ability to perform functional activities and contributing to his other symptoms.[9] As discussed in later chapters, the adequacy of the treatment provided can be monitored on an ongoing basis through regular reexamination of the client's status. This will provide the clinician with several opportunities for refining the treatment regimen and for enhancing the technical process of care delivery.

INTERPERSONAL ASPECTS OF CARE DELIVERY
The list of interpersonal aspects of the process of care in Table 1-2 can serve as a reminder of the importance of the therapeutic relationship and the impact that it can have on clinical outcomes. Three components compose the interpersonal aspect of care delivery. At the heart of clinical care lies the client and all of the things that he or she brings into treatment, such as physical and psychological characteristics, family history, lifestyle, work and home environment, and belief systems. Furthermore, the client enters treatment with expectations for treatment and outcomes that will affect the treatment process whether or not the clinician inquires about them. The clinician's interpersonal manner is the second component. A clinician's primary purpose is not just to implement plans of care; indeed, the clinician's ability to engage, educate, motivate, and support the client throughout the treatment process is as important as his or her technical skill. The interaction between client and clinician is the third component. The quality of this interaction can shape the level of client adherence, client motivation, and in many ways, the results of the plan of care. Therefore, the clinician is wise to engage the client in the therapeutic process, to solicit and respect the client's input on the plan of care and treatment outcomes, to consider the context in which the client lives and works, and to seek the client's feedback throughout the course of treatment. This is particularly true in the clinical use of massage techniques, because the use of touch can raise issues related to personal vulnerability, emotional responses to treatment, and the need to set appropriate boundaries between the client and clinician.

OUTCOMES OF CARE

The outcomes of care are the results of an intervention or the treatment regimen as a whole.[2] Outcomes of care can be measured in a myriad of ways. Administrators may be more concerned with cost-effectiveness, the efficiency of care, and client satisfaction. Clinicians, on the other hand, may look at the short-term and long-term effects of care on the client's physical and psychological impairments, functional limitations, and disability. In addition, more clinicians are considering the effect of care on the client's overall quality of life. Clients, in turn, bring their own perspective on the relevant effects of care on their impairments, functional limitations, disability, and quality of life.

The impairment-oriented and functional limitations approaches discussed earlier in this chapter result in different types of clinical outcomes (Table 1-3). The impairment-oriented approach sets outcomes that are related to the impairments that are being assessed and treated. In some professions, these impairment-level outcomes are referred to as treatment goals.[7] By contrast, although impairments are also assessed and treated in the functional limitations approach, the client's functional limitations are addressed in the functional outcomes of care, or treatment outcomes.[10] In other words, the latter approach uses functional outcomes of

Table 1-3
Comparison of Impairment-Level and Functional Outcomes of Care

Impairment-Level Outcomes of Care	*Functional Outcomes of Care*
· Client reports that he experiences no pain	· Client initiates functional activity readily without fear of pain
· No edema present in the region of the carpal tunnel	· Client is able to keyboard for 20 min without wearing wrist splint and without an increase in edema
· Client reports that he experiences no numbness or tingling	· Client is able to write with a pen for 15 min without wearing wrist splint with no complaints of paresthesia
· Full range of motion at wrist and fingers; extensibility of the flexor retinaculum within normal limits	· Client is able to carry out filing activities (open/closing filing cabinet drawers and lifting/manipulating file folders) without wearing wrist splint, without complaints of reduced range of motion restricting his ability to perform these activities
· Grade 5 (full) strength of hand (especially thenar muscles and lumbricals) and wrist muscles	· Client is able to lift 5-lb box of files or groceries with both hands from floor to waist level without wearing wrist splint, without complaints of his wrist giving out or his hand being weak

care as the primary outcomes, with impairment-level outcomes of care playing a secondary role.

Regardless of the type of outcome selected, the clinician needs to be cautious in overemphasizing the outcomes of care to the exclusion of structure and process. In reality, a clinician needs to understand and evaluate the structure and process of care to ascertain how much of the achieved outcome can be attributed to the care she provided or to understand why the intervention was successful or not. Furthermore, the danger always exists that a clinician may discard a potentially effective intervention because the outcomes achieved were poor, when in fact the fault lay in the manner in which the intervention was delivered (process of care). A holistic, client-centered treatment regimen will, therefore, consider the structure, process, and outcomes of care.

Conceptual Frameworks for Massage

Massage techniques are used within the process of clinical care as a component of the interventions that the clinician provides to the client. Clinicians can use conceptual frameworks about the practice of massage and the classification of massage techniques to guide their training and their selection and application of massage techniques within their interventions.

INTELLIGENT TOUCH

The conceptual framework of Intelligent Touch defines the learned skills that the authors propose to be essential for successful clinical use of massage: attention and concentration, discrimination, identification, inquiry, and intention. The premise of this conceptual framework is that clinicians who lack, or are deficient in, their ability to perform any of these skills may be unable to consistently achieve the identified outcomes of care. Consequently, the authors suggest that to be effective, a clinician should not only learn these skills, but also practice them continuously.

ATTENTION

Attention refers to the clinician's capacity to focus on the sensory information that she receives primarily, but not exclusively, through her hands. Clinicians must learn to focus awareness on selected aspects of the sensory field at hand and to constantly analyze and organize the many types of information that they obtain. The most basic characteristics that a clinician can sense through multiple tissue layers and in different anatomical structures are tissue temperature, texture, and tension. Massage that is performed mechanically or mindlessly—without continuous attention to the broad spectrum of sensory information that is available—produces less-than-optimal results.

DISCRIMINATION

Discrimination, within the context of outcome-based massage, refers to the clinician's ability to distinguish fine gradations of sensory information. With practice, the clinician can begin to identify and compare more refined types of sensory information, such as tissue characteristics and responses to movement or applied force. Discriminative ability varies widely among novice clinicians and can be improved through education. Furthermore, although good discriminative ability is a fairly common gift, novice clinicians may require numerous hours of practice performing massage techniques before their discriminative ability is adequate for independent clinical practice.

IDENTIFICATION

Clinicians must be able to distinguish between healthy and dysfunctional tissue states. In addition, they must be able to identify structures and their responses to applied forces. Identification is the component of Intelligent Touch that benefits the most from formal training in anatomy that includes examining skeletons, palpating live bodies, and ideally, exploring cadavers while referencing a well-illustrated anatomical atlas.

INQUIRY

Intelligent Touch is inquiring touch. A good clinician is constantly asking questions, and the use of massage is no exception to this requirement. The use of inquiring touch does not imply that the clinician's touch feels tentative to the client or that it lacks firmness when required. Instead, it reflects the never-ending set of questions that inform Intelligent Touch, such as the following: What is this tissue? How does the feel of this tissue relate to the client's history? How does this relate to the client's symptoms? How does this compare to the feel of this type of tissue in other places in the client's body? How does this compare with other healthy and dysfunctional tissues that have been palpated in the past? The process of inquiry entails a constant comparison of the tissue being palpated to other tissues in the client's body and to the clinician's memory of other tissues that she has palpated.

INTENTION

The final element of Intelligent Touch is intention. Intention refers to the clinician's aim of using massage techniques to produce a more normalized response of the client's tissues or other structures. Consequently, intention depends on the clinician having a clear notion of the feel of improvements in the function of tissue and of structures, which can arise during the application of any given technique. The clinician also needs to understand how this improved feel relates both to impairment-level outcomes and functional outcomes of treatment. The clinician who has clear intentions knows how both healthy and dysfunctional tissues respond to massage and works to produce as close to the ideal tissue response as possible, given the constraints of the client's characteristics and the clinical setting.

Table 1-4
General Therapeutic Effects and Impairment-Level Outcomes of Massage Techniques

Effect[a]	Description	Example
Mechanical[b]	Effects are caused by physically moving the tissues by compression, tension (stretch), shearing, bending, or twisting	Increased lymphatic return Mobilized bronchial secretions
Reflex[b]	Functional change is mediated by the nervous system	Sedation or arousal Facilitation of skeletal muscle contraction
Physiological[b]	Involves a change in biochemical body processes	Improved modeling of connective tissue Reduced muscle spasm
Psychological	Effect occurs in the mind, emotions, or behavior	Improved social interaction Improved physical self-image
Psychoneuro-immunological	Altered feeling state is accompanied by changes in hormone levels or immune function; this term emphasizes that "mere" feeling states like relaxation represent complex multisystem phenomena	Decreased anxiety and cortisol levels Improved T-cell function

[a]Any given massage technique produces multiple effects, and outcomes are usually achieved through several mechanisms operating simultaneously.
[b] Effects may be local, occurring only on the site of manipulation, or general, occurring throughout the body.

CLASSIFICATION OF MASSAGE TECHNIQUES

Conceptual frameworks also provide the foundation of the classification systems of clinical techniques. Clinicians, in turn, use these classification systems to guide their selection of the treatment techniques they provide in their interventions. In recent decades, massage techniques have been organized on the basis of conceptual frameworks that categorize techniques in terms of the distinction between "classical" and "modern" methods or on the basis of the therapeutic effects of the techniques.[3,11] The classification system proposed for the perspective of outcome-based massage in this text seeks to avoid some of the limitations of these two approaches to classification.

This text intentionally avoids the division into "classical" and "modern" service-marked methods and has attempted to reflect this in the chosen structure and nomenclature. In doing so, the authors recognize that several innovative approaches to massage or "body work" have influenced the contemporary practice of massage substantially and give these approaches their due acknowledgment. Nevertheless, the authors suggest that these approaches represent an elaboration and refinement of older techniques that can be organized into the six categories they have proposed for massage techniques. This categorization reflects the authors' belief in the importance of consolidating the wide variety of available methods into a coherent classification system that supports a contemporary outcome-based approach to massage.

The therapeutic effects of massage may be defined as being mechanical, physiological, and psychological.[3] To this list, some authors add reflex effects and energetic effects.[11] The therapeutic effects or possible impairment-level outcomes of massage cannot be ignored, because the structured, purposeful touch of massage is applied in very precise ways to maximize treatment outcomes that have been indicated for the client's presenting condition.

Massage techniques cannot, however, be classified solely on the basis of their therapeutic effects, because a given technique can produce multiple effects. For example, even light incidental touch, which stimulates local nerve receptors, can produce a cascade of physiological and psychological effects. For this reason, this text presents a framework for classifying and ordering the presentation of techniques based only in part on the defined therapeutic effects or impairment-level outcomes of the techniques shown in Table 1-4.

The proposed classification system for massage techniques and the order in which these techniques are presented are based on anatomical, operational, and heuristic concerns, in addition to therapeutic effects and outcomes. The anatomical categorization of techniques results in techniques being organized in terms of the tissues that they engage. In this instance, "engage" means that the clinician palpates and directs the mechanical force of the manipulation to a particular type of tissue. On this basis, techniques that are directed toward superficial tissues are presented first, those affecting deeper tissues are presented later, and those that affect multiple tissue layers are presented last. From an operational perspective, those techniques that require the clinician to palpate and observe similar phenomena are grouped together. Finally, the heuristic approach orders techniques that require the acquisition of simpler skills before techniques that require complex skills.

These criteria can be used to define four broad categories of massage techniques that engage particular types of tissue: superficial reflex techniques, superficial fluid techniques, neuromuscular techniques, and connective tissue techniques. It also produces two categories of techniques that engage multiple tissue layers: passive movement techniques and percussive techniques. Techniques in each of these categories have specific therapeutic effects; in addition, the first four categories may produce psychoneuroimmunological effects, such as the reduction of anxiety[12] (see the details of effects in the individual techniques chapters).

1. Superficial reflex techniques: These techniques engage only the skin and produce reflex effects, such as counterirritant analgesia, but no mechanical effects.
2. Superficial fluid techniques: These techniques engage skin, superficial fascia, and subcutaneous fat down to the investing layer of the deep fascia. They produce mechanical effects on superficial lymphatics and possibly the venous circulation.
3. Neuromuscular techniques: These techniques engage muscle and the tissues it contains. They affect the function of the contractile element, hydration of connective tissue, and lymphatic return and may also produce complex reflex effects.
4. Connective tissue techniques: These techniques engage superficial and deep layers of connective tissue. They mechanically affect the hydration, extensibility, and modeling of connective tissue and may also produce complex reflex effects.
5. Passive movement techniques: These techniques produce substantial tissue or joint motion without effort on the part of the client. They engage multiple tissues and structures and have wide-ranging effects on fluid flow, connective tissue, and the neural control of muscle tone.

Box 1-3
Major Categories of Massage Techniques

1. Superficial reflex techniques
   Static contact
   Superficial stroking
   Fine vibration
2. Superficial fluid techniques
   Superficial effleurage
   Superficial lymph drainage technique
3. Neuromuscular techniques
   Broad contact compression
   Petrissage
   Stripping
   Specific compression

4. Connective tissue techniques
   Skin rolling
   Myofascial release
   Direct fascial technique
   Friction
5. Passive movement techniques
   Shaking
   Rhythmical mobilization
   Rocking
6. Percussive techniques
   Percussion

---

6. Percussive techniques: These techniques deform and release tissues quickly. They engage different tissues, depending on the force with which they are applied. They are used primarily in cardiopulmonary rehabilitation to mechanically assist bronchial drainage and airway clearance. They may also produce useful reflex neuromuscular effects.

These categories and selected techniques within each category are summarized in Box 1-3 and will be explored in depth in their own chapters. This presentation includes a wide spectrum of clinically useful massage techniques that are supported by research.

Conclusion

The NCMMR[1] model of disablement, Donabedian's framework of the components of clinical care, the concept of Intelligent Touch, and the proposed classification system of massage techniques intersect to provide the conceptual framework for outcome-based massage. In this framework, clinicians evaluate a client's impairments, functional limitations, and social limitations and use this information to define which impairments need to be addressed in their intervention.[10] They use the information on the client's functional status to define functional outcomes that they can reasonably expect to achieve through treatment. Clinicians treat the client's impairments as a means of enhancing the client's functional ability and decreasing the client's impairments. They reevaluate impairments to refine their selection of treatment techniques, and they reevaluate functional limitations to determine when the identified functional outcomes of care have been met and treatment can be terminated. Throughout the course of their interventions, clinicians using the outcome-based massage approach take the structure and process of care into consideration in planning and delivering care. As they incorporate massage techniques into the clinical care

they deliver, these clinicians also use the framework of Intelligent Touch that fosters their development of skills that will facilitate their successful use of massage techniques. Finally, clinicians using outcome-based massage enhance their ability to effectively achieve the identified outcomes of care by basing their selection of techniques for their interventions on the proposed classification system of massage techniques that organizes techniques in terms of the tissues that they engage, the phenomena that they observe during application, and the outcomes that they can achieve.

References

1. National Institute of Child Health and Human Development. Research plan for the National Center for Medical Rehabilitation Research. Public Health Service NIH Publication no. 93-3509. Bethesda, MD: National Institutes of Health, US Department of Health and Human Services, 1993.
2. Donabedian A. Evaluating the quality of medical care. Milbank Q 1966;3:166–206.

3. deDomenico G, Wood EC. Beard's Massage. 4th ed. Philadelphia, PA: WB Saunders, 1997.

4. Portney L, Watkins M. Foundations of clinical research: applications to practice. East Norwalk, CN: Appleton & Lange, 1993.

5. Earp J, Ennett S. Conceptual models for health education research and practice. Health Educ Res 1991:6(2):163–171.

6. Nagi S. Disability concepts revisited: implications for prevention. Executive summary. In: Pope A, Tarlov A, eds. Disability in America, Washington DC: National Academy Press, p 1.4, 1991.

7. American Physical Therapy Association. Guide to physical therapist practice. Phys Ther 1997;77(11):ix–xii.

8. Jette AM. Using health-related quality of life measures in physical therapy outcomes research. Phys Ther 1993;73:528–537.

9. Maitland G. Peripheral manipulation. 2nd ed. London: Butterworths, 1981.

10. Sullivan P, Markos P. Clinical decision-making in therapeutic exercise. East Norwalk, CT: Appleton & Lange, 1995.

11. Tappan FM, Benjamin P. Tappan's handbook of healing massage techniques. 3rd ed. Stamford, CT: Appleton & Lange, 1998.

12. Field TM. Massage therapy effects. Am Psychol 1998;53(12):1270–1281.

2

The Clinical Decision-Making Process

*T*he clinical decision-making process guides the clinician through the examination, treatment, and discharge of the client. The decision-making process proposed for outcome-based massage addresses issues that are specific to the integration of massage techniques into clinical practice. This chapter discusses the technical and interpersonal aspects of the process of care[1] for outcome-based massage that occur over four phases: the Evaluative Phase, the Treatment Planning Phase, the Treatment Phase, and the Discharge Phase. It provides guidelines for enhancing the appropriateness and adequacy of the examinations performed, the plans of care outlined, and the interventions planned and provided by clinicians. This chapter also describes how clinicians can address the client's ethical, emotional, and educational needs that arise during the course of clinical care.

The Clinical Decision-Making Process

Clinical decision-making, clinical reasoning, and *clinical problem-solving* are terms that have been used by various authors to describe their models of the process by which clinicians synthesize and analyze information on their clients' conditions and use the results of their analysis to formulate and progress a therapeutic regimen for their clients.[1–5] The clinical decision-making model for outcome-based massage discussed integrates clinical reasoning models with the conceptual frameworks for massage discussed in the previous chapter. This model outlines the components of the clinical decision-making process related to the integration of massage techniques into clinical care in four phases: the Evaluative Phase; the Treatment Planning Phase, the Treatment Phase, and the Discharge Phase. Although this model, like all clinical decision-making models, is presented graphically as a series of steps, it is not intended to be used in a linear, sequential manner. Instead, clinicians' use of this model should be guided by the research findings on clinical decision-making. First, researchers have observed that clinicians who were engaged in the clinical decision-making process often performed several steps of the process concurrently.[4] In addition, these clinicians used an iterative decision-making process rather than a linear process. In other words, they cycled through the same steps of the decision-making process several times, and each time that they repeated the steps, they expanded on the information that they possessed and further refined their hypotheses.

Overview of the Process of Clinical Care

The process of care, or the clinical process, is the manner in which care is delivered—the activities that take place within and between the clinician and the client.[1] This encompasses the interpersonal aspects of the client–clinician interaction and the technical aspects of how the clinician provides care. The technical aspects of the process of care refer, in part, to the appropriateness and adequacy of the examination performed, the plan of care outlined, and the intervention planned and provided by the clinician (see Table 1-2). The interpersonal aspects of the process of clinical care involve three components: the client, the clinician, and the client–clinician interaction, often referred to as the therapeutic relationship (see Table 1-2). The decision-making model for outcome-based massage describes the technical and interpersonal aspects of the process of care that occur over four phases: the Evaluative Phase, the Treatment Planning Phase, the Treatment Phase, and the Discharge Phase.

Social Context of the Process of Clinical Care

The client and the clinician are typically the central players in the process of clinical care. They engage in a clinical relationship, often referred to as the therapeutic relationship. Clinicians bring their clinical knowledge, manual skills, and interpersonal style to the relationship and use their clinical decision-making process to guide them through the process of clinical care. Clients bring their interpersonal style to the relationship, as well as their psychological and physical response to their condition and the treatment process. Yet rarely is the process of clinical care limited to the interactions that occur between these two people; typically, this process occurs within a larger social context (Fig. 2-1). First, the health care setting may include a variety of health care professionals with whom both clinician and client may interact. In addition, the client has a social network of caregivers, relatives, and others who may participate in, or have an impact on, the process of clinical care.

The complexity of the interactions involved in the process of clinical care will vary with the clinical setting, the client, and the client's presenting medical condition. For example, a clinician who is treating a geriatric client with a stroke in a rehabilitation setting will have to manage numerous interactions over the course of treatment. These may include interactions with the client, the client's family, the other members of the health care team (neurologists, neurosurgeons, nurses, physical therapists, occupational therapists, respiratory therapists, social services, orthotist, recreational therapists), health care team members in the rehabilitation setting, and possibly some community-based resources for the family. On the other hand, a clinician who is treating an adult with plantar fasciitis in an outpatient clinic will only have to interact with the client and, possibly, the referring physician.

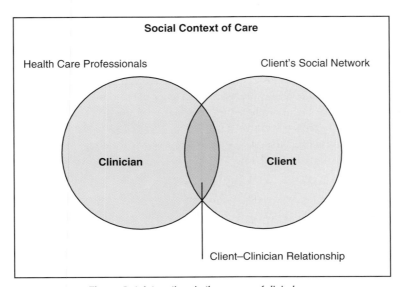

Social Context of Care

Health Care Professionals

Client's Social Network

Clinician

Client

Client–Clinician Relationship

Figure 2-1. Interactions in the process of clinical care.

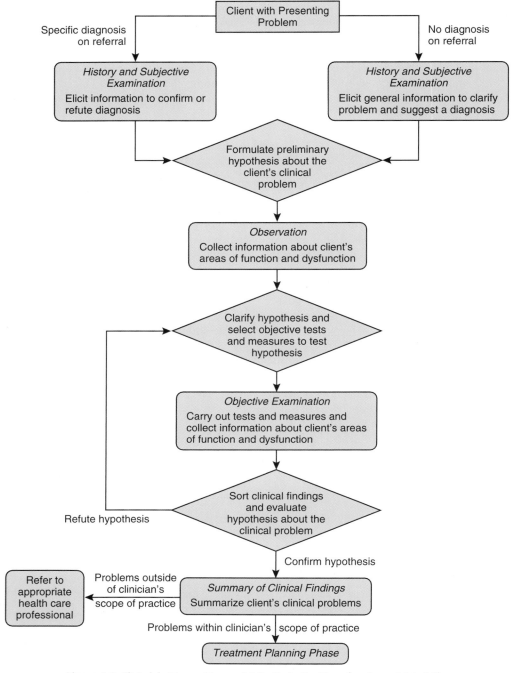

Figure 2-2. Clinical decision-making model: the Evaluative Phase (see Boxes 2-1 to 2-7).

Technical Aspects of the Process of Clinical Care

EVALUATIVE PHASE

The Evaluative Phase provides the foundation of the clinical treatment process. The steps in the Evaluative Phase (Fig. 2-2) revolve around the formulation and confirmation of a hypothesis about the client's clinical problem. This phase begins with data gathering through the client examination and also involves the confirmation of the clinical problem, the creation of a summary of clinical findings, and the decision of whether to pursue treatment.

The importance of the evaluative phase cannot be emphasized enough. When a client presents for clinical care, it is often an acknowledgment of the fact that a problem exists. Through the client examination and the evaluation of the clinical findings, the clinician clarifies the client's clinical problem and identifies the client's relevant impairments, functional limitations, and disability on which he will base outcome identification and treatment planning. Consequently, an appropriate, accurate, and comprehensive implementation of the steps in the evaluative phase can assist in maximizing the potential effectiveness of a treatment regimen.

CLIENT EXAMINATION

The evaluative phase begins with the client examination: the collection of information on the client's health status and clinical condition through history taking, a general systems review, and tests and measures.[6] The scope of the examination performed by the clinician is determined by the clinician's scope of practice; the clinician's area of specialization; the type of examination being conducted; the client's diagnosis; the acuity, severity, complexity, and stability of the client's condition; the client's general health status; and the nature of the clinical setting (Table 2-1). The initial multidisciplinary neurological examination for a geriatric client with Parkinson's disease in a home health setting, for example, would include a detailed history of present and prior health status and functional level; a systems review of the client's communication status and overall physiological status; and tests and measures to evaluate range of motion, motor function, reflex activity, sensory integrity, gait, locomotion, balance, integumentary integrity, assistive and adaptive devices, and activities of daily living. This would be broader in scope and cover the issues in more detail than would an interim examination of an adolescent with chondromalacia patellae in an outpatient orthopedic clinic. The latter would involve tests and measures related to the impairments in the areas of muscular performance, joint integrity and

mobility, and activities of daily living that were specified as the focus of treatment.

History Taking and Subjective Component of the Examination

Prior to taking the client history, the clinician determines whether or not the client has a specific diagnosis on the referral. If there is a specific diagnosis, then the clinician's history taking and subjective examination will include questions relating to that condition and will focus on eliciting information to confirm or refute the client's presenting diagnosis. If, on the other hand, the client has a referral without a medical diagnosis, the clinician begins by eliciting general information that will serve to clarify the client's presenting problem and suggest a clinical diagnosis (Box 2-1). Chapter 3, Review of Client Examination Concepts for Massage, provides suggestions for issues to consider in history taking for massage. The client's history can be documented within the written plan of care or separately.

Preliminary Clinical Hypothesis

Existing clinical decision-making models all include some form of data gathering and the formulation and testing of a clinical hypothesis.[1–5] In the current model, the clinician forms a preliminary clinical hypothesis (the clinician's hypothesis about the client's key clinical problems) based on the diagnosis on the client's referral and the information gathered from the history and subjective examination (Box 2-2).

Client Observation

Once this preliminary clinical hypothesis is formed, the clinician will observe the client to see if there are any observational cues that may support his hypothesis (Box 2-3). At this early stage of the examination, the clinician needs to avoid having too narrow a focus. The observation of the client should be general enough to provide data that may suggest an alternative hypothesis, yet still enable the clinician to identify specific clinical signs that are consistent with the clinician's hypothesis. This observation can include postural alignment, muscle bulk and contours, and other areas outlined in Chapter 3, Review of Client Examination Concepts for Massage, and the individual techniques chapters. Based on his observations, the clinician may be able to refine his hypothesis about the client's clinical problem.

Objective Tests and Measures

The clinician then proceeds to the next step in gathering data to confirm or refute the clinical hypothesis: the selection and application of objective tests and measures (Box 2-4). The types of tests and measures used and the

Table 2-1
Scope and Content of Client Examinations

	Initial Examination	*Interim Examination or Reexamination*	*Discharge Examination*	*Follow-Up Examination*
Scope	Detailed exploratory examination	Focused examination related to the identified impairment-level outcomes (treatment goals) and functional outcomes of care (outcomes)	Detailed examination related to the treatment provided and the impairment-level outcomes (treatment goals) and functional outcomes of care (outcomes) achieved	Focused examination related to *(a)* the maintenance of previously achieved impairment-level outcomes (treatment goals) and functional outcomes of care (outcomes) or *(b)* the identification of ongoing treatment needs
Timing	Performed prior to the initiation of treatment	Performed at intervals following the initiation of treatment	Performed at the end of the treatment period prior to discharge of the client	Performed following discharge from an episode of care
Objectives	· Confirm/refute the client's presenting diagnosis · Identify and measure the client's impairments, functional limitations, and functional areas to provide a basis for treatment planning and a baseline for interim examinations · Identify and measure the client's prior and presenting level of function to provide a basis for identifying reasonable functional outcomes	· Identify and measure changes in the client's impairments and functional level from the baseline established at the initial examination · Determine client's achievement of goals and outcomes · Determine the client's readiness for treatment progression · Determine the need to modify the plan of care or outcomes	· Determine the client's readiness for discharge through measurement of progress on goals and outcomes · Identify and measure the client's discharge needs · Identify and measure changes in the client's impairments and functional level from the baseline established at the initial examination	· Identify and measure changes in the client's health status, impairments, and functional disability from the baseline established at the most recent discharge examination · Determine the client's level of safety and adaptation to her environment · Determine the client's ongoing treatment needs
Components	· History—elicit information to confirm/refute diagnosis or to establish a diagnosis if none is given · Tests and measures to *(a)* confirm/refute diagnosis or to establish a diagnosis if none is given and *(b)* identify and measure impairments, functional limitations, disability, and quality of life	· Tests and measures to determine changes in impairments, functional limitations, and disability	· History—summary of treatment · Discussion of the client's perceived discharge needs · Tests and measures to determine the client's impairments, functional level, disability, and quality of life at discharge	· History—elicit information on changes in health status, safety, adaptation to the environment · Tests and measures to determine changes in impairments, functional limitations, disability, and quality of life

Box 2-1
History Taking and Subjective Examination

The client is a 28-year-old woman who works as a cashier in a supermarket with a 2-month history of neck pain of gradual onset. Her referral states "Neck pain—evaluate and treat." Since the referral does not provide a specific diagnosis, the clinician includes questions aimed at clarifying whether the client has a radiculopathy or a soft-tissue injury, including radiation of pain, 24-hour pain behavior, effect of position on pain, and presence of paresthesia. The client's responses about her neck pain do not include radiating pain below the elbow, paresthesia, or pain increasing with cervical extension or side flexion. Instead, she reports an insidious onset of localized neck and shoulder pain, with stiffness, decreased active cervical range of motion, neck muscle tightness, neck muscle spasm, and transient headaches.

Box 2-2
Preliminary Clinical Hypothesis

Based on the findings of the history and subjective examination, the clinician hypothesizes that the client's symptoms are due to the presence of active myofascial trigger points.

A myofascial trigger point is a hyperirritable spot within a skeletal muscle that is associated with a hypersensitive palpable nodule in a taut band.[15] Trigger points may refer pain, create nerve entrapment, contribute to muscle weakness, and significantly limit range of motion.

Active trigger points, which are painful even when they are not being palpated, contribute to the following:

- Decreased muscle flexibility and muscle strength
- Increased referred pain during compression; in this case, they will produce referred pain in a pain pattern specific to that trigger point and can produce referred motor and autonomic responses
- Local twitch response in the muscle fibers in the area of the active trigger point if stimulated enough

Box 2-3
Observation of the Client

The clinician gathers observational data to initiate his identification of whether the client has myofascial neck pain rather than a radiculopathy. Based on his observations that there is no muscle wasting and that the client has a forward head posture and muscle spasm in the region of the right upper trapezius, the clinician refines his clinical hypothesis to state that the client has active myofascial trigger points in the right upper trapezius and possibly levator scapulae muscles.

Box 2-4
Objective Tests and Measures

The clinician selects objective tests and measures that will provide information to help confirm or refute the presence of these myofascial trigger points. He palpates the client's trapezius and levator scapulae muscles for the presence of taut bands or nodules, the occurrence of a twitch response, levels of sensitivity to pressure, and patterns of pain referral during palpation of trigger point locations. He also measures range of motion and strength and notes that the client presents with decreased active cervical range of motion and decreased strength R trapezius and levator scapulae (scapular elevation and retraction). He tests upper extremity, dermatomes, myotomes, and cervical compression and distraction to refute the presence of a radiculopathy and records the negative findings. Since he can use the client's functional areas to compensate for areas of dysfunction, he records the client's normal upper-extremity range of motion and strength. He also documents the client's inability to adequately perform the functional tasks associated with her job as a cashier: driving to work, lifting and transferring objects with her right arm, and reaching objects above her head.

order in which they are conducted differ with the client's characteristics and condition. Specifically, there are differences in the approaches to client examination that clinicians use for neurological, musculoskeletal, cardiopulmonary, and psychological conditions. For example, a musculoskeletal examination in physical therapy may consist of postural analysis, visual inspection, range-of-motion testing, muscle performance testing, and palpation, performed in that order. By contrast, a cardiopulmonary examination in physical therapy may consist of visual inspection, palpation, percussion, and auscultation. Furthermore, variations in examination approach also exist among adult practice, pediatrics, and geriatrics.

The selection of appropriate tests and measures is one of the most difficult components of the examination. The problem lies not in a lack of information, but in the possibility of being overwhelmed by the considerable information on special tests and clinical signs in the numerous texts on clinical assessment. The clinician faces the challenge of recalling appropriate examination techniques, noting the client's response, and making a correct interpretation of the findings. Having one or two hypotheses about the client's problem can assist the clinician in refining his choice of examination techniques. To keep data at a manageable level, the clinician may find it effective to first select and carry out a few tests that are commonly used to confirm or refute a given condition. If the findings are positive, the clinician can then collect more-general information about the client's impairments, functional limitations, and areas of function. If the findings from these confirmatory tests are negative, the clinician can decide whether additional tests are needed or whether to change hypotheses. In situations in which the clinician does not have a clear clinical hypothesis, scanning examinations provide a means of quickly determining the integrity of several systems and assessing the nature of the client's symptoms.[7] Chapter 3, Review of Client Examination Concepts for Massage, provides information on some of the examination techniques that are relevant to massage that the reader can use to guide the selection of examination techniques.

EVALUATION OF FINDINGS

Confirmation of the Clinical Hypothesis

At the conclusion of the client examination, the clinician analyzes the impairments stemming from the client's clinical condition and either confirms or refutes his clinical hypothesis (Box 2-5). In some health care professions, such as physical therapy, the process and result of analyzing and organizing the findings from the client examination into clusters or syndromes is called the diagnosis.[6] If the findings from the client examination do not support the clinician's clinical hypothesis, he will have to reformulate his hypothesis and repeat the pro-

cess of selecting and carrying out appropriate tests and measures. There are situations in which the client may not present with a clearly defined clinical condition. It may be appropriate in these cases for the clinician to focus the treatment planning process on the general goal of remediating the client's presenting impairments, functional limitations, and disability rather than on the identification and treatment of a specific clinical condition.[6]

Summary of Pertinent Clinical Findings

Once the clinician confirms the clinical hypothesis, he produces a summary of pertinent clinical findings: the impairments, functional limitations, and disabilities with which the client presents (Box 2-6). This summary can be documented within the written plan of care or separately. In outcome-based massage, as with other clinical approaches, failure to identify the impairments that are contributing to the client's functional limitations can lead to the development of a treatment regimen that is not effective in achieving the desired functional outcomes of care. In the clinical example, had the clinician erroneously assumed that the client was presenting with functional limitations secondary to a radiculopathy, he would have provided a regimen that would have neither relieved the client's symptoms nor improved the client's functional level.

Appropriateness for Treatment

Not all clients who are referred to a clinician will require treatment. Clinicians must, therefore, review the findings from the client examination and determine whether the client would benefit from treatment, such as the direct application of treatment techniques, education, or coordination of services (Box 2-7). Once the clinician has confirmed that treatment is appropriate, and before he begins treatment planning, he needs to address the issues of whether he has a legal right and the clinical competence to treat the client's clinical condition.

Legal right to treat refers to whether the treatment of the presenting clinical problem, the examination techniques, and the treatment techniques that the clinician wishes to use are within the clinician's professional

---

> ### Box 2-5
> ### Confirmation of Clinical Hypothesis
>
> The clinician identifies the critical impairments stemming from the client's medical condition. He also confirms his clinical hypothesis that the presence of pain (neck pain and headaches), spasm, muscle tightness, decreased range of motion, decreased strength, and inability to lift and reach were secondary to active myofascial trigger points in the R upper trapezius and R levator scapulae.

Box 2-6
Summary of Pertinent Findings for Client with Myofascial Cervical Pain

Subjective Information

- Neck pain at rest, at end of range of motion, and during functional activity
- Reported pain intensity of 8 on Visual Analog Scale
- Reported inability to drive or check out groceries at the cash register for >10 min because of increased neck pain
- Tightness of neck muscles on waking and with fatigue
- Transient headaches (temporal region)

Objective Information
Areas of dysfunction

- Forward head posture
- Palpable muscle spasm in right (R) trapezius
- Palpable taut bands in trapezius and levator scapulae
- Reported positive pattern of pain referral on palpation of R trapezius trigger point
- Reported positive pattern of pain referral on palpation of R levator scapulae trigger point
- Twitch response on palpation of trigger point locations in upper trapezius and levator scapulae
- Decreased active cervical range of motion: flexion 50%, extension 75%, R rotation 75%, L side-flexion 50%
- Tightness of R trapezius and R levator scapulae
- Decreased strength: R levator scapulae—scapular elevation = grade 4–, R trapezius—scapular elevation, scapular retraction = grade 4–
- Active trigger points in R upper trapezius and R levator scapulae: grade 2 trigger point (a difference >4 kg/cm^2 but <6 kg/cm^2 between the involved and normal sides)[15];R upper trapezius pressure algometer reading = 1; R levator scapulae pressure algometer reading = 0.8
- Inability to drive for >10 min because of increased neck pain
- Inability to perform repetitive upper extremity movements in standing using right arm for >10 min (as required for checking out groceries at the cash register) because of neck pain
- Inability to reach objects placed 1 ft above head with right arm (as required for retrieving items from overhead shelves) because of neck pain
- Inability to lift 5-lb object above shoulder level using right arm (as required for placing boxes of dried goods on overhead shelves) because of neck pain
- Inability to lift and transfer a 15-lb object using right arm (as required for placing customers' purchases into shopping carts) because of neck pain
- Inability to perform more than three repetitions of lifting and transferring a 3-lb object at waist level using right arm (as required for checking out customers groceries and placing them in shopping bags) because of neck pain

Relevant functional areas

- Range of motion of shoulder, elbow, wrist, and hand within normal limits
- Strength of shoulder flexors, extensors, abductors, adductors; elbow flexors, extensors, pronators, supinators; wrist flexors, extensors, radial and ulnar deviators; thumb flexors, extensors, abductors, adductors; finger flexors, extensors within normal limits

scope of practice. Professional scope of practice is
dictated in the laws of the jurisdiction in which the
clinician practices. Health care professions have practice
acts that protect public health and safety by regulating
the qualifications, registration, and discipline of members of the profession. For each profession, these
practice acts outline the qualifications, licensing or
registration requirements, treatments that can be applied,
grounds for discipline, and sanctions that will be applied
to violators of the practice act.

Legal right to treat can be a gray area where the
practice of massage is concerned, since some massage
techniques can be used by clinicians from a range of
health care professions for the management of different
conditions within their scope of practice and without
advanced training or certification, while others cannot.
Superficial stroking applied to facilitate relaxation, can
be incorporated into the treatment regimens provided by
athletic trainers, massage therapists, nurses, occupational
therapists, physical therapists, chiropractors, and other
bodyworkers for clients with a variety of clinical conditions. By contrast, the application of superficial lymph
drainage technique for the management of lymphoedema may be outside the scope of practice of several of
these health care professionals.

Another aspect of scope of practice relates to the
clinician's need to determine whether the client also has
therapeutic needs that are more appropriately addressed
by another health care profession. This situation would
warrant a referral to another health care professional for
treatment of the clinical problems that are outside the
clinicians scope of practice. In light of the complexity
of issues related to scope of practice, clinicians are
referred to the practice acts for their professions to
determine their legal right to use massage techniques for
the different clinical conditions they encounter in clinical
practice.

In addition to the legal issues, the clinician has an
ethical decision to make regarding his competence to
treat the client's presenting clinical problems. This is a
subjective decision that requires a balance of confidence
in one's clinical skills and a realization of the limitations
of one's clinical expertise. In other words, it is not
sufficient that the clinician's practice act permits the
provision of interventions for a condition or the
application of selected techniques; the clinician must
also have sufficient training to administer this care
appropriately, safely, and effectively.

Common Errors in Hypothesis Generation

The research on clinical decision making can provide
some guidance on how to avoid some common errors in
hypothesis generation and verification. Comparisons of
master and novice clinicians have shown that master
clinicians included in their data gathering both objective
data and information on their clients' perception of their
medical condition and functional limitations.[2] This
integration of findings from different sources assisted the
master clinicians in confirming the clinical hypotheses.
Unlike novice clinicians, master clinicians were selective
in the data that they gathered and were able to depart
from a standard examination framework to seek clarification on issues that arose during the examination. This
strategy prevented the problem that novice clinicians
frequently encountered of becoming overwhelmed by a
large amount of irrelevant data. Generating a few hypotheses about the client's clinical problem early in the
examination appeared to give the clinician more opportunities for refining the hypothesis and arriving at a
hypothesis that was supported by the clinical findings.[3,4]

On the other hand, there were several common
errors made by clinicians during an examination. Having
too many hypotheses made it difficult for the clinician to
use a focused set of tests and measures and resulted in
the gathering of divergent information. Making hypotheses very general so that they would fit inconsistent
findings led the clinicians to arrive at incorrect conclusions about the client's clinical condition. Incorrect
conclusions also occurred when the clinicians made the
error of exaggerating findings to justify an existing
hypothesis rather than acknowledging that the existing
hypothesis was incorrect and seeking a new hypothesis.

TREATMENT PLANNING PHASE

The steps in treatment planning involve the identification
of impairments that are appropriate for treatment and the
selection of treatment techniques that are most likely to
result in improvements in the client's impairments and
the functional limitations to which they contribute.[5] The
treatment-planning phase for outcome-based massage
(Fig. 2-3) begins with the summary of clinical findings
from the evaluative phase and ends with a written plan
of care.

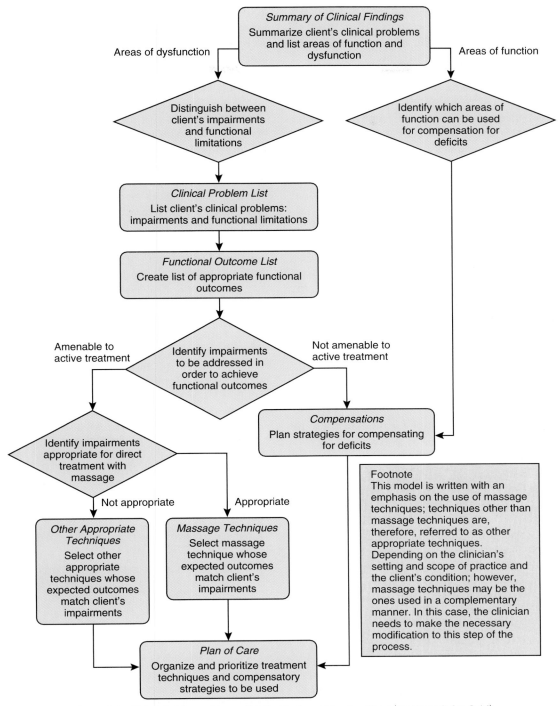

Figure 2-3. Clinical decision-making model: the Treatment Planning Phase (see Boxes 2-6 to 2-14).

CLINICAL PROBLEM LIST

Before the clinician can begin selecting treatment techniques, he needs to organize the clinical findings on the client's impairments, functional limitations, and disabilities into the clinical problem list that he will use as the basis of the treatment planning. First, it is important for the clinician to distinguish between the client's areas of function and dysfunction or those areas that will respond to the direct application of treatment techniques and those that will not. Rather than dismissing areas that are functional as not being in need of treatment, the clinician is wise to identify which of these areas can be used to compensate for impairments that are not amenable to active treatment. An example of this strategy is presented during the discussion of the identification of impairments that are not amenable to treatment.

Once the clinician has identified the areas of dysfunction, it is important for him to differentiate between the client's impairments and functional limitations. The strategy used in treatment planning for outcome-based massage will be to select treatment techniques to treat the identified impairments and to use the identified functional limitations as a baseline for setting functional outcomes of care. The reader is reminded that an *impairment* is a loss or abnormality of the affected individual's physiological, anatomical, cognitive, or emotional structure or function that occurs as a result of the initial or subsequent pathophysiology.[8] *Functional limitations* are restrictions of the individual's ability to perform actions or activities within the range considered normal for the organ or organ system. Once the clinician completes the above-mentioned tasks he can compile the clinical problem list (Box 2-8).

IDENTIFICATION OF FUNCTIONAL OUTCOMES OF CARE

The clinician can now focus on identifying relevant functional outcomes of care in collaboration with the client and predicting the amount of time needed to achieve these outcomes (Box 2-9). These outcomes should be consistent with the functional limitations that were documented during the client examination. Examples of functional outcomes are given in Table 2-2. The outcomes and the time needed to achieve them will also be based on a consideration of the client's current and prior level of function; the severity, complexity, stability, and acuity of the client's condition; the client's discharge destination; the literature on the prognosis for an individual with that condition; and the clinician's judgment, from clinical experience, of what the client has the potential to achieve.[6] In addition, clinicians can seek guidance from articles on clinical practice and research in professional journals; clinical texts; general practice guidelines for professions, such as the American Physical Therapy Association's "Guide to Physical Therapist Practice";[6] or the numerous practice guidelines that are available for specific clinical conditions. In some health care professions, such as physical therapy, this process of predicting the client's level and timing of improvement is known as the prognosis.[6]

It is not sufficient to identify the long-term functional outcomes of care for the client; the clinician must also identify short-term outcomes and predict what level of improvement the client can achieve within a given time frame. This is necessary because long-term functional outcomes of care can be used to gauge the client's readiness for discharge but are of little value in evaluating

---

Box 2-8
Clinical Problem List

Impairments

- Pain: Neck pain and temporal headaches
- Decreased muscle extensibility: Tightness of trapezius and levator scapulae
- Postural malalignment: Forward head posture
- Muscle spasm in R trapezius
- Decreased active cervical range of motion
- Decreased muscular performance

    Decreased R trapezius and R levator scapulae strength and endurance

    Decreased muscle integrity: Active trigger points in R upper trapezius and levator scapulae

Functional Limitations

- Inability to drive for >10 min because of increased neck pain
- Inability to perform repetitive upper extremity movements in standing using right arm for >10 min (as required for checking out groceries at the cash register) because of neck pain
- Inability to reach objects placed 1 ft above head with right arm (as required for retrieving items from overhead shelves) because of neck pain
- Inability to lift 5-lb object above shoulder level using right arm (as required for placing boxes of dried goods on overhead shelves) because of neck pain
- Inability to lift and transfer a 5-lb object using right arm (as required for placing customers' purchases into shopping carts) because of neck pain
- Inability to perform >3 repetitions of lifting and transferring 3-lb object at waist level using right arm (as required for checking out customers' groceries and placing them in shopping bags) because of neck pain

Box 2-9
Functional Outcomes of Care

The clinician identifies the functional outcomes of care outlined below on the basis of *(a)* the client's presenting functional limitations and *(b)* the observation that the client is a young woman who is in good health other than the myofascial neck pain and who had normal functional ability before the onset of pain 2 months prior to the examination.

Functional Limitations

- Inability to drive for >10 min because of increased neck pain
- Inability to perform repetitive upper extremity movements in standing using right arm for >10 min (as required for checking out groceries at the cash register) because of neck pain
- Inability to reach objects placed 1 ft above head with right arm (as required for retrieving items from overhead shelves) because of neck pain
- Inability to lift 5-lb object above shoulder level using right arm (as required for placing boxes of dried goods on overhead shelves) because of neck pain
- Inability to lift and transfer a 15-lb object using right arm (as required for placing customers' purchases into shopping carts) because of neck pain
- Inability to perform more than three repetitions of lifting and transferring 3-lb object at waist level using right arm (as required for checking out customers groceries and placing them in shopping bags) because of neck pain

Functional Outcomes of Care
Short-term outcomes (2 weeks)

- Able to drive for ½ hr without complaints of pain
- Able to work checking out groceries at the cash register for ½ hr, with appropriate breaks, without complaints of pain
- Able to lift 5-lb object and place it on shelf at shoulder level—one repetition without complaints of neck pain
- Able to reach objects placed 1 ft above head with right arm without complaints of neck pain
- Able to lift and transfer an 8-lb object at waist level with right arm without complaints of pain
- Able to perform five repetitions of transferring a 5-lb object at waist level using right arm without complaints of pain

Long-term outcomes (discharge: 4 weeks)

- Able to drive for 1.5–2 hr without complaints of neck pain
- Able to work checking out groceries at the cash register for 2 hr, with appropriate breaks, without complaints of pain
- Able to lift an 8-lb object and place it on shelf at shoulder level—five repetitions without complaints of neck pain
- Able to reach objects placed 2 ft above head with right arm without complaints of neck pain
- Able to lift and transfer a 15-lb object at waist level with right arm without complaints of neck pain
- Able to perform 15 repetitions of transferring a 5-lb object at waist level using right arm without complaints of neck pain

the client's immediate and ongoing response to treatment. A short-term outcome that can be achieved within a few sessions provides a useful early benchmark of the effectiveness of the treatment regimen and can, thus, be an invaluable aid to the ongoing modification and progression of treatment. The time period for achieving these short-term outcomes of care will vary with the acuity, severity, complexity, and stability of the client's condition; the expected rate of change in the client's functional level; the frequency of interventions; the anticipated duration of the treatment; and the clinical

setting. The aim is to set outcomes in measurable and meaningful increments that can be reasonably achieved in the allocated time. It may be appropriate, for example, to set weekly outcomes for a client in an acute-care or outpatient setting who is expected to have significant functional gains over a short course of treatment. By contrast, monthly outcomes may be more meaningful for a geriatric client in a skilled nursing setting who is being treated for a chronic condition.

A common question is "How can the clinician determine whether the functional outcomes of care are

Table 2-2
Sample Functional Outcomes of Care

Activities of Daily Living	*General Outcomes*
· Increased ability to perform grooming tasks, such as bathing and dressing · Increased ability to perform work-related tasks, such as lifting and keyboarding · Increased ability to perform leisure tasks · Increased ability to perform transfers, such as sit to stand · Increased ability to perform bed mobility tasks, such as rolling side to side or scooting · Increased ability to perform gait, locomotion tasks · Increased ability to perform functional mobility tasks, such as toilet and bath transfers · Increased ability to perform cooking tasks · Improved quality or quantity of movement during functional activity · Improved safety during functional activity · Decreased level of supervision required for task performance · Increased tolerance for positions and activities	· Improved self-management of condition · Decreased risk of recurrence of condition · Improved decision-making regarding health issues · Reduced utilization and cost of health care services · Decreased need for adaptive, assistive, supportive, protective, or orthotic equipment or devices · Ability to recognize and seek intervention for a recurrence of the clinical condition · Decreased intensity of care required

Data from American Physical Therapy Association. Guide to physical therapist practice. Phys Ther 1997;77(11):3–14.

appropriate for massage?" In reality, the issue is whether the impairments that must be addressed to achieve the functional outcome are appropriate for treatment with the use of massage as the primary treatment technique. This decision about the relevance of the impairments for the use of massage comes later in this phase of the decision-making process.

IDENTIFICATION OF TREATABLE IMPAIRMENTS AND IMPAIRMENT-LEVEL OUTCOMES OF CARE

Once the functional outcomes of care have been established, the clinician works backward to identify *(a)* which impairments need to be treated to facilitate the achievement of the functional outcomes of care, *(b)* which of these impairments are amenable to active treatment, *(c)* which impairments require compensations because they are not amenable to active treatment, and *(d)* the predicted outcome for each impairment that will be treated (Box 2-10).

Traditionally, clinicians established treatment goals and selected treatment techniques solely on the basis of the impairments that they observed during the client examination. The adoption of disablement models in health care has resulted in the focus on the impact of treatment on the client's identified functional limitations and disability. Nevertheless, clinicians must still identify and treat the clients' underlying impairments, in addition

to addressing their functional limitations.[5] What remains unclear is whether there is a direct relationship between improved impairments and improvements in functional level. A balanced approach to treatment planning would identify and treat the client's impairments as a means of facilitating the achievement of the functional outcomes of care, rather than focusing solely on impairments or functional limitations.

The clinician also distinguishes between the impairments that are amenable to active treatment and those for which he must plan a means of compensation. The clinical case of the client with myofascial cervical pain (Box 2-1) is admittedly a straightforward one in which all of the client's impairments are amenable to active treatment. A more complex case would be, for example, a 65-year-old who is 3 months post a right-sided cerebrovascular accident. The therapists treating this client have identified a left drop foot, left-sided weakness, primitive movement patterns, increased tone in the trunk and involved extremities, painful left shoulder subluxation, and edema in the left hand as the primary impairments. Of these, the drop foot has shown no further signs of recovery and no longer appears amenable to active treatment. Consequently, the therapists consider the drop foot to be an impairment that will need to be compensated for with an ankle-foot orthosis and ambulatory aids. The therapist can also use one of the client's available functional areas to compensate for this impairment in addition to using external orthoses and devices. For example, the physical therapist could use gait training in the use of more functional pelvic and lower extremity muscle groups to compensate for the drop foot as a means of facilitating effective locomotion.

Although the clinician will use the identified functional outcomes of care as the primary means of judging the client's progress, it is still beneficial for him to identify impairment-level outcomes of care (Box 2-11). The clinician can then use the client's progress, or lack thereof, with respect to the impairment-level outcomes as a basis for determining whether the client is responding to the treatment techniques that are being applied. Table 2-3 contains some examples of impairment-level outcomes.

IDENTIFICATION OF IMPAIRMENTS APPROPRIATE FOR MASSAGE

In the clinical decision-making model for outcome-based massage, the treatment-planning phase also includes the identification of those impairments that are most appropriate for the application of massage techniques. This decision is based on the clinician's knowledge of the expected impairment-level outcomes of care of the

massage techniques and whether massage techniques can have a direct or secondary effect on the impairment. There are three possible options: massage has a direct effect on the impairment, massage has a secondary effect on the impairment, or massage has no effect on the impairment. Distinguishing between the impairments that can be treated with massage techniques as the primary treatment technique and those that cannot can assist the clinician in *(a)* creating a treatment regimen that will result in improved functional outcomes of care and *(b)* prioritizing treatment techniques and the use of time during interventions.

Since the decision regarding the relevance of impairments for the use of massage is a critical one, here are further examples of how clinicians can make this decision. Consider the case of a client who presents with the impairments of pain, adhesions, and decreased muscle extensibility in the later stages of therapy following surgical repair of the Achilles tendon. Connective tissue and neuromuscular techniques can be used to increase muscle extensibility and to promote remodeling of dense connective tissue; therefore, adhesions and decreased muscle extensibility are impairments that are appropriate

---

Box 2-10
Functional Limitations and Associated Impairments

Functional Limitation	Associated Impairments
Inability to perform driving tasks	• Pain: Neck pain and temporal headaches • Postural malalignment: Forward head posture • Decreased active cervical range of motion • Muscle spasm in right (R) trapezius • Decreased muscle integrity: Active trigger points in R upper trapezius and levator scapulae
Inability to perform repetitive upper extremity movements in standing	• Pain: Neck pain and temporal headaches • Postural malalignment: Forward head posture • Decreased active cervical range of motion • Muscle spasm in R trapezius • Decreased muscular performance: Decreased R trapezius and R levator scapulae strength and endurance • Decreased muscle integrity: Active trigger points in R upper trapezius and levator scapulae
Inability to perform lifting tasks	• Pain: Neck pain and temporal headaches • Decreased muscle extensibility: Tightness of trapezius and levator scapulae • Muscle spasm in R trapezius • Decreased muscular performance: Decreased R trapezius and R levator scapulae strength and endurance • Decreased muscle integrity: Active trigger points in R upper trapezius and levator scapulae

Box 2-11
Impairment-Level Outcomes of Care

- Normalized cervical and head posture
- No palpable muscle spasm in R trapezius
- No signs of active trigger points on palpation of trapezius and levator scapulae: palpable taut bands, positive pattern of pain referral, or twitch signs; a difference of <2 kg/cm^2 between the involved and normal sides using pressure algometry[15]
- Active cervical range of motion: flexion 100%, extension 100%, R rotation 100%, L side-flexion 100%
- Normal extensibility of R trapezius and R levator scapulae
- Muscle strength: R levator scapulae—scapular elevation = grade 5, R trapezius—scapular elevation, scapular retraction = grade 5

Table 2-3
Impairments Amenable to Treatment with Massage and Related Impairment-Level Outcomes of Care

Impairment	*Outcome*
Musculoskeletal	
· Adhesions/scarring	· Increased tissue mobility · Decreased scarring

· Impaired connective tissue integrity
  Fascial restrictions
  Abnormal connective tissue density
  Decreased mobility of skin, superficial, and deep fascia
	· Separation and lengthening of fascia
	· Promotion of dense connective tissue remodeling
	· Increased connective tissue mobility

· Impaired joint integrity
  Inflammation of joint capsule or ligaments
  Restrictions of joint capsule and ligaments
	· Decreased signs of inflammation of joint capsule, tendons, or ligaments
	· Decreased capsular and ligament restrictions
	· Increased joint mobility
	· Increased joint integrity

· Impaired joint mobility Decreased voluntary range of motion	· Increased joint mobility

· Impaired muscle integrity
  Decreased muscle extensibility
  Tendinopathies
  Trigger points
	· Increased muscle extensibility
	· Decreased signs of inflammation and promotion of healing of tendons
	· Increased joint mobility
	· Decreased trigger point activity

· Muscle strains and tears	· Decreased signs of inflammation and promotion of healing of muscle
· Impaired muscle performance (strength, power, endurance)	· Enhanced muscle performance secondary to the enhancement of muscle extensibility, reduction of pain, reduction of muscle spasm, enhancement of joint mobility, normalization of joint integrity, reduction of trigger point activity, etc. · Balance of agonist/antagonist muscle function
· Abnormal muscle-resting tension and muscle spasm	· Decreased muscle spasm · Normalized muscle-resting tension · Increased joint mobility

Table 2-3 *(continued)*

Impairment	*Outcome*
· Pain	· Pain reduction through primary treatment of dysfunction, e.g., active trigger points · Counterirritant analgesia · Systemic sedation resulting in decreased perception of pain
· Postural malalignment	· Normalized postural alignment · Increased postural awareness
· Impaired sensation secondary to entrapment neuropathy or nerve root compression	· Normalized sensation secondary to the reduction of nerve and nerve root compression due to fascial restrictions and trigger points
· Swelling Edema, joint effusion, lymphoedema	· Increased lymphatic return · Increased venous return · Decreased joint effusion · Decreased edema · Increased joint integrity · Increased joint mobility

Neurological

· Abnormal neuromuscular tone: Spasticity, rigidity, clonus	· Normalized neuromuscular tone · Alteration of movement responses through proprioceptive and exteroceptive stimulation techniques · Balance of agonist/antagonist muscle function

Cardiopulmonary

· Impaired airway clearance	· Increased respiration/gaseous exchange · Increased airway clearance/mobilization of secretions · Decreased dyspnea
· Dyspnea	· Decreased dyspnea due to increased airway clearance · Decreased dyspnea due to increased perceived relaxation
· Decreased rib cage mobility (other than bony abnormality)	· Increased rib cage mobility · Increased muscle extensibility · Increased ventilation

Psychoneuroimmunological

· Stress	· Systemic sedation · Increased perceived relaxation · Decreased levels of cortisol, epinephrine, and norepinephrine
· Anxiety	· Decreased perceived anxiety · Increased perceived relaxation · Decreased levels of cortisol, epinephrine, and norepinephrine
· Depression	· Decreased cortisol levels
· Immune suppression	· Stimulated immune function through decreased cortisol levels

Gastrointestinal

· Gastrointestinal immobility secondary to sedentary status	· Stimulated peristalsis

Central nervous system

· Athletic preperformance needs	· Systemic arousal and enhanced alertness
· Failure to thrive in high-risk infants	· Promoted weight gain and development through increased vagal activity, sensory organization
· Lethargy	· Sensory arousal and enhanced alertness

for treatment with massage as a primary treatment technique (Box 2-12). In this situation, the massage technique will have a direct effect on the impairment, and other techniques can be used in a complementary manner.

There are also circumstances in which massage techniques can have a secondary or indirect effect on an impairment, for example, a client who presents with decreased muscle performance because of pain, guarding, and muscle spasm following the reduction of a glenohumeral dislocation. In this situation, superficial reflex techniques can be used to reduce pain, guarding, and muscle spasm and thus facilitate improvements in muscle performance. If a massage technique has a secondary effect on the impairment, the clinician may choose to use that technique in a complementary manner within the intervention. In this case, the primary treatment techniques to address decreased muscle performance would be therapeutic exercise.

Finally, if the client presented with the impairment of muscle weakness secondary to a metabolically induced peripheral neuropathy, then the impairment would not be appropriate for massage, since massage techniques do not have a documented effect on neurologically based muscle weakness. If the massage technique has no

documented or demonstrated effect on the impairment, the clinician has little justification for including it in the treatment regimen. A general summary of the expected impairment-level outcomes of care of massage techniques is presented in Table 2-3 to assist the clinician in determining whether impairments are appropriate for treatment with massage.

At this point in the decision-making process, as mentioned above, the clinician is able to ascertain whether the identified functional outcomes related to the impairments are appropriate for massage.

SELECTION OF TREATMENT TECHNIQUES

Once the clinician has identified the impairments for which massage techniques have a direct or secondary effect, he can proceed with the selection of the techniques to be used in the treatment regimen (Box 2-13). The clinician matches appropriate massage techniques to impairments by considering three factors: match of expected impairment-level outcome of the massage technique to the client's impairment; identification of contraindications or cautions in the application of that technique given the client's clinical condition; and the clinician's legal right and competence to use the technique. The techniques chapters and Chapter 11, The

---

Box 2-12
Appropriateness of Impairments for Massage

Impairments	Role of Massage
Pain: Neck pain and headaches	• Direct effect on pain due to presence of active trigger points
Decreased muscle extensibility of trapezius and levator scapulae	• Direct effect on muscle extensibility
Postural malalignment: Forward head posture	• Direct effect on lengthening of shortened anterior neck and trunk muscles; there will also be a secondary effect resulting from the inactivation of the trigger point, since the decrease in pain will minimize the compensatory postural changes that are due to trigger point pain
Spasm in R trapezius	• Direct effect on muscle spasm
Decreased active cervical range of motion	• Direct effect on lengthening of shortened anterior neck and trunk muscles that contribute to decreased range of motion; there will also be a secondary effect from the inactivation of the trigger point, since the decreased range may be due in part to a combination of trigger point pain and compensatory muscle guarding
Decreased muscular performance: Decreased R trapezius and R levator scapulae strength	• Secondary effect since weakness is likely to be due to trigger point pain and disuse
Decreased muscle integrity: Active trigger points in R upper trapezius and levator scapulae	• Direct effect on the active myofascial trigger point

---

Box 2-13
Selection of Treatment Techniques

Massage Techniques

- Superficial stroking
- Superficial effleurage
- Broad-contact compression
- Petrissage
- Stripping
- Specific compression
- Self-care specific compression with a handheld massage device

Other Appropriate Treatment Techniques

- Moist heat for trigger point pain
- Ice for acute spasm
- Specific stretches for trapezius and levator scapulae
- Postural reeducation
- Active range-of-motion exercises
- Strengthening exercises
- Self-care education
- Functional activity

Treatment Process and Discharge Planning (see Table 11.1) of this text describe the expected impairment-level outcomes of care of each of the techniques presented, to facilitate the clinician's selection of massage techniques.

Simply matching impairment to impairment-level outcomes of care of the massage techniques is not, however, sufficient to guarantee that a technique is appropriate for that client's condition. Before performing any massage technique, the clinician needs to consider the general cautions and contraindications to the application of that technique for the client's clinical condition.[9–12] Some of the suggested general cautions and contraindications for the application of massage techniques to various clinical conditions are summarized in Table 2-4. The cautions and contraindications for specific massage techniques are also reviewed in the relevant techniques chapters.

While this list is a necessary starting point for the consideration of cautions and contraindications to treatment, clinicians should use their judgment about the application of massage techniques to the client at hand. A useful rule of thumb is that if a client's condition requires ongoing medical management, then it is appropriate for the clinician to consult the clinician who is responsible for that medical management for guidelines regarding cautions and contraindications to treatment.

The clinician also needs to consider whether there are any anatomical structures that can be damaged during the application of massage techniques.[8,9,10,13] For example, the application of friction or specific compression over a peripheral nerve in a location where it is close to the skin may produce a neuropraxia.[14] While some sources describe "endangerment sites" (Table 2-5) as areas of the human body over which the use of direct or sustained pressure is contraindicated,[9,13] clinicians may use their judgment in determining whether these areas

are contraindicated for other massage techniques. Students and novice clinicians who are not experienced in applying treatment techniques should take a conservative approach to the application of massage techniques in situations that are cautions or contraindicated and in "endangerment sites."

ARTICULATION OF THE PLAN OF CARE

It is unlikely that a plan of care will consist only of massage techniques. The clinician must also select other treatment techniques, such as therapeutic exercise, electrotherapeutic modalities, education, and training on functional activity, that will be needed to achieve the identified outcomes of care. The treatment techniques available to the different health care professionals are well documented in current clinical texts.

A list of treatment techniques does not constitute a plan of care; the clinician also needs to specify and document the treatment parameters within the client's written plan of care (Box 2-14). The duration of the episode of care (the current treatment period) and the frequency of interventions should be consistent with the severity, stability, complexity, and acuity of the client's clinical condition; the client's treatment tolerance; the client's prognosis; and the identified outcomes of care. Other factors that can influence the duration of care and frequency of interventions include the client's cognitive status, preexisting conditions, potential discharge destination, overall health status, and probability of prolonged impairment.[6] The clinician must also determine the scope and duration of massage in each intervention, as well as the duration and frequency of each technique that is used. Chapter 11, The Treatment Process and Discharge Planning, provides further information about these issues. Finally, the clinician also needs to consider the client's home or work environment, social context, and personal goals for treatment, to

Table 2-4
Suggested Cautions and Contraindications for Reflex and Mechanical Massage Techniques

Local Conditions

Contraindications

Acute flare-up of inflammatory arthritis: rheumatoid arthritis, systemic lupus, Reiter's syndrome, etc.
Acute neuritis
Aneurysms
Areas of altered or impaired sensation
Baker's cyst
Ectopic pregnancy
Esophageal varicosities
Frostbite
Local contagious skin condition
Local infection
Local irritable skin condition
Malignancy
Open wound or sore
Peripheral neuropathy
Phlebitis, thrombophlebitis, arteritis
After anti-inflammatory injection (24–48 hr)
Recent burns
Undiagnosed lump

Cautions

Acute disk herniation
Acute inflammatory condition
Allergies to lubricants and cleansers
Antiinflammatory injection site
Buerger's disease
Chronic abdominal or digestive disease
Chronic arthritic conditions
Chronic diarrhea
Chronic or long-standing superficial thrombosis
Contusion
Endometriosis
Flaccid paralysis
Fracture—while casted and immediately after cast removal
Hernia
Joint instability or hypermobility
Kidney infection or stones
Mastitis
Minor surgery
Pelvic inflammatory disease
Pitting edema
Portal hypertension
Presence of pins, staples
Prolonged constipation
Recent abortion or vaginal birth
Trigeminal neuralgia

General Conditions

Contraindications

Acute conditions requiring first aid: anaphylaxis, epileptic seizure, pneumothorax, myocardial infarction, syncope, status asthmaticus, cerebrovascular accident, diabetic coma, insulin shock, appendicitis
Advanced kidney failure
Advanced respiratory failure
Anemia (depending on the cause)
Diabetes with complications
Eclampsia
Hemophilia
Hemorrhage
Highly metastatic cancers
Intoxication
Liver failure
Sepsis
Severe atherosclerosis
Shock
Significant fever (>101.5°F or 38.3°C)
Systemic contagious/infectious condition
Unstabilized cerebrovascular accident
Unstable hypertension
Unstabilized myocardial infarction

Cautions

Asthma
Atherosclerosis
Cancer
Chronic congestive heart failure
Chronic kidney disease
Client taking medications that alter neurological, cardiovascular, psychological, or renal function
Coma
Drug withdrawal
Emphysema
Epilepsy
Hypertension
Hypotension
Immunosuppression
Inflammatory arthritis
Major or abdominal surgery
Multiple sclerosis
Osteoporosis
Post–cerebrovascular accident
Post–myocardial infarction
Pregnancy and labor
Psychiatric conditions
Recent head injury
Spasticity or rigidity

Data from references 9–12.

Note: A technique that is not contraindicated is not necessarily appropriate for the treatment of a given condition.

Table 2-5
Selected Endangerment Sites

Head and Neck	*Trunk*	*Extremities*
· Neck, including anterior and posterior triangle · Eye · Trachea · Styloid process of the temporal bone	· Axilla · Xiphoid process · 12th (floating) rib · Kidneys in the area of the 12th rib · Umbilicus · Linea alba · Sciatic notch	· Ulnar nerve at medial epicondyle · Femoral artery, nerve, and vein in the area of the inguinal triangle

Data from references 9, 10, and 13.

Box 2-14
Plan of Care

History	**History of present illness:** 2 months ago, client had insidious onset of localized neck and shoulder pain right (R) > left (L), with stiffness, decreased active cervical range of motion, neck muscle tightness, neck muscle spasm, and transient headaches; seen by an MD and given muscle relaxants with little effect; referred to physical therapy; is right-handed Current medication: Acetaminophen for pain Current functional status: On reduced hours because of neck pain and difficulty performing job-related tasks **Past medical history:** Unremarkable; no prior history of neck or upper extremity injuries; no prior physical therapy **Prior functional level:** Full-time cashier at supermarket; able to perform all job-related tasks without difficulty
Examination Findings	**Subjective** *Pain*: Neck pain at rest, at end of range of motion and during functional activity; reported pain intensity of 8 on Visual Analog Scale; transient headaches (temporal region) *Muscle tightness:* Tightness of neck muscles on waking and with fatigue *Functional limitations:* Reported inability to drive or check out groceries at the cash register for more than 10 min because of increased neck pain **Objective** *Posture:* Forward head posture *Palpation:* Palpable muscle spasm in R trapezius; palpable taut bands in trapezius and levator scapulae; reported positive pattern of pain referral on palpation of R trapezius trigger point; reported positive pattern of pain referral on palpation of R levator scapulae trigger point; twitch response on palpation of trigger point locations in R upper trapezius and R levator scapulae *Muscle sensitivity:* Grade 2 trigger points in R upper trapezius and R levator scapulae (difference >4 kg/cm^2 but <6 kg/cm^2 between the involved and normal sides);[15] R upper trapezius pressure algometer reading = 1; R levator scapulae pressure algometer reading = 0.8 *Range of motion:* Decreased active cervical range of motion: flexion 50%, extension 75%, R rotation 75%, L side-flexion 50% with pain at end of range of motion; other ranges full and pain free; full and pain-free active range of motion of shoulder, elbow, wrist, and hand bilaterally *Muscle extensibility*: Tightness of trapezius and levator scapulae **Strength:** Decreased strength of R levator scapulae—scapular elevation = grade 4–; decreased strength of R trapezius—scapular elevation, scapular retraction = grade 4–; strength of shoulder flexors, extensors, abductors, adductors; elbow flexors, extensors, pronators, supinators; wrist flexors, extensors, radial and ulnar deviators; thumb flexors, extensors, abductors, adductors; finger flexors, extensors bilaterally = grade 5

continued

Box 2-14 (continued)
Plan of Care

Functional limitations:
· Inability to drive for >10 min because of increased neck pain
· Inability to perform repetitive upper extremity movements in standing using right arm for >10 min (as required for checking out groceries at the cash register) because of neck pain
· Inability to reach objects placed 1 ft above head with right arm (as required for retrieving items from overhead shelves) because of neck pain
· Inability to lift 5-lb object above shoulder level using right arm (as required for placing boxes of dried goods on overhead shelves) because of neck pain
· Inability to lift and transfer a 15-lb object using right arm (as required for placing customers' purchases into shopping carts) because of neck pain
· Inability to perform more than three repetitions of lifting and transferring a 3-lb object at waist level using right arm (as required for checking out customers' groceries and placing them in shopping bags) because of neck pain

Outcomes of Care

Impairment-level outcomes of care
· Normalized cervical and head posture
· No palpable muscle spasm in R trapezius
· No signs of active trigger points on palpation of trapezius and levator scapulae muscles; palpable taut bands, positive pattern of pain referral, or twitch signs; a difference of < 2 kg/cm^2 between the involved and normal sides using pressure algometry
· Active cervical range of motion: flexion 100%, extension 100%, R rotation 100%, L side-flexion 100%
· Normal extensibility of R trapezius and R levator scapulae
· Muscle strength: R levator scapulae—scapular elevation = grade 5, R trapezius—scapular elevation, scapular retraction = grade 5

Functional outcomes of care
Short-term outcomes (2 weeks)
· Able to drive for ½ hr without complaints of pain
· Able to work checking out groceries at the cash register for ½ hr, with appropriate breaks, without complaints of pain
· Able to lift 5-lb object and place it on shelf at shoulder level—one repetition without complaints of neck pain
· Able to reach objects placed 1 ft above head with right arm without complaints of neck pain
· Able to lift and transfer an 8-lb object at waist level with right arm without complaints of pain
· Able to perform five repetitions of transferring a 5-lb object at waist level using right arm without complaints of pain
Long-term outcomes (discharge: 4 weeks)
· Able to drive for 1.5–2 hr without complaints of neck pain
· Able to work checking out groceries at the cash register for 2 hr, with appropriate breaks, without complaints of pain
· Able to lift an 8-lb object and place it on shelf at shoulder level—five repetitions without complaints of neck pain
· Able to reach objects placed 2 ft above head with right arm without complaints of neck pain
· Able to lift and transfer a 15-lb object at waist level with right arm without complaints of neck pain
· Able to perform 15 repetitions of transferring a 5-lb object at waist level using right arm without complaints of neck pain

Treatment Plan

Treatment qd, 2 × week for 4 weeks; discharge to self-care program and full-time employment

Massage techniques
· Superficial stroking
· Superficial effleurage
· Broad-contact compression
· Petrissage
· Stripping
· Specific compression
· Self-care specific compression with a handheld massage device

Box 2-14 *(continued)*

Therapeutic exercise
· Specific stretches for trapezius and levator scapulae muscles
· Postural reeducation
· Active range-of-motion exercises
· Strengthening exercises
· Modalities
· Moist heat in the location of the trigger points to reduce trigger point activity and pain
· Ice for acute muscle spasm

Functional training
· Functional training in lifting tasks required for effective job performance as a cashier

Education
· Self-care education in pain and trigger point management

ensure that the treatment regimen adequately addresses these factors. Failure to do so may have a negative impact on the level of the client's adherence with self-care and participation in the plan of care.

TREATMENT PHASE

The treatment phase is best described as an ongoing cycle of treatment, reexamination, and treatment progression that begins after the clinician completes the plan of care (Fig. 2-4). The end of this phase is not clearly delineated; instead, there is a gradual transition from treatment phase to discharge phase.

SELECTING TREATMENT AND REEXAMINATION TECHNIQUES

The clinician is ready to initiate treatment once he has completed the plan of care. First of all, he selects a subset of the prioritized massage and complementary treatment techniques from the plan of care as a starting point. Since the aims of the first stage of treatment are to gauge the client's treatment tolerance and to ascertain whether the treatment techniques can affect the client's impairments, it is advisable to select those techniques that are most likely to have a direct effect. At the outset of the episode of care, the clinician also identifies which subjective and objective examination techniques he can use to determine whether the client is having a positive response to treatment. In doing so, he includes questions that seek the client's perspective on her progress and the intervention. This information is invaluable, since these factors can signal problems that the client is having with the intervention and can provide the clinician with guidance on how to improve client adherence to or participation in the plan of care.

FIRST STAGE OF TREATMENT AND REEXAMINATION

As mentioned above, during the first stage of treatment the clinician is evaluating the appropriateness of the plan

of care and gauging the client's treatment tolerance. He bases the intensity of the interventions on the level of acuity of the client's condition; that is, he uses a less intense level for a more acutely ill client and vice versa. In addition, he is cautious not to introduce too many treatment techniques at once, since that will make it difficult for him to identify the techniques to which the client had a positive or adverse response (Box 2-15). The clinician also conducts formal and informal client examinations to determine the client's response to treatment.

The clinician can perform informal client examinations at any time during the interventions. As Chapter 3, Review of Client Examination Concepts for Massage, describes, palpation and the massage techniques themselves can provide information on the client's response to the technique being applied and to the intervention as a whole. These informal examinations can be interspersed throughout the interventions. Once the client has reached a point at which the clinician can reasonably expect a measurable clinical change, the clinician carries out a more formal reexamination using the tests and measures he selected for this purpose (Box 2-16). The reexamination is focused on the identification and measurement of changes in the client's impairments and functional level from the baseline established at the initial examination (see Table 2-1). The clinician uses the reexamination as a means of determining the client's progress toward the achievement of the identified outcomes and the client's readiness for treatment progression. He can use this information as the basis for the decision on whether to modify the plan of care or the identified outcomes.

If the result of the client reexamination is that the client does not demonstrate any clinical change, the clinician must first determine whether it may be too early to observe a change. If this is the case, he reattempts treatment with the original set of techniques and may

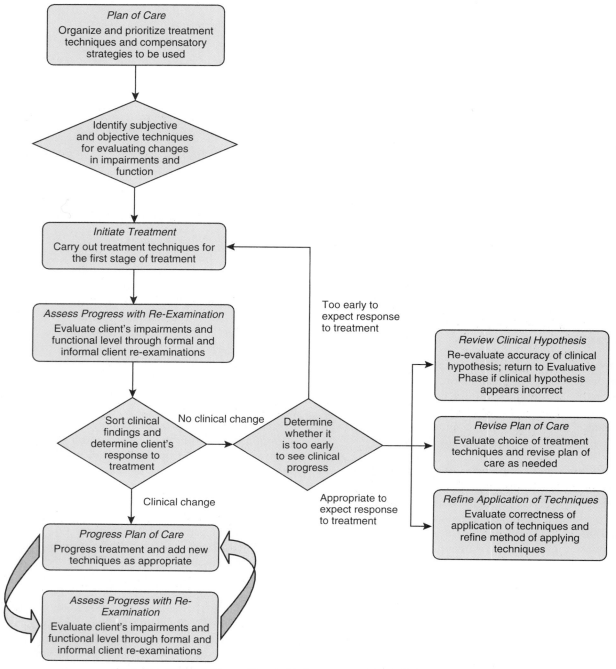

Figure 2-4. Clinical decision-making model: the Treatment Phase (see Boxes 2-14 to 2-17).

consider the addition of another treatment technique before the next formal reexamination. If, however, the clinician believes that the client has had ample time to demonstrate a clinical change, then the clinician must reevaluate the appropriateness of the plan of care. Possible causes for the client's failure to respond to interventions for the clinician to consider are *(a)* the

clinician's clinical hypothesis was incorrect; *(b)* the treatment technique was not appropriate for the client's condition; or *(c)* the clinician did not apply the technique correctly. If the clinician's clinical hypothesis was incorrect, he will need to revisit the evaluative phase and repeat the process of the client examination to identify the client's clinical condition. The clinician can remedy the choice of inappropriate treatment techniques by selecting more-appropriate techniques and modifying the plan of care. Finally, if the clinician's choice of clinical hypothesis and treatment techniques appears to be accurate, then he needs to refine his application of the treatment techniques.

ONGOING PROGRESSION AND REEXAMINATION

Once the clinician is confident that the direction of the plan of care is appropriate, then the cycle of treatment progression and informal or formal reexamination begins (Box 2-17). Throughout this cycle, the clinician ensures that he assesses both the client's impairments and functional level at appropriate intervals. Ideally, each intervention should incorporate an element of informal examination and progression or modification of either the treatment techniques or client education. Chapter 11, The Treatment Process and Discharge Planning, discusses these issues in greater detail. During the application of each treatment technique, the clinician

---

Box 2-15
Initial Treatment and Examination Techniques

Massage Treatment Technique
- Superficial stroking on the site of the acute spasm
- Broad-contact compression around the site of spasm

Complementary Technique
- Specific stretches for trapezius and levator scapulae
- Ice for spasm
- Self-care education for pain control

Examination Techniques
Subjective
- Pain reports
- Perceptions of treatment and progress made

Objective
- Muscle spasm
- Trigger point sensitivity
- Trigger point pain referral pattern
- Range of motion

Box 2-16
Client's Response to Initial Interventions (1 week)

Treatment Technique	· Superficial stroking on the site of the spasm · Broad-contact compression on the location of the trigger points and off the site of the spasm · Petrissage off the site of the spasm · Specific stretches for trapezius and levator scapulae · Ice on the location of the muscle spasm · Self-care education for pain control
Results of Informal Examination	· Client had negative response to use of ice for spasm, this exacerbated trigger point pain; superficial stroking used for spasm · Moist heat applied to the trigger point location may be more effective for pain relief · Client's trigger points initially too sensitive to tolerate specific compression; broad-contact compression used · Client able to perform specific stretches for trapezius and levator scapulae appropriately
Results of Formal Examination	· Decreased reports of pain during functional activity—reported pain intensity of 6.5 on Visual Analog Scale · Decreased trigger point sensitivity—pressure algometer reading trapezius = 1.4, levator scapulae = 0.9 · Decreased muscle spasm · Pattern of pain referral—unchanged
Clinician's Conclusions	· Client is responding to treatment; trigger point therapy is appropriate

continued

Box 2-17
Treatment Progression and Reexamination

	Week 2	Week 3
Treatment Techniques	**Massage techniques**	**Massage techniques**

Week 2

Massage techniques
- Broad-contact compression
- Petrissage
- Specific compression

Other appropriate treatment techniques
- Specific stretches for trapezius and levator scapulae muscles
- Heat to location of trigger points for pain
- Postural reeducation
- Active range-of-motion exercises
- Functional activity
- Self-care education—add home range of motion and stretching program

Week 3

Massage techniques
- Broad-contact compression (decreased duration)
- Petrissage (decreased duration)
- Stripping (increased duration and depth)
- Specific compression (increased duration and depth)

Other appropriate treatment techniques
- Specific stretches for trapezius and levator scapulae muscles
- Heat for preparation for stretching
- Postural reeducation
- Functional activity
- Strengthening exercises
- Self-care education—add self-care specific compression with a handheld massage device

Results of Client Reexamination

Week 2

Functional outcomes of care
- Reports being able to drive for 0.5 h without complaints of neck pain
- Able to perform repetitive upper extremity movements while standing 0.75 h without complaints of neck pain
- Able to lift a 5-lb object and place it on shelf at shoulder level—five 5 repetitions without complaints of neck pain
- Able to reach objects placed 1 foot above head with right arm without complaints of neck pain
- Able to lift and transfer a 5-lb object at waist level with right arm without complaints of neck pain
- Able to perform 10 repetitions of transferring a 5-lb object at waist level using right arm without complaints of neck pain

Other examination findings
- Reported recent flare-up of pain following attempts to increase work time
- Reported pain intensity of 5 on Visual Analog Scale by end of week
- Decreased trigger point sensitivity—pressure algometer reading trapezius = 2, levator scapulae = 1.5
- Pattern of pain referral—decreased intensity of pain on palpation of trigger points
- Active cervical range of motion: flexion 75%, extension 90%, R rotation 90%, L side-flexion 75%
- Strength: R levator scapulae—scapular elevation = grade 4, R trapezius—scapular elevation, scapular retraction = grade 4

Week 3

Functional outcomes of care
- Reports being able to drive for 1 hr without complaints of neck pain
- Able to perform repetitive upper extremity movements while standing 1.25 hr without complaints of neck pain
- Able to lift a 10-lb object and place it on shelf at shoulder level—one repetition without complaints of neck pain
- Able to reach objects placed 1.5 ft above head with right arm without complaints of neck pain
- Able to lift and transfer a 10-lb object at waist level with right arm without complaints of neck pain
- Able to perform 15 repetitions of transferring a 5-lb object at waist level using right arm without complaints of neck pain

Other examination findings
- Reported pain intensity of 3.5 on Visual Analog Scale
- Decreased trigger point sensitivity—pressure algometer reading trapezius = 2.5, levator scapulae = 1.8
- No pain referral on palpation of upper trapezius trigger point, minimal reports of pain for levator scapulae trigger point
- Active cervical range of motion: flexion 90%, extension 100%, R rotation 100%, L side-flexion 75%
- Strength: R levator scapulae—scapular elevation = grade 4+, R trapezius—scapular elevation, scapular retraction = grade 4+

informally evaluates the client's response and uses this information as the basis of fine-tuning the intervention and his application of the treatment techniques. These informal examinations can also be used to identify when the client has a flare-up of her clinical condition that results in an increase in her impairments and functional limitations. Timing of formal examinations of the client's progress with the established functional outcomes of care will depend on the timing of the outcomes of care defined by the clinician.

DISCHARGE PHASE

Discharge involves the transition of the client from the care of the clinician to care by another clinician or to self-care. The discharge phase begins before the date on which the client is discharged; it spans the period from the initiation of discharge planning to the actual discharge date (Fig. 2-5).

There is, unfortunately, no exact formula to use to determine when to initiate the discharge process;

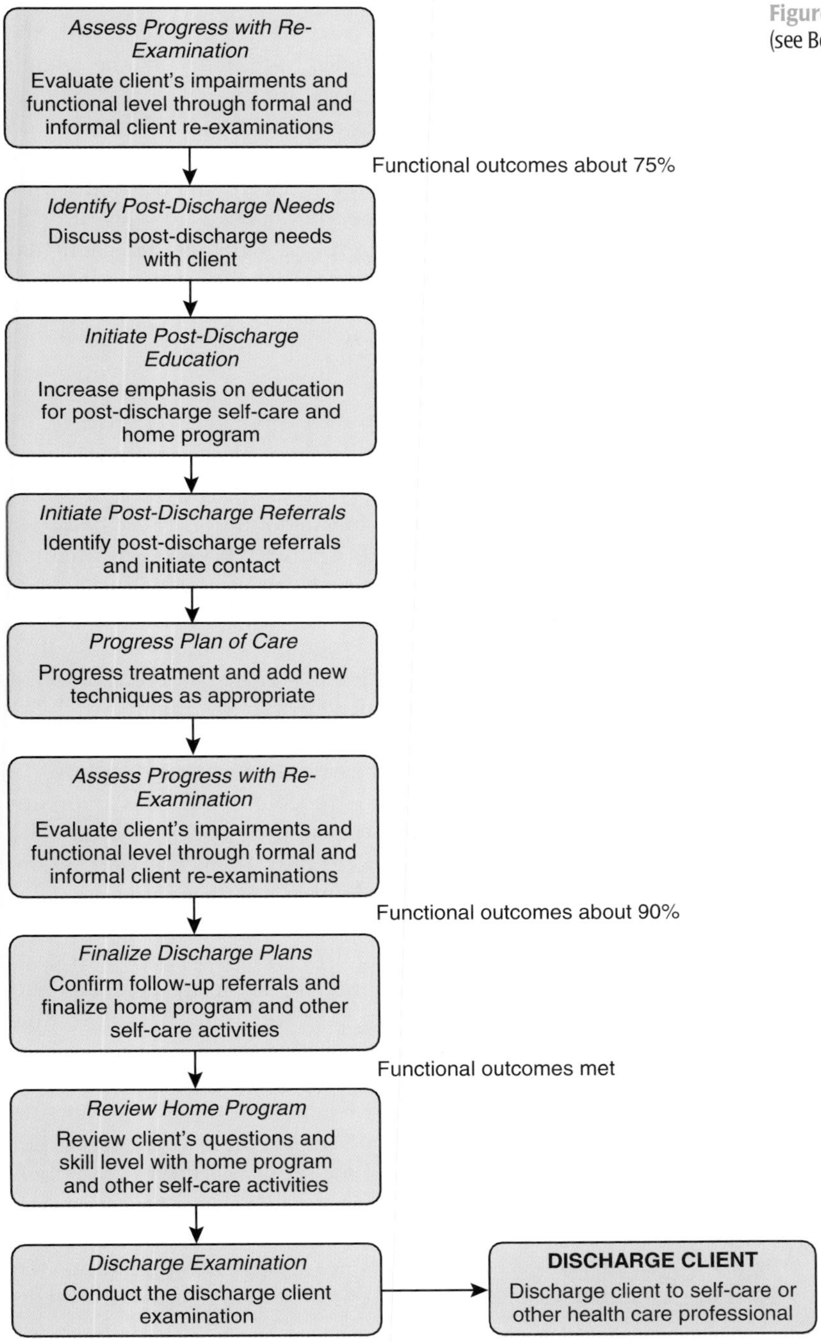

Figure 2-5. Clinical decision-making model: the Discharge Phase (see Boxes 2-17 and 2-18).

Assess Progress with Re-Examination
Evaluate client's impairments and functional level through formal and informal client re-examinations

Functional outcomes about 75%

Identify Post-Discharge Needs
Discuss post-discharge needs with client

Initiate Post-Discharge Education
Increase emphasis on education for post-discharge self-care and home program

Initiate Post-Discharge Referrals
Identify post-discharge referrals and initiate contact

Progress Plan of Care
Progress treatment and add new techniques as appropriate

Assess Progress with Re-Examination
Evaluate client's impairments and functional level through formal and informal client re-examinations

Functional outcomes about 90%

Finalize Discharge Plans
Confirm follow-up referrals and finalize home program and other self-care activities

Functional outcomes met

Review Home Program
Review client's questions and skill level with home program and other self-care activities

Discharge Examination
Conduct the discharge client examination

DISCHARGE CLIENT
Discharge client to self-care or other health care professional

discharge planning may be initiated as early as the first session or much later in the treatment process. In the clinical example, clinicians may begin discharge planning in earlier sessions because of the relative brevity of the episode of care. Many factors can influence the clinician's decision on when to begin the discharge phase. First, the clinician must also consider the client's characteristics, such as the client's progress with her functional outcomes of care, her psychological and educational readiness for discharge, and the resources needed and available to the client following discharge. In addition, the clinician cannot ignore the constraints to discharge planning imposed by the nature of the clinical setting and the predicted length of the episode of care. While one can argue that every intervention is preparing the client for discharge, there are specific activities that are associated with facilitating an effective discharge. As the client approaches achievement of her functional outcomes of care (approximately 75% achieved), the clinician needs to initiate a discussion of the client's discharge concerns and needs. This may occur earlier if the client appears to have complex needs that will require more discharge planning or the clinical setting dictates shorter episodes of care. Although all of the client's discharge needs may not be appropriate for the clinician to address, this information is valuable for planning self-care education, referrals to other health care professionals, and other resources.

By the time the client is close to achieving her functional outcomes of care, the clinician should have initiated referrals, identified equipment needs, initiated equipment purchases, and finalized the content of home programs, and begun discharge self-care education. The emphasis of the final sessions prior to discharge will shift to include a larger educational component (Box 2-18). If the client is being referred to another clinician, for example, a subacute unit or home health care, the discharge process will also include written and verbal communication with the other clinician.

Can you discharge a client if her functional outcomes of care are not met? There is much discussion and controversy about whether clinicians terminate an episode of care based on the achievement of functional outcomes of care or on other factors, such as end of reimbursement or the client's request. Ideally, the clinician will use the extent to which the client achieves her functional outcomes of care as the guide for discharge. There are circumstances, however, in which the client need not meet the established functional outcomes of care before discharge. These situations include *(a)* when the clinician recognizes that the outcomes were not achievable given the client's condition and health status; *(b)* when the client's functional level reaches a plateau before achieving the outcomes, but she carries out her

daily activities well enough to justify discharge; *(c)* when the client is unable to progress toward the outcomes because of medical or psychological complications; *(d)* when the client refuses ongoing treatment; and *(e)* when the clinician believes that the client cannot benefit from more treatment.[6] Ultimately, the clinician must use his clinical judgment, input from the client, and examination findings to guide his decisions about the timing of discharge. In all situations, appropriate documentation of the rationale for discharge is necessary.

Can you justifiably continue to treat a client after her identified outcomes of care have been met? If the identified outcomes of care were consistent with the severity, complexity, stability, and acuity of the client's clinical condition and appropriate for her discharge needs, then continued treatment cannot be justified on an ethical basis. If a clinician who is approaching the end of treatment is uncertain that treatment should end, he should reevaluate the predicted outcomes and his scope of practice to determine whether the client has ongoing therapeutic needs that he can address or whether he needs to refer the client to another health care professional.

ONGOING CARE

Clinicians must modify the four-phase clinical decision-making process for clients who require ongoing episodes of care because of their clinical condition or the nature of the care being provided. Clients who require ongoing episodes of care include pediatric clients with developmental disabilities; clients with chronic or terminal conditions who are at risk for deterioration of health status; geriatric clients who are at risk for falls or deterioration of health status; and clients who have ongoing disability and health care needs as a result of spinal cord injury, head injury, amputation, or other traumatic injury. In addition, clients who are receiving wellness interventions may also require ongoing episodes of care. The clinical decision-making process does not end at the discharge phase when a client requires ongoing episodes of care. First, the clinician's discharge planning must include organization, or at the very least a discussion, of the follow-up care. Secondly, the clinician must plan and implement a follow-up client examination and thus initiate the evaluative phase once more.

The follow-up examination is a focused client examination in which the clinician determines whether the client demonstrates deterioration of the status of her impairments, functional limitations, disability, and quality of life from the level that was documented at the last discharge examination (see Table 2-1). Based on the clinical findings he obtains from this examination, the clinician determines whether the client has new treat-

Box 2-18
Discharge Planning and Discharge

Treatment Techniques	*Week 4: Intervention 1*

Week 4: Intervention 1
Massage techniques
· Petrissage (decreased duration)
· Broad-contact compression (decreased duration)
· Specific compression (increased duration and depth)
· Stripping (increased duration and depth)

Other appropriate treatment techniques
· Postural reeducation
· Functional activity
· Strengthening exercises
· Self-care education—add ergonomics education, reviewed education on identifying and managing flare-ups

Week 4: Intervention 2
Other appropriate treatment techniques
· Review of self-care education: pain management, ergonomics, home stretching, home range of motion, and self-care specific compression with a handheld massage device
· Discharge to home self-care program

Results of Client Reexamination

Reexamination findings
· Discharge concerns: cashier station not ergonomically correct, this aggravates pain, concerned about how to manage flare-ups
· Able to demonstrate all self-care activities correctly
· Reported pain intensity of 1 on Visual Analog Scale
· Decreased trigger point sensitivity—pressure algometer reading trapezius = 2.7, levator scapulae = 2.0
· No pain referral on palpation of upper trapezius or levator scapulae trigger point

Discharge examination findings
Functional outcomes of care
· Able to drive for 2.5 hr without complaints of neck pain, using stretches and postural checks
· Able to work checking out groceries at the cash register for 2 hr without complaints of neck pain; takes appropriate breaks and uses stretches and postural checks; has had ergonomic adjustments to cashier station; occasional complaints of neck tightness with fatigue
· Able to perform lifting tasks required for work as a cashier:
  1. Able to lift an 8-lb object and place it on shelf at shoulder level—five repetitions without complaints of neck pain
  2. Able to reach objects placed 2 ft above head with right arm without complaints of neck pain
  3. Able to lift and transfer a 15-lb object at waist level with right arm without complaints of neck pain
  4. Able to perform 20 repetitions of lifting and transferring a 5-lb object at waist level using right arm without complaints of neck pain

Other examination findings
· Reported pain intensity of 0.5 on Visual Analog Scale
· Normalized cervical and head posture
· No palpable muscle spasm in R trapezius muscle
· No signs of active trigger points on palpation of trapezius and levator scapulae: palpable taut bands, positive pattern of pain referral, or twitch signs; a difference of >2 kg/cm^2 between the involved and normal sides using pressure algometry
· Maintained level trigger point sensitivity—pressure algometer reading trapezius = 2.7, levator scapulae = 2.0
· Active cervical range of motion: flexion 100%, extension 100%, R rotation 100%, L side-flexion 100%
· Normal extensibility of R trapezius and R levator scapulae
· Muscle strength: R levator scapulae—scapular elevation = grade 5, R trapezius—scapular elevation, scapular retraction = grade 5

ment needs. If the client does not require ongoing care, the clinician documents this finding and organizes further follow-up if this is warranted. On the other hand, if the client does demonstrate deterioration in status, the clinician initiates the treatment-planning phase of the clinical decision-making process and then moves onto the treatment and discharge phases. In the case of wellness interventions, the need for ongoing care is not based on a deterioration of health status but on the identification of the client's need for further treatment (direct application of treatment techniques, education, or coordination of services) as a means of maintaining or improving his or her current health status.

The Interpersonal Aspects of the Process of Clinical Care

EVALUATIVE PHASE

The interpersonal aspects of the evaluative phase are concerned with adequate clinician preparation and appropriate engagement of the client into the clinical process (Fig. 2-6).

TREATMENT PLANNING PHASE

The interpersonal aspects of the Treatment Planning Phase focus on obtaining informed consent to evaluate and treat, on appropriately eliciting the client's perception of her illness, and on negotiating a plan of care with the client (Fig. 2-7).

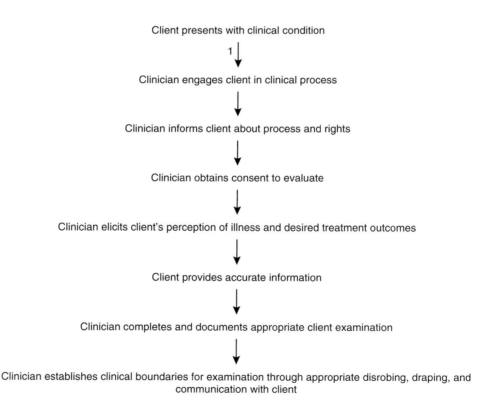

Client presents with clinical condition

1 ↓

Clinician engages client in clinical process

↓

Clinician informs client about process and rights

↓

Clinician obtains consent to evaluate

↓

Clinician elicits client's perception of illness and desired treatment outcomes

↓

Client provides accurate information

↓

Clinician completes and documents appropriate client examination

↓

Clinician establishes clinical boundaries for examination through appropriate disrobing, draping, and communication with client

1   Steps are sequential

Figure 2-6. Process of care: Evaluative Phase.

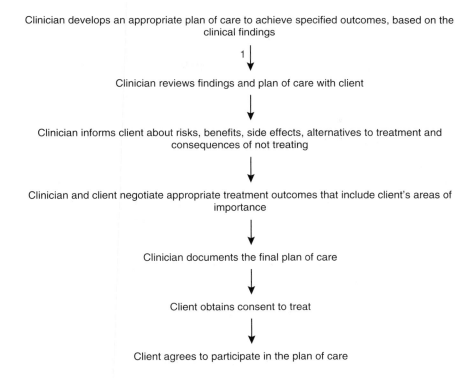

Figure 2-7. Process of care: Treatment Planning Phase.

TREATMENT PHASE

The interpersonal aspects of the Treatment Phase focus on maintaining an ethical and clinically appropriate therapeutic relationship and ensuring appropriate, on-going self-care on the part of the clinician (Fig. 2-8). The end of this phase is not clearly delimited; instead, there is a gradual transition from Treatment Phase to Discharge Phase.

DISCHARGE PHASE

The Discharge Phase begins before the date on which the client is discharged: it spans the period from the initiation of discharge planning to the actual discharge date. The interpersonal issues addressed during this phase concern achieving appropriate closure to the therapeutic relationship (Fig. 2-9).

Relevant Issues for All Phases

There are three critical aspects of the process of clinical care that are relevant for all four of the phases in the clinical decision-making process proposed in this chapter. The first involves the ethical considerations that should guide the clinician's practice and the client–clinician relationship. The client's emotional response to treatment and the clinician's approach to addressing this

response compose the second issue. Lastly, there is client adherence to treatment and the strategies that the clinician can use to enhance adherence. All of these issues can have an impact on the extent to which the outcomes of care are achieved. The clinician would, therefore, be wise to integrate strategies for addressing these issues into all aspects of the process of clinical care.

ETHICAL ISSUES

The client–clinician relationship is complicated by the imbalance of power that is associated with the clinician's presumed role of "healer" and his possession of information and skills that are needed by the client, and the client's vulnerability and dependence on the clinician. Consequently, ethical issues are not confined to any particular phase of the process of clinical care; instead, these issues must be addressed at all points during and beyond the client–clinician interaction. Both the client and the clinician have rights and responsibilities that result from their participation in the process of clinical care. The importance of these rights and responsibilities is underscored by the fact that health care professions have a clearly articulated set of guidelines for ethical conduct in clinical practice to which they expect all members of their profession to adhere.[16–24]

The client comes into the client–clinician relationship with rights that are intended to protect her from being victimized or harmed by the clinician, as well as to ensure that she receives a high standard of care. The client's rights summarized in Box 2-19 revolve around issues of autonomy, privacy, information, confidentiality, and respect.

Clinician adheres to guidelines for ethical conduct

1 ⟶

Clinician maintains clinical boundaries during the intervention through appropriate draping and communication with client

⟶

Clinician performs appropriate preparations of materials for each intervention

⟶

Clinician uses appropriate physical and psychological self-care during the course of treatment

⟶

Clinician uses appropriate body mechanics and manual techniques and delivers treatment in a safe manner

⟶

Clinician demonstrates responsible caring and concern for the client

⟶

Clinician appropriately delegates care to and supervises adjunct staff

⟶

Clinician appropriately responds to client's emotional reaction to treatment

⟶

Clinician facilitates client participation in and adherence to treatment

⟶

Clinician elicits client's ongoing feedback on progress with clinical outcomes

⟶

Clinician provides client with appropriate education

⟶

Clinician maintains updated documentation on the treatment provided and the client's response

⟶

Clinician maintains communication with referring clinician as appropriate

⟶

Client participates in care in a responsible manner or accepts the consequences of refusing to participate

⟶

1 Steps are concurrent

Figure 2-8. Process of care: Treatment Phase.

Clinician elicits client's perceived discharge needs

1 ↓

Clinician informs client of post-discharge treatment requirements

↓

Clinician prepares appropriate initial discharge plan based on clinical findings

↓

Clinician and client negotiate discharge goals and arrangements

↓

Clinician documents final discharge plan

↓

Clinician prepares client for discharge by addressing client's physical and psychological needs

↓

Client participates in pre-discharge education and preparation

↓

Clinician completes and documents pre-discharge examination and determines whether client has achieved the identified functional outcomes

↓

Clinician facilitates appropriate closure to client–clinician relationship

↓

Clinician transfers the client to another clinician or caregivers for follow up care as appropriate. In the case of wellness massage, the clinician arranges for a follow-up visit at an appropriate interval.

↓

Clinician provides other clinicians or caregivers with appropriate documentation for follow-up care

1   Steps are sequential

Figure 2-9. Process of care: Discharge Phase.

Yet, the client is not without responsibility in the client–clinician interaction. As the client's responsibilities outlined in Box 2-20 suggest, the client must bear the responsibility of acting on her rights and must, in turn, treat the clinician with respect.

The clinician bears the burden of most of the responsibility in the client–clinician relationship because of the need to ensure that he does not abuse the power that he holds within this relationship. Not only does the clinician have the responsibility for seeing that the client's rights are met (Boxes 2-21 and 2-22), but he also has responsibilities to his profession and society as a whole that are beyond the scope of this chapter.

Unfortunately, the clinician's rights are rarely discussed. With increasing erosion of the clinician's autonomy in practice, it is important not to lose sight of the clinician's right to exercise his best clinical judgment and to work in an environment in which he can practice without coercion, conflict of interest, undue influence, or inappropriate scheduling demands (Box 2-23).

CLIENT'S EMOTIONAL RESPONSE TO TREATMENT

Clinicians are often unprepared for the client's emotional response to the application of massage techniques. The information in this chapter is intended to serve as an

---

Box 2-19
Client's Rights

- Accessible and impartial access to care
- Autonomy: Freedom of choice of practitioner; right to participate in decision-making during treatment; right to refuse or leave treatment regardless of the clinician's opinion; right to a consultation with another practitioner
- Care in a safe health-care environment
- Confidentiality, specifically no disclosure of any information about the client without her written consent
- Continuity of care
- Dignity, including the right not to remain disrobed longer than necessary
- Privacy, both visual and auditory; this includes not having to disclose any information that is not relevant to the care being received
- Respect for her values and cultural beliefs
- Right to be informed of her rights
- Timely and accurate information on the status or background of clinician providing care, the treatment provided, risks, side effects, alternatives, whether research is being conducted, postdischarge treatment needs, and consequences of not treating

---

Box 2-20
Client's Responsibilities

- Accept the consequences of refusing care, altering care, or choosing an alternative option to care
- Act with consideration and respect for clinicians and others in that setting
- Adhere to instructions provided by the clinician
- Ensure that financial obligations to the clinician or facility are met
- Follow rules of conduct of the health care setting
- Provide accurate information to the clinician

Box 2-21
Clinician's Responsibilities to the Client (Issues Related to Interactions with Client)

- Demonstrate responsible caring and concern for the client
- Do not guarantee a cure or misrepresent the potential effects of the treatment
- Do not treat clients when under the influence of any substance that would impair the ability to treat safely
- Listen to and respect client's values, beliefs, and needs
- Maintain appropriate clinical boundaries and avoid sexual interaction of any sort with clients
- Provide client-centered, preventative care
- Provide the client with an opportunity to give voluntary and informed consent
- Respond appropriately to client's emotional reaction to treatment
- Use draping to maintain the client's privacy and appropriate clinical boundaries

---

Box 2-22
Clinician's Responsibilities to the Client (General Issues)

- Act in the client's best interests
- Act without conflict of interest
- Assume responsibility for and provide appropriate examination, treatment, progression of care, and discharge planning
- Communicate information on the client's care to the referring clinician (within restraints of maintaining confidentiality)
- Delegate care to and supervise adjunct staff or students appropriately and take responsibility for the care they provide
- Document all of the client's findings accurately and appropriately
- Ensure and maintain a high level of competence
- Maintain confidentiality of records and information and obtain a signed release prior to disclosure
- Not refuse a client care on the basis of race, etc.
- Not treat unless the client's clinical condition (prevention, curative, maintenance, wellness) warrants it and thus avoid the overutilization of services
- Provide client-centered, preventative care
- Provide services to meet the client's needs, rather than for financial gain
- Provide the highest standard of care possible
- Request consultation from other clinicians as appropriate
- Take responsibility for the care provided to a client
- Transfer the client to another clinician as appropriate when the client–clinician relationship is ended or the client is discharged
- Use sound judgment
- Work within his or her scope of practice and refer to another clinician when the client's condition requires treatment that is beyond his or her legal scope of practice or level of competence

---

Box 2-23
Clinician's Rights

- To make independent clinical judgments
- To decline to treat a client if it would compromise his or her ethics, dignity, or values
- To work in an environment in which he or she can practice without coercion, conflict of interest, or undue influence, including being pressured into overutilization of services for the facility's financial gain
- To be treated with respect and consideration by the client and colleagues

overview of emotional responses to treatment and some basic strategies for responding to the client. The principles discussed in the section "Appropriateness for Treatment" above in this chapter also apply to the client's psychosocial needs. The clinician should ensure that he remains within the limits of his professional scope of practice and clinical training when he is addressing the client's emotional needs that arise during an intervention.

In particular, the clinician should recognize when it is appropriate to refer the client to a physician or health care professional who can provide psychosocial care.

THE PHYSICAL BASIS OF EMOTIONAL CONTROL

There are many different approaches to understanding and working with the connection between the body and the emotions. These approaches include bodyworkers who integrate psychological aspects into their therapeutic approach (energy work and chakras),[25] somatoemotional release,[26] traditional Chinese medicine,[27] psychotherapists who integrate bodywork into their approach (Reichian),[28] Bioenergetics,[29] Core-energetics,[30] other neo-Reichian and body-centered psychotherapies,[31] Jungian therapy,[32] Gestalt therapy,[33] and Primal Therapy.[34] The clinicians who integrate bodywork with psychotherapy/emotional work in these approaches draw from numerous theoretical perspectives. While the language and concepts of these approaches may differ, they are not mutually exclusive and can be seen as illustrating the diversity of human experience.

The approach described here is based, to a large degree, on the work of Wilhelm Reich, a student of

Freud's who correlated patterns of chronic muscular tension with psychological disorders. Reich[35–37] recognized that these patterns of muscular tension were not merely symptoms of his clients' neuroses, but actually the means by which they avoided experiencing emotions that were connected with childhood psychological traumas and maintained their psychological disorders. By incorporating bodywork into his psychoanalytic practice, he found that treating patterns of chronic muscular tension resulted in emotional and psychological responses that enabled his clients to become aware of the feelings that they were avoiding. Based on this observation, he formed a theory about the connection between the body and the emotions.

Reich proposed that the bodies of all living organisms vibrate or "pulsate" in an ongoing cycle of expansion and contraction. During normal levels of nervous system activity, these "pulsations" are difficult to observe; however, the intensity of these "pulsations" increases with increases in the intensity of an individual's emotional response. For example, an individual will shake when she experiences intense excitement or fear, or her chest will heave when she sobs. Furthermore, Reich theorized that people can learn to control their emotions by learning to control their physical reactions or "pulsations," even when the reasons for avoiding these emotions are unconscious.

Essentially, individuals can control the "pulsations" in their bodies by tensing groups of opposing muscles around a specific skeletal structure that is related to the emotion that they are trying to control.[38] This controlled tensing of the muscles can be short term or long term and habitual—not even relaxing in sleep. This muscle tension reduces the spontaneous movement in that part of the body and can result in that skeletal structure being generally held in a stiff and relatively fixed position known as "holding," or "armoring." Eventually, the posture of the entire body can reflect a psychological attitude. Not all muscle tension, however, is the result of an attempt to achieve emotional control. An individual's patterns of muscular tension may also be related to genetic predispositions, compensatory changes, injuries, and physical occupational stresses. Furthermore, not only can psychological attitudes affect muscular tension but the opposite may also be true. In traditional Chinese medicine,[39] imbalances in the organ systems are thought to give rise to energetic imbalances in psychoemotional states that, in turn, result in tension and imbalance in the musculoskeletal system (Fig. 2-10).

GENERAL IMPLICATIONS OF CHANGING BODY STRUCTURE

Rolf[40] and others[29–30] maintained that a change in myofascial length or tension that changes the structure of an individual's body shifts the way he or she is in the world. They believed that individuals become accustomed to a specific way of feeling their bodies

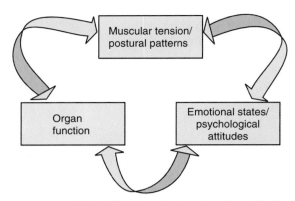

Figure 2-10. Relationship between body and emotions in traditional Chinese medicine.

and experiencing their usual physical sensations. In addition, during regular states of consciousness, individuals have their usual repertoire of emotional reactions with which they can identify. When the structure of their bodies is changed, they can experience new physical experiences—feelings of warmth and tingling—or sensations in areas of which they were previously unaware. These changes in their physical structure can also be accompanied by an enhanced potential to have thoughts and feelings other than the ones that they normally recognize. These thoughts and feelings may be so subtle that they are difficult to recognize, such as a delicate feeling of openness or a momentary feeling of vulnerability. On the other hand, the change in their bodies' structure might evoke an emotional response that is so strong that it makes it temporarily difficult for them to function socially.

Clinicians, therefore, should recognize that the application of a massage technique always has the potential to evoke an emotional response that stems from a change in the structure of the client's body. They also need to distinguish between the emotional response to a release of the client's tissues and the usual emotional response to being touched. Touch by its very nature tends to have emotional associations, especially for clients with traumatic touch or body associations, such as those with a history of physical or sexual abuse or anorexia. A release of chronic fascial tension will not; however, always evoke an emotional response, since humans have numerous ways of controlling emotional responses other than by controlling somatic "pulsations." These conscious and unconscious strategies for regulating emotional responses include refusing to recognize emotionally upsetting stimuli, "tuning out," holding one's breath, and substituting one emotion for another. Moreover, the types of stimuli that are needed to evoke an intense and difficult emotional reaction tend not to exist in the context of general massage treatment. Finally, individuals who are feeling emotionally fragile may consciously or unconsciously avoid situations like massage, which might evoke such an emotional response.

RECOGNIZING THE CLIENT'S EMOTIONAL PROCESS

In a Reichian theoretical perspective, there is a continuum of emotional release—from overt to subtle—in which signs of overt emotional release are easily recognized and those of subtle release less so. The signs and sensations of the usual vibratory and spontaneous movements in the body that accompany a subtle emotional release in the body include an increase in the rate of breathing, gurgles in the throat and abdomen, swallowing, tearing, the production of sounds such as sighing or moaning, spontaneous jerking of musculature, itches, sensations of heat and cold, and the movement of energy. These are usually simply signs and sensations of physical release—the movement from a tense state of sympathetic nervous system activation to a relaxed state of parasympathetic nervous system activation. When massage is used in a clinical setting, typically the occurrence of these signs and sensations in the client do not lead to anything other than a state of physical relaxation. When the client's physical signs and sensations are accompanied by thoughts and beliefs that form the psychological content of an emotion, however, an emotional release occurs.

The client can also manifest the physical and behavioral signs of limiting or containing, rather than releasing, emotions. These attempts to limit the vibratory or spontaneous movement in the body lead to reactions such as going still and silent, holding one's breath, exhibiting a rigidity in the musculature, focusing one's attention on an unrelated situation, or making distracting conversation. The individual will be able to maintain a distance from emotional content as long as these strategies are successful. The client's need to prevent emotional release can be in conflict with the massage-related treatment goals. For example, if she needs to maintain a certain degree of muscular tension to limit the vibratory and spontaneous movement in her body, this may be in conflict with the goal of deep relaxation of her tense musculature. If the clinician views the client's need to prevent emotional release and control her physical reactions as a reflection of her fear of unresolved and difficult emotional terrain, then he may be better able to respect the client's need for these strategies.

DEALING WITH EMOTIONAL RELEASE

The most appropriate response for a clinician untrained in working with emotional and psychological issues is to provide an atmosphere in which the client feels comfortable and safe to express emotions as they arise. This can be achieved by using the strategies outlined below.

Encouraging the Client to Give Feedback

Creating an open, accepting environment by encouraging the client to talk about what doesn't work for her during a session facilitates the development of open lines of communication. In addition, asking the client for her consent to treat both before and during a session can reaffirm her right to refuse any aspect of the treatment and contribute to her sense of safety.

Respecting the Client's Need to Avoid or Contain Her Emotions

There are times when the client needs to use strategies to avoid or contain her emotions, and the clinician finds that this need is in conflict with the goal of relaxation. Paradoxically, acceptance of the client's need to avoid or contain her emotions can reduce the tension associated with it and allow her to achieve greater relaxation.

Dealing with Containment

Unless the clinician has discussed a "contract" with the client that involves the exploration of her emotions, then he must simply be with whatever arises when the client experiences an emotional release. While everyone has his own unique way of being with someone who is experiencing intense emotions, within the context of a general massage context, this usually involves avoiding any actions that might intensify the client's emotional reaction. For example, engaging in the content of the emotion by asking the client questions can not only intensify her emotional reaction, but also lead to difficult interpersonal dynamics if the clinician's questions are not attuned to the client's emotional state and needs. In addition, moving to an area of the client's body where the emotional reaction is focused can also potentially intensify her emotional reaction. While intensifying the client's emotional reaction may be desirable, asking for the client's consent before doing so allows the client to control what she feels is appropriate for her and, in turn, helps her contain the level of her emotional reaction to what is suitable for the situation.

Knowing One's Comfort Level with Emotional Expression

Being comfortable with clients' expression of a range of emotions is a skill that develops with repeated exposure to clients' emotions. It is important for the clinician to acquire this skill and to learn his level of comfort with clients' emotions in preparation for a situation in which he encounters a client who starts to express her emotions. When a clinician exceeds his comfort level and pretends to be comfortable with his client's emotional expression, it can erode the client–clinician relationship for several reasons. The client may feel a lack of safety as a result of the clinician's falseness, or the clinician may feel that the proper boundaries of the client–clinician relationship have been transgressed by the client's emotional need.

When the clinician becomes aware that he has passed his acceptable comfort level, he must communicate to the client what level of emotions he can and cannot respond to within the session. Communicating one's limits appropriately is an interpersonal skill that can result in the client feeling good about herself and understanding where the limits are with regard to emotional expression and emotional processing within a clinical session. This skill not only involves the clinician knowing ways of phrasing and rephrasing the necessary information, but also requires that the clinician is aware of when the discomfort begins so he has time to convey the information to the client in a calming and accepting manner. Appropriate communication can help to avoid the interpersonal disconnection that can occur when the clinician suddenly feels overwhelmed and withdraws. This is important, since these disconnections can leave the client feeling that there is something wrong about her emotions and can result in interpersonal dynamics that are difficult to work through.

Being with Emotional Expression

Ideally, the clinician will allow the client's emotions to arise without encouragement or discouragement but with acceptance. An excellent way to communicate this acceptance to the client is through "mirroring"[41]—feeding back to the client through verbal statements or physical touch an empathetic understanding or perception of her present emotional state. This can range from the use of rephrasing or repeating the client's communications to the application of sensitive massage movements that are consistent with the client's expression of her emotions. In some cases, it may even mean respectfully stopping the massage while the client expresses her emotional state.

Regardless of the strategy used, the clinician needs to ensure that he attunes his response to the state and level of intensity of the client's emotional expression rather than engaging in the actual content of these emotions. This becomes particularly important when the client is in the middle of an intense emotion, since problems may arise when the clinician fails to match the client. For example, if the clinician noticeably lowers the intensity of his engagement when the client is increasing the intensity of her emotional expression, then the client may feel that her emotional expression is somehow not accepted. If, on the other hand, the clinician noticeably raises the intensity of his engagement beyond the intensity of the client's emotional expression, the client may feel pressured into expressing something more. This may result in transference dynamics when the client feeling that she has failed the clinician or that the clinician doesn't care about her true self. With practice, it is possible for the clinician to develop a repertoire of phrases that he can use to ask the client what she needs from the clinician. While both the timing and phrasing of these statements improve with practice, it is important for the novice to attempt these communications, even if somewhat awkwardly, so that the client can have an open line of communication with the clinician.

Emotions generally have an intensity that peaks and then passes, followed by a more reflective period. A general rule of thumb is to allow clients "space" that is unfettered by a large amount of verbal communication and difficult physical manipulations while they are in the intense phase of the emotional expression. Clients often appreciate the invitation—even if they chose not to accept—to talk about their experience after the intensity of it has passed. If she feels inclined to do so, talking about emotions can help the client to integrate the experience more deeply, while the clinician's empathetic listening and monitoring help to maintain a sense of interpersonal connectedness.

Finally, clinicians always need to be aware of the appropriate roles of the client–clinician relationship. While a small amount of sharing by the clinician may help reduce a client's sense of isolation, appropriate sharing is perhaps the most difficult art to master. The biggest danger faced by the clinician is the subtle, or not so subtle, reversal of the client–clinician role. As sharing by the clinician is not required for empathetic attunement, it is better to err on the side of not sharing anything too personal. When clinicians find that they have an emotional response to something that arises out of a clinical session, it is important for them to seek an appropriate means of dealing with those feelings, such as talking with a supportive colleague, supervisor, or mentor.

STRATEGIES TO ENHANCE CLIENT ADHERENCE

The client's adherence to the plan of care is the final component of the interpersonal aspects of the process of clinical care addressed in this chapter. Adherence has been defined in the literature in a variety of ways. Responsibility is placed on the client in the definition that adherence is the extent to which clients follow the instructions for care that they negotiate with their health care providers.[42] Adherence can also be viewed as being influenced by the clinician when it is defined as a positive behavior that occurs when a client is motivated by the clinician to adhere to the negotiated plan of care because of a perceived positive outcome or benefit.[43] However it is defined, adherence to a prescribed plan of care is necessary for the attainment of positive outcomes.[44] Based on research, various authors have suggested a variety of strategies for increasing clients' adherence to prescribed plans of care, which are outlined below.[45–54] These strategies revolve around the client's ability to understand the regimen and to follow the directions that were provided, the type of instructions provided by the clinician, and the extent to which the clinician tailors the regimen to the client's needs.

Unfortunately, the types of information that are least likely to be remembered are instructions and advice. The more information clients receive, the more likely they are to forget. Clients generally remember what they are told first and what they consider to be the most important. There is no correlation between the amount of information that is remembered and age or intelligence, although clients with more medical knowledge will recall more information. Furthermore, moderately anxious clients will recall more information than highly anxious clients or clients who are not anxious.

Adherence decreases when clinicians give unclear instructions; conversely, specific advice may increase adherence. For this reason, simple, direct, and repetitive instructions are most effective. For example, "You must do this exercise 10 times when you get out of bed every morning" will be recalled more readily than "Do this exercise several times each day." Furthermore, clients have difficulty complying when they are unclear why the various aspects of the regimen are important, even if the regimen is relatively simple. For example, the addition of the explanation "Putting ice on your ankle and elevating it by putting it up on a chair will help relieve the pain and swelling that you have in your ankle" as a precursor to instructions for the application of ice may clarify for the client why it would be beneficial to adhere to those instructions.

Modification of the characteristics of the prescribed regimen can increase adherence. Since adherence decreases with increasing duration of the treatment program and with increasing complexity of the treatment regimen, clinicians should simplify complex treatment regimens by breaking the plan of care into sequential steps. Clinicians can also tailor treatment programs to clients' activities and lifestyles in light of the findings that treatments that are perceived to intrude into the client's daily activities are less likely to be adhered to and that the simplest treatment regimen that is compatible with the client's lifestyle is most effective. Furthermore, clients respond positively when clinicians appear to accept that problems arise in integrating a regimen into a client's lifestyle and are available to help the client make modifications.

Clients place a high value on information, although clinicians often underestimate the extent to which they do so. Consequently, client education can become an intervention, not merely an adjunct to treatment. When a clinician is using client education as a primary intervention, small groups can be an effective approach. A small-group format allows clients to hear information repeated several times and provides opportunities for reinforcing that knowledge. Other clients may ask questions that a client may be hesitant to ask, either in a group setting or one-on-one with the clinician. Group participation may contribute to a sense of community by allowing the client to be with others with similar conditions. The proficiency in specific skills that is often required for successful self-management of chronic conditions can be gained through small-group sessions. If the skill acquisition is the primary goal of a small group, then most of the time should be spent on practice and the provision of feedback to the clients. In this context, breaking clients into pairs to practice skills and to develop action plans can be beneficial.

Conclusions

The clinical decision-making process proposed for outcome-based massage can be used to guide the clinician through the evaluative, treatment-planning, treatment, and discharge phases of clinical care. The aim of this process is to enable the clinician to integrate massage techniques into clinical care effectively, as the primary or complementary treatment techniques. Although the steps in this process are presented in a linear sequence, the process is an iterative one in which the clinician may perform several steps concurrently.

The decision-making model proposed in this chapter outlines both the technical aspects of how the clinician provides care and the interpersonal aspects of the client–clinician interaction. In doing so, it provides guidelines for enhancing the appropriateness and adequacy of the examinations performed, the plans of care outlined, and the interventions planned and provided by clinicians. In addition, the discussion of the interpersonal aspects of the process of clinical care outlines a variety of strategies that clinicians can use to conduct clinical interactions appropriately and to address the clients' ethical, emotional, and educational needs that arise during the course of clinical care. Since both technical and interpersonal factors can have an impact on the outcomes of care that are achieved, clinicians would be wise to attend to both of these aspects in the planning and delivery of care to their clients.

References

1. Donabedian A. Evaluating the quality of medical care. Milbank Q 1966;3:166–206.
2. Jensen GM, Shepard KF, Gwyer J, Hack LM. Attribute dimensions that distinguish master and novice physical therapy clinicians in orthopedic settings. Phys Ther 1992;72:711–722.

3. May B, Dennis J. Expert decision-making in physical therapy—a survey of practitioners. Phys Ther 1991;71:190–206.

4. Payton O. Clinical reasoning process in physical therapy. Phys Ther 1985;65:924–928.

5. Sullivan P, Markos P. Clinical decision-making in therapeutic exercise. East Norwalk, CT: Appleton & Lange, 1995.

6. American Physical Therapy Association. Guide to physical therapist practice. Phys Ther 1997;77(11):3–14.

7. Magee D. Orthopedic physical assessment. 3rd ed. Philadelphia: WB Saunders, 1997.

8. National Institute of Child Health and Human Development. Research plan for the National Center for Medical Rehabilitation Research. Public Health Service NIH Publication no. 93-3509. Bethesda, MD: National Institutes of Health, US Department of Health and Human Services, 1993.

9. Fritz S. Fundamentals of therapeutic massage. St. Louis: Mosby-Lifeline, 1995.

10. Tappan FM, Benjamin P. Tappan's handbook of healing massage techniques. 3rd ed. Stamford, CT: Appleton & Lange, 1998.

11. Werner RE, Benjamin BE. A massage therapist guide to pathology. Baltimore: Williams & Wilkins, 1998.

12. de Domenico G, Wood EC. Beard's massage. 4th ed. Philadelphia: WB Saunders, 1997.

13. Salvo SG. Massage therapy. Philadelphia: WB Saunders, 1999.

14. Herskovitz S, Strauch B, Gordon MJV. Shiatsu-induced injury of the median recurrent motor branch. Muscle Nerve 1992;October:1215 (letter).

15. Simons DG, Travell JG, Simons LS. Travell and Simons' myofascial pain and dysfunction: the trigger point manual, vol 1: Upper half of body. 2nd ed. Baltimore: Williams & Wilkins, 1999.

16. Canadian Occupational Therapy Association. CAOT code of ethics. Ottawa: Canadian Occupational Therapy Association, 1996.

17. Quality Assurance Committee of the College of Massage Therapists of Ontario. Code of ethics and standards of practice. Toronto: College of Massage Therapists of Ontario, 1999.

18. American Association of Drugless Practitioners. Code of ethics. Gilmer, TX: American Association of Drugless Practitioners, 1990.

19. Canadian Physiotherapy Association. The code of ethics and rules of conduct. Toronto: Canadian Physiotherapy Association, 1989.

20. Commission on Standards. Occupational therapy code of ethics. Bethesda, MD: American Occupational Therapy Association, 1994.

21. International Chiropractors Association. ICA code of ethics. Arlington, VA: International Chiropractors Association, 1985.

22. Ethics and Judicial Committee. Guide for professional conduct. Alexandria, VA: American Physical Therapy Association, 1999.

23. American Massage Therapy Association. Code of ethics for massage therapists. Evanston, IL: American Massage Therapy Association, 1995.

24. Nursing Practice Division. Code of ethics. Washington, DC: American Nursing Association, 1985.

25. Brennan BA. Hands of light: a guide to healing through the human energy field. Toronto: Bantam Books, 1988.

26. Updledger J. Somatoemotional release and beyond. Palm Beach Gardens, FL: UI Publishing, 1990.

27. Raheem A. Soul return: integrating body, psyche and spirit. Lower Lake, CA: Aslan Publishing, 1987.

28. Baker EF. Man in the trap. New York: MacMillan, 1967.

29. Lowen A. Bioenergetics. New York: Penguin Books, 1976.

30. Peirrakos JC. Core energetics. Mendocino, CA: LifeRhythm, 1987.

31. Kurtz R. Body-centered psychotherapy: the Hakomi method. Mendocino, CA: LifeRhythm, 1990.

32. Mindell A. Dreambody: the body's role in revealing the self. Boston: Sigo Press, 1982.

33. Smith EW. The body in psychotherapy. Jefferson: McFarland, 1985.

34. Janov A. The primal scream; primal therapy: the cure for neurosis. New York: GP & Putnam's Sons, 1970.

35. Reich W. The function of the orgasm. New York: Orgone Institute Press, 1942.

36. Reich W. Character analysis. 3rd ed. New York: Simon and Schuster, 1972.

37. Goring S. Relational characterology and embodiment (an interpersonal interpretation of the characterological and somatic theories of Alexander Lowen and Stephen Johnson). Unpublished masters thesis. Vermon College of Norwich University, 1994.

38. Keleman S. Emotional anatomy. Berkeley, CA: Center Press, 1985.

39. Seam M. Bodymind energetics: towards a dynamic model of health. Rochester, NY: Healing Arts Press, 1989.

40. Rolf IP. Rolfing®: the integration of human structure. New York: Harper and Row, 1977.

41. Wolf E. Treating the self: elements of clinical self psychology. New York: Guildford Press, 1988.

42. Hulka BS. Patient-clinician interactions and compliance. In: Haynes RB, Taylor DW, Sackett DL, eds. Compliance in health care. Baltimore: The Johns Hopkins University Press, 1979:62–77.

43. Bond WS, Hussar DA. Detection methods and strategies for improving medication compliance. Am J Hosp Pharm 1991;48:1978–1987.

44. Sluijs EM. A checklist to assess patient education in physical therapy practice: development and reliability. Phys Ther 1991;71(8):561–569.

45. Strategies to promote self management of chronic disease. Atlanta, GA: Center for Health Promotion and Education and Centers for Disease Control, 1982.

46. Ice R. Long-term compliance. Phys Ther 1985;65(12):1832–1839.

47. Turk DC, Salovey P, Litt MD. Adherence: a cognitive-behavioral perspective. In: Gerber KE, Nehemkis AM, eds. Compliance: the dilemma of the chronically ill. New York: Springer, 1986:44–72.

48. Becker MH. Theoretical models of adherence and strategies for improving adherence. In: Shumaker SA, Schron EB, Ockene JK, eds. The handbook of health behavior change. New York: Springer, 1990:5–43.

49. O'Brien MK, Petrie K, Raeburn J. Adherence to medication regimens: updating a complex medical issue. Med Care Rev 1992;49(4):435–453.

50. Haynes RB. Determinants of compliance: the disease and the mechanics of treatment. In: Haynes RB, Taylor DW, Sackett DL, eds. Compliance in health care. Baltimore: The Johns Hopkins University Press, 1979:49–61.

51. Meichenbaum D, Turk DC. Facilitating treatment adherence: a practitioner's guidebook. New York: Plenum Press, 1987:41–68.

52. Grueninger UJ. Arterial hypertension: lessons from patient education. Patient Educ Counsel 1995;26:37–55.

53. Sluijs EM, Kok GJ, van der Zee J. Correlates of exercise compliance in physical therapy. Phys Ther 1993;73(11): 771–782.

54. Donovan JL. Patient decision making: the missing ingredient in compliance research. Int J Technol Assess Health Care 1995;11(3):443–455.

3

Review of Client Examination Concepts for Massage

*T*his chapter reviews selected concepts that must be considered when conducting a client examination with a view to using massage as a primary or complementary treatment modality. These topics include the focus of an examination for massage; impairments that are relevant for massage; client reports that arise during the course of history taking that can suggest soft-tissue dysfunction; and the use of palpation and nonpalpatory approaches to assess impairments, functional limitations, and disability issues that are relevant to the use of massage. The clinician can integrate these

concepts into the approach to client examination that is appropriate for the client's condition and the clinician's professional scope of practice and area of specialization. Since numerous clinical texts document client examination techniques for musculoskeletal, neurological, cardiopulmonary, and psychological conditions for the various health care professions, this chapter assumes that the reader will consult those texts for details on the client examination approach and techniques that are within the reader's scope of practice.

Focus of the Client Examination for Massage

Chapter 2, The Clinical Decision-Making Process, outlined the purpose of, and steps involved in conducting, a client examination. Conducting a client examination with a view to using massage as a primary or complementary treatment modality requires more than the addition of a few soft-tissue examination techniques to one's customary approach to examination. To be effective, the clinician needs to expand the focus of the examination to include the following objectives:

1. Identification of soft-tissue dysfunction related to the client's clinical condition
2. Identification of other primary and secondary impairments that are amenable to treatment with massage
3. Identification of functional limitations and disability that are associated with the impairments that are amenable to treatment with massage

The assessment of soft-tissue function and dysfunction can involve the use of tests and measures, such as palpation, that directly assess soft tissue. In addition, the clinician can extend her interpretation of the findings from standard musculoskeletal, neurological, cardiopulmonary, or psychological tests and measures to include an analysis of the contribution of soft-tissue dysfunction. The extent to which the clinician will have to modify her customary approach to the client examination will depend on the pertinence of soft-tissue dysfunction to the client's clinical condition. For example, the inclusion of a strong focus on soft-tissue dysfunction and impairments that are relevant to massage is less appropriate in the case of a clinician who is examining a client with a long-standing below-knee amputation who has been referred for gait training following a change in prosthesis than it would be for a clinician whose client presents with chronic neck and shoulder pain and has "failed" multiple treatments. Nevertheless, clinicians are wise always to consider, even briefly, the role of soft-tissue dysfunction and potential uses of massage during their examinations of their clients.

Relevant Impairments for Massage

In the disablement models discussed in Chapter 1, Conceptual Frameworks for Outcome-Based Massage, the pathophysiology associated with a given clinical condition determines the specific impairments that can occur.[1,2] These impairments, in turn, result in functional limitations and disability. During the client examination, the clinician identifies and measures the client's impairments. However, not all of the impairments that the clinician notes will be amenable to treatment with massage techniques. Conversely, if the clinician fails to identify impairments that are directly related to the client's functional outcomes that can be treated using massage techniques, the effectiveness of the treatment may be compromised. Although the task of sorting impairments into those that are or are not amenable to treatment with massage techniques comes later in the treatment-planning process, it is useful to consider whether a reported or observed impairment may involve soft-tissue dysfunction. Table 3-1 summarizes some of the impairments that are relevant to the use of massage techniques and examples of relevant examination techniques. Issues relating to the examination of these impairments and the associated functional limitations and disabilities, with a view to using massage techniques, are discussed later in the chapter.

Issues in the Client History for Massage

The nuances of history taking for the various health care professions are described in detail in numerous clinical texts. During the course of taking the standard client history, the clinician can integrate questions that can elicit information that may suggest a condition for which the use of massage techniques is appropriate. Box 3-1 contains a brief list of issues that may prompt further exploration of a soft-tissue lesion.

Using Palpation to Assess Impairments for Massage

Skilled palpation is an art, a required component of many client examination techniques, and a prerequisite skill for the effective execution of all massage techniques.[3–5] Palpation can be used to assess and reassess the client's impairments throughout the client examination and treatment process. Furthermore, continuous palpation during massage provides an enormous advantage over nonmanual treatment techniques, since the clinician can use the client's response to the massage to guide the continuous refinement of the intervention as it proceeds.

There are many ways to perform palpation that are determined by the purpose of palpation, the object being palpated, the client's condition, and, to some degree, the clinician's abilities.[6–8] Nevertheless, regardless of how the palpation is being performed, all types of palpation share common characteristics. Palpation focuses the clinician's discriminative skill, or ability to distinguish fine gradations of sensory information, on a selected object being palpated and seeks to characterize and distinguish between normal and abnormal findings.[3,9–13] Palpation is also comparative in nature and thus involves movement, either of the contact surface or of the clinician's attention.[9,14] Although the emphasis of this chapter is on the client examination, the comments on palpation are as germane to the process of treatment as they are to the process of client examination.

Table 3-1
Outcomes and Examination Techniques for Impairments Relevant to Massage

Impairment	Outcome	Tests and Measures
Musculoskeletal		
Adhesions/scarring	Increased tissue mobility Decreased scarring	· Visual inspection · Measurement of dimensions · Palpation · Ultrasonography · Magnetic resonance imaging · Arthroscopy

Impaired connective tissue integrity
  Fascial restrictions
  Abnormal connective tissue density
  Decreased mobility of skin, superficial and deep fascia
	Separation and lengthening of fascia
	Promotion of dense connective tissue remodeling
	Increased connective tissue mobility
		· Visual inspection of static and dynamic postural alignment
		· Palpation
		· Skin mobility

Impaired joint integrity
  Inflammation of joint capsule or ligaments
  Restrictions of joint capsule and ligaments
	Decreased signs of inflammation and promotion of healing of joint capsule, tendons, or ligaments
	Decreased capsular and ligament restrictions
	Increased joint mobility
	Increased joint integrity
		· Palpation
		· Selective tissue tension testing
		· Ligament stability tests
		· Magnetic resonance imaging
		· Arthroscopic examination
		· Arthrography
		· Stress radiography
		· Ultrasonography
		· Also see impaired joint mobility

Impaired joint mobility Decreased voluntary range of motion	Increased joint mobility	· Universal goniometer · Parallelogram goniometer · Visual estimation of range of motion · Fingers-to-floor distance · Schoeber (tape measure) method · Passive accessory motion testing · Palpation of end feel on overpressure · Two- and three-dimensional computer-aided motion analysis · Computerized six-degree-of-freedom electromagnetic tracker · Self-report range of motion measures · Cervical Range of Motion (CROM) instrument · Single and double inclinometer · Electrogoniometers · Pelvic Palpation Meter · Arthrometer

Impaired muscle integrity
  Decreased muscle extensibility
  Muscle strains and tears
  Tendinopathies
  Trigger points
	Increased muscle extensibility
	Decreased signs of inflammation and promotion of healing of tendons
	Decreased signs of inflammation and promotion of healing of muscle
	Decreased trigger point activity
	Increased joint mobility
		· Muscle extensibility tests
		· Selective tissue tension testing
		· Palpation
		· Trigger point tests: twitch response, presence of taut bands, patterns of pain referral, electromyography
		· Pressure sensitivity testing (pressure algometer)
		· Universal goniometer
		· Isokinetic dynamometer
		· Dynamic ultrasonography

Table 3-1 (continued)

Impairment	Outcome	Tests and Measures
Impaired muscle performance (strength, power, endurance)	Enhanced muscle performance secondary to the enhancement of muscle extensibility, reduction of pain, reduction of muscle spasm, enhancement of joint mobility, normalization of joint integrity, reduction of trigger point activity, etc. Balance of agonist/antagonist muscle function	· Manual muscle testing · Handheld dynamometer · Repeated isotonic motion · Modified sphygmomanometer · Pinch meter · Self-report measures of perceived exertion · Isokinetic dynamometer · Isoinertial devices · Pedaling devices · Electromyogram · Kinematic and kinetic gait analysis with two- or three-dimensional computer-assisted motion analysis and force analysis
Abnormal muscle resting tension and muscle spasm	Decreased muscle spasm Normalized muscle resting tension Increased joint mobility	· Palpation · Tissue compliance meter · Continuous electromyogram · Thermography
Pain	Pain reduction through primary treatment of dysfunction, e.g., active trigger points Counterirritant analgesia Systemic sedation resulting in decreased perception of pain	· Pain behavior · Interview regarding location, quality, and behavior of pain · Pain diagram (used in conjunction with interview) · Self-report measures of pain intensity and affective component · Self-report measures of the impact of pain on function · Palpation · Pressure sensitivity testing (pressure algometer) · Selective tissue tension testing · Tests and measures of pain syndromes · Neural tissue tension tests · Neural provocation tests · Trigger point tests: twitch response, presence of taut bands, patterns of pain referral, electromyography · Dynamic surface electromyography · Electrophysiological studies · Thermography
Postural malalignment	Normalized postural alignment Increased postural awareness	· Visual inspection of static and dynamic posture · Postural grid · Posture analysis forms · Universal goniometer · Plumb line · Inclinometer · Tape measure · Photography · Video image and frame analysis · Two- or three-dimensional computer-assisted motion analysis · Three-dimensional electrogoniometers · X-ray line-drawing analysis · Force platforms · Functional postural analysis measures

continued

Table 3-1 (continued)

Impairment	*Outcome*	*Tests and Measures*
Impaired sensation secondary to entrapment neuropathy or nerve root compression	Normalized sensation secondary to the reduction of nerve and nerve root compression due to fascial restrictions and trigger points	· Dermatome testing: light touch, pin prick, temperature · Filament testing (pressure) · Palpation of nerve · Neural tension testing · Myotome testing · Electrophysiological (nerve conduction) testing · Electroneurotomy · Single-frequency vibrometry tests · Magnetic resonance imaging
Swelling: edema, joint effusion, lymphoedema	Increased lymphatic return Increased venous return Decreased joint effusion Decreased edema Increased joint integrity Increased joint mobility	· Visual inspection · Volumetric analysis · Girth measurements: tape measure, wire, jeweler's ring · Palpation · Multiple-frequency bioelectrical impedance analysis · Magnetic resonance imaging laser-Doppler flowmetry

Neurological

Abnormal neuromuscular tone Spasticity, rigidity, clonus	Normalized neuromuscular tone Alteration of movement responses through proprioceptive and exteroceptive stimulation techniques Balance of agonist/antagonist muscle function	· Palpation · Graded passive range of motion tests, e.g., Ashworth Scale · Quick stretch tests · Reflexes · Pendulum test · Isokinetic dynamometer · Handheld dynamometer · Electromyogram with isokinetic dynamometer · Electrophysiological testing · Standardized measures of motor control · Standardized measures of self-care

Cardiopulmonary

Impaired airway clearance	Increased respiration/gaseous exchange Increased airway clearance/mobilization of secretions Decreased dyspnea	· Interview regarding frequency and effectiveness of cough · Visual inspection of effectiveness of cough · Visual inspection of quality and quantity of sputum · Visual inspection and palpation of respiration rate and pattern · Auscultation of breath sounds · Pulse oximetry · Self-report dyspnea rating scales · Arterial blood gases · Pulmonary function tests · Self-report measures of quality of life · Standardized measures of self-care

Table 3-1 *(continued)*

Impairment	Outcome	Tests and Measures
Dyspnea	Decreased dyspnea because of increased airway clearance Decreased dyspnea because of increased perceived relaxation	· Visual inspection of respiratory pattern and effort of breathing · Self-report perceived exertion and dyspnea rating scales · Self-report measures of outcome of dyspnea · Respiration rate · Oxygen saturation · Arterial blood gases · Capnography
Impaired rib cage mobility (other than bony abnormality)	Increased rib cage mobility Increased muscle extensibility Increased ventilation	· Visual inspection and palpation of lateral costal, sternal, and diaphragmatic motion during respiration · Palpation of rib cage motion during respiration · Changes in girth of rib cage during respiration
Psychoneuroimmunological		
Stress	Systemic sedation Increased perceived relaxation Decreased levels of cortisol, epinephrine, and norepinephrine	· Interview regarding perceived stress levels and symptoms of stress · Self-report stress measures · Galvanic skin response · Heart rate · Blood pressure · Finger pressure · Blood work: lipid peroxide, prolactin, cortisol, testosterone, glycated hemoglobin · Salivary cortisol levels

Box 3-1
Issues in a Client History That Suggest Soft-Tissue Dysfunction

· Reports of any long-standing musculoskeletal condition, since this may result in chronic soft-tissue tightening
· A history of prolonged infection
· Reports of a change in pain over time from an initially specific, localized pain to a more diffuse, generalized pain
· A history of chronic pain
· A history of pain that is combined with anxiety or stress
· Idiopathic pain with a complex history of multiple injuries or multiple surgeries, i.e., events that would predispose the client to scarring
· A history of ambiguous symptoms, particularly when motion testing yields inconclusive results and subjective reports of symptoms are vague or ambiguous
· A history of multiple conflicting assessments or multiple ineffective treatments
· A history of a gradual onset of symptoms with a clearly perceived alteration of posture over approximately the same period
· A history of having a relief of symptoms through massage or stretching
· When prior treatments that are reported do not include comprehensive treatment of soft-tissue lesions, e.g., treatment with ultrasound but not frictions for tendinitis
· During history taking, the client refers to the texture of his soft tissue as "tight," "hard," or "wired" and makes a connection between this texture and his symptoms
· A history of bony malalignment, such as a leg-length discrepancy, scoliosis, or dental malocclusion
· A history of emotional trauma

BASIC PRINCIPLES OF PALPATION

Palpation is moving inquiry that requires a unhurried, nonabrupt manner and a quiet, listening mind.[3] The limits of palpation reflect the limits of the clinician's knowledge of form and function and how these are related in each client.[3] As the clinician performs palpation, she seeks answers to a variety of questions that form the background to effective palpation, such as What is this structure or quality? How does this finding differ from other structures or qualities that I have palpated? How does this finding relate to the client's history? How does this structure reflect the client's demonstrated and reported function? After extensive practice, the clinician becomes more adept at the practice of the different components of Intelligent Touch, as described in Chapter 1, Conceptual Frameworks for Outcome-Based Massage.

CONTACT SURFACES USED FOR PALPATION

The clinician's hands must be supple and relaxed at all times during palpation. Since the clinician's dominant hand is generally the more sensitive of the two,[15] it should be used for palpating very subtle objects. As palpation is performed, the two hands may be used to do similar things, such as comparing left and right sides, or they may be used to perform different tasks, as is the case when one hand moves a body segment and the other evaluates the motion that is being produced.

Virtually any surface of the hand can be used to palpate: fingers and thumbs, the whole palmar surface, the thenar and hypothenar eminences, or the back of the hand. The surface selected by the clinician should be related to the particular aim of palpation. For example, the finger and thumb tips and pads have the greatest discriminatory ability[3] and should be used for palpating subtle objects. On the other hand, grasping forms of palpation may use the index finger and thumb together like a pincer[16] or the whole hand.

FORCE OF PALPATION

As with massage techniques, the manner in which force is applied to the tissues during palpation should be related precisely to the task at hand. There are several ways in which this force can be varied: rate, pressure, direction, and duration.[3]

RATE

Different rates of palpation can be used to obtain different types of information.[3,4] A scanning or stroking type of palpation moves relatively quickly over a large area. Consequently, it is used when the clinician wants to collect information from a wide area, such as when comparing bilateral tissue contours or assessing resting muscular tone of the client's entire back. A scanning or stroking type of palpation is also used when a static palpation would distort findings. By contrast, static palpation involves no movement on the part of the clinician and is used when palpating moving phenomena, such as the rhythms of pulse and respiration.

PRESSURE

Clinicians generally use the minimum pressure required to contact the chosen tissue or structure. Therefore, lighter forces are used to palpate more superficial layers and greater forces are used to palpate deeper layers. The clinician does not need to apply pressure slowly; however, regardless of the rate of application of pressure, the clinician's touch should not be tentative nor abrupt. There will be occasions when the clinician needs to apply a considerable amount of compression to the client's tissues. In this situation, the clinician needs to gauge the extent to which the client's compressed tissues are deforming under this controlled application of the clinician's body weight. Since the clinician's entire body is being used to sense the movement of tissues, this type of palpation might be termed "proprioceptive palpation," as opposed to strict manual palpation.

DIRECTION

The force of palpation can be applied in a direction that is perpendicular or parallel to the client's tissues or as a shearing force. When the clinician applies the force of palpation in a direction that is perpendicular to the client's tissues, a vertical compression results. This is used, for example, when palpating a pulse or pitting edema or when measuring the sensitivity of a trigger point.

The clinician can apply the force of palpation in a direction that is parallel to the client's tissues (horizontal force), to exert tension along a particular tissue layer and produce drag. *Drag* is a term that is used to describe both the clinician's action of applying a force along a particular tissue layer in a direction that is parallel to the tissues and the resistance to lengthening that occurs in the tissue layer in response to the force that was applied. External and internal factors can result in increase or decrease of the amount of drag that occurs during palpation. For example, external factors include the presence of moisture on the skin, which can increase or decrease drag, and the presence of skin oil or lubricant, which can generally decrease it. On the other hand, tissue dystrophy is an internal factor that affects drag.[17] The assessment of drag is an integral part of the examination of connective tissues such as skin and fascia.

Clinicians can also use palpation to exert a shearing force on the client's tissue. Shear involves adjacent and parallel tissue layers sliding over one another, resulting in the displacement of adjacent laminar elements.[18] When drag is applied to a specific tissue layer, shear occurs between that tissue layer and the layer that is adjacent and parallel to it. Clinicians can use shearing forces, in combination with compression, when assessing muscle tone and bulk.

In practice, any palpation technique or massage technique combines elements of compression, drag, and shear. Not surprisingly, the direction of the force that the clinician applies during the palpation of a particular tissue is often the same as the direction of force that she would use to treat that tissue.

DURATION

Although the performance of palpation should not be hurried, the palpation of most objects does not need to be prolonged beyond a few seconds. Indeed, the effects of prolonged palpation on tissues can confound the client examination. This occurs because maintaining a position or pressure can result in the adaptation of tissue receptors in the clinician's hands[9] and can also induce changes in the client's tissues that alter the nature of the condition.[3] For example, these would both be factors when palpating a myofascial trigger point located in a deep layer, since the sustained pressure would overlap in function with the specific compression technique used for treatment of this condition. An exception to the need for a brief period of palpation is the palpation of barriers in connective tissue, which can take longer than a minute because of the biochemical nature of the tissue.[4] In this case, palpation merges into treatment.

INTEGRATION OF INFORMATION FROM OTHER SENSES

The clinician's eyes may be useful in corroborating some of the types of findings of palpation, such as posttraumatic swelling.[21] Visual inspection may, however, interfere with the clinician's attention when palpating more-subtle objects, such as the small intrinsic movements of connective tissue under traction.[28] Effective palpation is the result of appropriate interplay of the clinician's senses.

OBJECTS BEING PALPATED

The clinician identifies the client's impairments through palpation of specific "objects." The object being palpated is the chosen portion of the sensory field on which the clinician focuses her attention during palpation. The object being palpated is not necessarily a physical object; instead it may be a characteristic, such as temperature, or a phenomenon, such as resistance to movement. The clinician's choice of method of palpation is influenced by the nature of the object being palpated. For example, it is difficult to palpate skin temperature using deep thumb pressure or to palpate barriers in the superficial fascia using a fast scanning palmar contact. Consequently, the clinician should specify the object(s) of inquiry prior to beginning palpation and select a palpation technique that is suited to the object of palpation.

TEMPERATURE

The palpation of temperature can provide information about the status of inflammation,[21] circulation, and organ function.[15] There are several approaches to palpating temperature. In one method, the clinician places the back of her hand in direct contact with the client's skin.[21] The pressure used for this method must be very light; otherwise, vasodilatation will occur and confound the findings.[17] Another method is to use the palm of the dominant hand to scan approximately 4 inches (10 cm) off the surface of the client's body.[15] In this technique, the motion of the clinician's hand must be continuous to avoid vasodilatation, insulation, and reradiation effects.[15,17]

CONTOUR AND BULK

Contour and *bulk* refer to the gross shape and size of the client's body, which the clinician can best examine with a relatively fast-moving scanning palpation using a large contact surface, such as the entire palmar surface of the hand. The clinician should correlate the information she obtains from the palpation of contour and bulk with the findings from her visual inspection of the client's body.

TEXTURE AND CONSISTENCY

Texture and *consistency* refer to variations in the density of tissues regardless of the depth of the layer in which they occur. In other words, it is appropriate to discuss the texture of both skin and the hamstring attachment to the ischial tuberosity.

The two general categories of tissue texture that are related to the presence of inflammation have significant clinical relevance. Acute inflammation generally produces different degrees of tissue softness that reflect the presence of extravasated fluid in the tissues. This texture is described using the terms "distended," "spongy," or "boggy." Conversely, chronic inflammation generally produces varying degrees of tissue "hardness," as a result of the deposit of collagen into the tissues. Some descriptors for the tissue hardness associated with chronic inflammation are "indurated," "ropy," and "stringy."

FLUID STATUS

The clinician can use palpation to measure turgidity, that is, fluid pressure or fluid tension. Fluid tests, such as the ballottement test, involve the use of large contact surfaces to palpate excess fluid and push it from one place to another. These tests enable the clinician to gauge the amount of excess fluid in an area, the pressure of the fluid, and whether it is located in the intra- or extraarticular space, that is, whether it is an edema or an effusion. In addition, the clinician can use sustained digital compression to determine whether "pitting" is present.

Viscosity refers to the "thickness" or "stickiness" of semiliquid materials. The clinician can assess viscosity by use of palpation. This is valuable, since muscle and connective tissue commonly become less viscous in response to interventions, such as the local application of heat and neuromuscular or connective tissue massage techniques.

SOFT TISSUE LAYERS ("LAYER PALPATION")[5,9,18]

Traditionally, the term *soft tissue* has been used to describe any tissue that is not bone or articular surface.[4] More specifically, soft tissue includes the epithelium, the connective tissues, and the contractile tissues. When palpating the client's body the clinician is frequently presented with a succession of layers of tissue that are oriented from surface to deep. The clinician can use differences between the characteristics of layers, such as hardness, density, texture, and mobility, to distinguish one layer from another. The tissue layers are as follows.

The epithelium is made up of closely packed columnar or squamous cells that have little intercellular material between them.[19] Connective tissue consists of several different types of cells, such as fibroblasts and fat cells, and elastin and collagen fibers embedded in a matrix of gelatinous material, the consistency of which varies in response to many factors. Nerves, blood vessels, and lymph vessels are found in the connective tissue. Contractile tissue is composed of muscle, its enveloping fascial layers, its associated tendon(s), and its periosteal attachments.

As Figure 3-1 shows, the skin consists of a layer of epithelium, the epidermis, and the dermis, which is the first layer of connective tissue.[19] Deep to the skin lies the superficial fascia, which houses fat and water, provides a path for nerves and vessels, and may contain, in certain areas of the body, striated muscle that controls the movement of the skin, such as the platysma muscle. The investing layer of the deep fascia is dense connective tissue that lies between the superficial fascia and muscle. The investing layer of the deep fascia is continuous with the superficial fascia and the deep fascia that lies between muscle fibers. The primary functions of the deep fascia are to allow muscles to move freely, to carry nerve and blood vessels, to fill the space between muscles, and to provide an origin for muscles. For example, aponeuroses, retinacula, and interosseous membranes are all deep fascia. The deep fascia around muscle is continuous with the periosteum. In areas in which no muscle is present, the investing layer of the deep fascia is continuous with the periosteum. Connec-

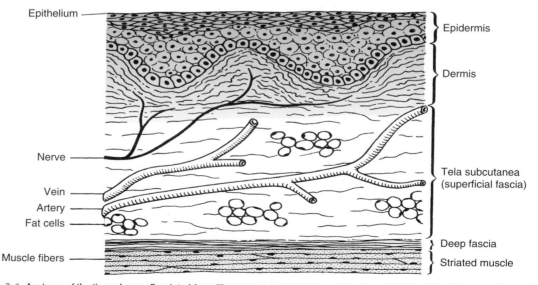

Figure 3-1. Anatomy of the tissue layers. Reprinted from Thomson JS. Core Textbook of Anatomy, 1977: p 15 with the permission of Lippincott Williams & Wilkins.

tive tissue is also found in synovial joints; for example, the synovial membrane and the extrinsic ligaments are modified connective tissue.

Skin

The clinician should use minimal force when palpating the client's skin.[4] In doing so, she should note normal variations in skin thickness, for example in the sole versus the dorsum of the foot; elastic rebound, which varies with age; and tightness of the attachment of the skin, for example the elbow versus the scalp.[17] The clinician can also assess the level of moisture on the skin surface and the hydration of the skin itself, since these may reflect the client's circulatory, trophic, or nutritional status. The clinician may also be able to distinguish the epidermis from the dermis by using gentle horizontal drag at the very surface of the skin.

The clinician can assess segmental or nerve root dysfunction[4] and imbalance of visceral function[3] by noting whether there is tightness or resistance during the following sequence of movements:[4]

1. Stretch the skin horizontally one direction at a time without gliding or engaging underlying issues.
2. Let the skin recoil.
3. Stretch the skin and sustain this position at the barrier.
4. Note how soon the skin begins to elongate.

Superficial Fascia

The clinician can engage the superficial fascia, and the fat deposits it contains, by increasing the compressive force applied. Because edema is often deposited into this tissue layer, the clinician can try to gauge the "turgor," or fluid pressure, of the tissues. She can also estimate the thickness of the superficial fascial layer by comparing different regions. The mobility tests outlined in steps 1 to 4 above are also appropriate for assessing the superficial fascia. In addition, the clinician can test the mobility of the superficial fascia by folding it[4] or by lifting and rolling it over the surface of the underlying tissues[18] (see "skin rolling" in Chapter 8, Connective Tissue Techniques). The clinician should compare the results she obtains for superficial fascia with those obtained for the skin.

The Investing Layer of the Deep Fascia

This smooth, firm, and continuous landmark lies between the superficial fascia and muscle and may take practice to locate precisely.[5] The assessment of the investing layer of the deep fascia is part of the client examination procedure for connective tissue massage.[3] The mobility of this connective tissue layer is assessed using techniques that are similar to those for the more superficial layers described above. The difference is that assessing the investing layer of the deep fascia requires more-refined palpation skills because there is more

intervening tissue. Tissue restrictions identified by the clinician will often correlate with those restrictions that are found in the more superficial layers. These restrictions may indicate underlying muscle tension, segmental dysfunction, or visceral imbalance.[3]

Muscle

The clinician assesses resting muscle tension during palpation by noting a muscle's response to the compressive and shearing forces delivered with her finger(s) or hand(s). During palpation, the hand(s) may simply compress the whole muscle or bow it,[4] or her fingers or thumbs can be used to slowly enter the muscle tissue and tease apart its fibers.[3] The higher the resting level of tone, the denser and harder the tissue will be on palpation. Increases and decreases in muscle resting tension are relative states, since degrees of tone vary greatly from one person to another and between one segment of an individual's body and another. Spasm and atonia—being more extreme—are more readily distinguished by the clinician. Elevated resting tone can result from a wide variety of clinical conditions, including injury, degenerative diseases, and stress.

In addition to assessing muscle resting tension during the palpation of muscle, the clinician can note whether high turgor (fluid distention) is present, since this can indicate a postexercise condition or an inflammatory condition.[17]

Periosteum

This tissue layer is only accessible to palpation in areas where there is no overlying muscle. The clinician can use compressive fingertip force to palpate a thin, dense, spongy layer that is superimposed on the hardness of the underlying bone.

TISSUE MOBILITY AND RESTRICTIVE BARRIERS

Normal Soft-Tissue Range of Motion

Soft tissues have an available range of motion that is analogous to the range of motion available in joints. Within this range of motion, normal soft tissue has three barriers or resistances that can limit movement (Fig. 3-2).[4,5] The clinician is "engaging" these tissue barriers at the point at which the clinician palpates a resistance to tissue motion.[4] The physiological barrier *(Pb)* is the resistance that determines the range of motion that is available under normal conditions. In other words, the range of motion lies between the two physiological barriers, with the least amount of resistance being apparent at the midrange *(M)*. The elastic barrier *(E)* is the resistance that the clinician feels at the end of the passive range of motion when she has taken the slack out of or has engaged the tissue. The anatomical barrier *(A)* is the final resistance to normal range of motion that can be provided by

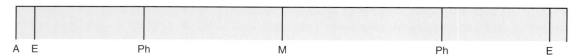

Figure 3-2. Normal tissue barriers. *A,* anatomical barrier; *E,* elastic barrier; *Ph,* physiological barrier; *M,* midrange. Reprinted with adaptations from Greenman PE. Principles of Manual Medicine, 2nd ed., 1996: p 43 with the permission of Lippincott Williams & Wilkins.

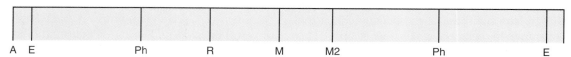

Figure 3-3. Restrictive tissue barriers. *A,* anatomical barrier; *E,* elastic barrier; *Ph,* physiological barrier; *R,* restrictive barrier; *M,* midrange; *M2,* pathological midrange. Reprinted with adaptations from Greenman PE. Principles of Manual Medicine, 2nd ed., 1996: p 43 with the permission of Lippincott Williams & Wilkins.

bone, ligament, or soft tissue. Motion beyond the anatomical barrier results in tissue damage.

Restrictive Barriers

Restrictive, or pathological, barriers are observed when soft-tissue dysfunction is present.[5] Restrictive barriers may occur in skin, fascia, muscle, ligament, or joint capsule or a combination of these tissues. They can be located anywhere between the normal physiological barriers, can limit the available range of motion within the tissues, and can alter the position of the midrange. Furthermore, the presence of a restrictive barrier will change the quality of the movement and the "feel" at the end of the tissue range of motion. This is analogous to the abnormal end feels observed in joints. An example of a restrictive barrier *(R)* and its impact on the position of the midrange *(M2)* is shown in Figure 3-3.

Barrier-Release Phenomenon

The clinician engages the tissue barrier at the point at which she palpates a resistance to tissue motion.[4] If the clinician sustains the pressure on the tissue barrier, a "release" may occur after a latency period that will vary with the nature and state of health of the tissue. This release results in a reduction of the resistance that will enable the clinician to move the tissue beyond the location of the original barrier without increasing the pressure of palpation. This phenomenon is known as the barrier-release phenomenon.

Different types of tissue will respond differently to sustained pressure. For example, connective tissue is most responsive to sustained pressure and will demonstrate a slow, palpable stretch of tissues called creep, or viscoelastic creep.[21] This stretch occurs beyond the elastic barrier *(E)* shown in Figure 3-3. In the case of pathological or restrictive barriers, this release can last for up to 30 seconds or longer and can result in

normalized tissue mobility and pain reduction. Since connective tissue forms a portion of all soft tissues, some creep will be evident in all soft tissues in proportion to the amount of connective tissue that is present in that tissue.

The barrier-release phenomenon can be observed during the application of horizontal drag, vertical compression, or shear forces[4] that are applied to the tissues with either small or large contact surfaces. Consequently, palpation can be used to identify the feel at the end of the available range of motion of tissue through more than digital compression. For example, assessment can be performed using a palmar drag on the superficial fascia. The barrier-release phenomenon is most useful when palpating connective tissue, but it can also be applied to any tissue or structure.

Palpation of Tissue Mobility

A clinician can apply a compression or drag force, or a combination of the two, to a given tissue or structure within a client's body and observe the resulting movement. In doing so, she can observe whether the normal range of motion is present in the tissues or whether restrictive barriers exist. If a restrictive barrier is palpated, the clinician must note the available range of motion, the quality of movement through the range of motion, and the feel of the point at which the restrictive barrier is engaged.[5]

ANATOMICAL STRUCTURES

The ability to systematically palpate anatomical structures is an absolute prerequisite for the clinician who uses massage, since this has a direct impact on the accuracy of the assessment using palpation and whether many treatment outcomes are achieved. The palpation of anatomical structures that is detailed in comprehensive texts on this topic involves the ability to discriminate between tissue types and to accurately distinguish one structure from surrounding structures. Through palpation, clinicians can identify bone, joint space (joint line), ligament, tendon (including junctions to both periosteum and to muscle), aponeurosis, fascia (septa, sheathes, retinacula), nerves, vessels, and viscera. Each of these has a characteristic "feel" that is related to its structure and histology. Palpation of anatomical structures requires that the clinician use compressive contact. Her choice of contact surface and pressure will depend on the structure that she is palpating.

BODY RHYTHMS

The clinician assesses pulses and respiration using static palpation with minimal-to-moderate compression and a contact surface of appropriate size. The amount of force applied during the palpation of pulses is important, since the use of excessive compression results in inaccurate findings. Pulses are assessed using a single hand; however, when palpating respiration, the clinician can use two hands, placed on opposite sides of the rib cage, to produce a three-dimensional test.[22] Both pulse and respiration can be palpated at a distance from the site although this technique sometimes confuses novices.

Clinicians with advanced skills or specialized training can palpate more-subtle pulsations of inherent tissue motions[5] using a broad-contact static palpation.

TREMORS AND FASCICULATIONS

Fasciculations are localized, subconscious muscle contractions that result from the contraction of the muscle cells innervated by a single motor axon and thus do not involve the entire muscle.[20] Tremors, by contrast, are rhythmic movements of a joint that result from involuntary contractions of antagonist and agonist muscle groups. Both tremors and fasciculations are palpated statically with minimal-to-moderate compression, using varying sized surfaces.

VIBRATION

The clinician can palpate two types of vibration: crepitus and fremitus. Crepitus is a vibration of variable fineness that is associated with roughened gliding surfaces of a tendon or its sheath or of the articulating surfaces of a joint.[21] Crepitus can sometimes be heard, as well as palpated. Another palpable vibration is fremitus, a pulmonary vibration that a clinician can palpate over the rib cage as the client speaks or vocalizes.[22]

CLIENT'S RESPONSE TO PALPATION

Palpation can evoke a variety of verbal and physiological responses from the client that the clinician must observe and interpret. Local reflex signs include discoloration of the skin (blanching or flushing)[3] or more-general autonomic responses, such as sweating and nausea. Neuromuscular responses include twitching,[16] spasm, or clonus. Clients may indicate that they are experiencing pain by grimacing, vocalizing, or making sudden involuntary movements.[16] Clinicians must remember that pain is a common response to palpation and should be respected and carefully observed, for example, Magee[20] suggests a four-point rating scale for grading tenderness. Types of pain responses differ in their significance and reliability. Tenderness to deep palpation, for example, is an unreliable finding,[21] since tenderness can be referred.[16] Pain on percussion may have specific meaning for certain musculoskeletal conditions.[23] Finally, during palpation, the clinician needs to be aware that palpation itself can sometimes produce tissue changes in the tissue that is being palpated, which can be either positive or negative.

In summary, Box 3-2 outlines some of the impairments that can be assessed using palpation.

Box 3-2
Selected Impairments Evaluated Through Palpation

- Abnormal connective tissue density
- Abnormal levels of resting muscle tension
- Abnormal neuromuscular tone
- Adhesions
- Impaired extensibility of contractile and noncontractile tissues
- Impaired integrity of contractile and noncontractile tissues
- Decreased rib cage mobility
- Fascial restrictions
- Muscle spasm
- Pain
- Scarring
- Swelling: edema, effusion, lymphedema
- Trigger points

Nonpalpatory Approaches to Assessing Impairments, Functional Limitations, and Disabilities for Massage

MUSCULOSKELETAL IMPAIRMENTS

ADHESIONS AND SCARRING

Definitions and Etiology

Scar

The fibrous tissue that replaces normal tissues that have been destroyed by a burn, wound, surgery, radiation, or disease.[24]

Adhesions

Like scars, adhesions result from the replacement of normal tissue that has been destroyed by burn, wound, surgery, radiation, or disease with connective tissue.[24,25] They involve a binding together with dense connective tissue of tissues that normally glide or move in relation to each other. The result is loss of mobility. Adhesions may be fibrous or fibrinous. Fibrinous adhesions have fine bands of fibrin that form as a result of an exudate of plasma or lymph or an extravasation of blood.[24] Fibrous adhesions come from the organization of fibrinous adhesions into fibrous strands. Unlike scarring, adhesions are distinguished by a loss of mobility of tissues that normally glide or move in relation to each other. Adhesions can contribute to impaired muscle, joint, and connective tissue integrity that is described in detail in other sections of this chapter.

Overview of Examination Techniques

Adhesions are of greater clinical significance than scars, since they are associated with impaired tissue mobility. The measurement of adhesions through observation and palpation is, unfortunately, less accurate than that of scars. The presence of scars can be confirmed through visual inspection, an important component to include in the measurement of scars, since many clients forget scars. Some strategies for measuring and describing scars and adhesions are described in Appendix B, Selected Soft-Tissue Examination Techniques. Ultrasonography, magnetic resonance imaging, and arthroscopy are more accurate, though clinically less practical approaches.[26,27] Visceral adhesions may be assessed more specifically by those trained in visceral manipulation.

IMPAIRED CONNECTIVE TISSUE INTEGRITY

Definitions and Etiology

Fascial Restrictions

The loss of mobility of one fascial layer with respect to another owing to a loss of fluid consistency and movement of collagenous cross-links. Fascial restrictions may result from repair of tissue damage and prolonged immobility.[25] Fascial restrictions may be caused by trauma; adhesion; postural malalignment, such as leg length discrepancy, pelvic malalignment, and dental malocclusion; inflammatory or infectious processes; osseous restrictions; chronic fascial compartment syndromes; or neurological or circulatory compression syndromes.[18,25,28-40] Fascial restrictions may cause pain, impaired motion, and general dysfunction throughout the body. Symptoms may occur at a distance from the restriction and may result in impaired cellular metabolism, nutrition, elimination, respiration, or lymphatic flow.[25,28]

Abnormal Connective Tissue Density

Irregular connective tissue remodeling that occurs during the consolidation and maturation stages of connective tissue healing.[41-50] This can be associated with chronic orthopedic injuries, including strains, and fractures, as well as for repetitive strain injuries, such as tendinitis, tenosynovitis, bursitis, and plantar fasciitis, in which there is ongoing microtrauma, low-grade inflammation, and tissue remodeling.

Overview of Examination Techniques

Techniques for evaluating connective tissue impairments include visual inspection of the client's static and dynamic postural alignment; palpation of tissue, skin mobility, and vasomotor response to palpation; and assessment of craniosacral rhythm characteristics.[3-5,18,25,28] The clinician is advised to evaluate the client's entire body, regardless of the client's complaint, since imbalances in the fascial system can have significant effects at locations other than the site of the restriction.[25] Selected techniques for assessing fascial restrictions are described in Appendix B, Selected Soft-Tissue Examination Techniques.

IMPAIRED JOINT INTEGRITY

Definitions and Etiology

Joint Integrity

The extent to which a joint conforms to the expected anatomical and biomechanical norms.[51]

Capsular Restrictions

Anatomical or pathological shortening of the joint capsule. Capsular restrictions occur as a result of a variety of clinical conditions, such as disuse and immobility, as well as venous congestion[52] and diabetes.[53] "Frozen shoulder," or adhesive capsulitis, for example, is a common capsular lesion seen in rehabilitation. This adherence of the shoulder capsule to the humeral head may be the consequence of alteration of the supporting structures of and around the shoulder and autoimmune, endocrine, or other systemic diseases.[54,55]

Capsular Laxity

Anatomical or pathological lengthening of the joint capsule. For example, global (anterior, inferior, and posterior) excessive laxity of the glenohumeral joint capsule leads to multidirectional instability of the shoulder.[56]

Capsulitis and Synovitis

Inflammation of the synovium and the joint capsule and associated internal ligaments.[57,58] This can be associated with capsular distention secondary to increased levels of fluid in the joint, for example as in rheumatoid arthritis.[59]

Ligament Insufficiency

Anatomical or pathological shortening of the capsular ligament. For example, anterior capsular ligament length insufficiency in the glenohumeral joint can contribute to altered glenohumeral joint mechanics and shoulder pain.[60]

Ligament Laxity

Anatomical or pathological lengthening of the capsular ligament. Anterior cruciate ligament laxity, for example, is a common cause of knee instability, pain, and functional limitations in athletes.[61–64]

Nonmyofascial Trigger Points

A hyperirritable spot in scar tissue, fascia, periosteum, ligaments, and joint capsules that is associated with a hypersensitive palpable nodule in a taut band.[16]

Overview of Examination Techniques

Cyriax[65] defined the "capsular patterns," clinical signs of capsular lesions that are demonstrated during selective tissue tension testing that are supported by recent research.[66] Selective tissue tension testing involves the performance of a specific sequence of active range of motion, passive range of motion, and resisted isometric testing of the joint in question, during which the clinician observes sequences of pain and limitations of motion.[65] Clinicians can identify clinical conditions with high levels of reliability (κ [kappa] = 0.875) using selective tissue tension testing.[67]

The integrity of ligaments is best assessed clinically using a variety of static stability tests that demonstrate the stability of the ligaments of selected joints.[68,69] An example of these tests is the Lachman test of knee anterior cruciate stability.[64] Laboratory or instrumented tests of impaired joint integrity include magnetic resonance imaging, arthroscopic examination,[70] arthrography, stress radiography, and ultrasonography.[70]

IMPAIRED JOINT MOBILITY

Definitions and Etiology

Joint Range of Motion

The capacity of the joint to move within the anatomical or physiological range of motion that is available at that joint on the basis of its arthrokinematics and the ability of the periarticular connective tissue to deform.[28,50] Range of motion reflects the function of the contractile, nervous, inert, and bony tissues and the client's willingness to perform a movement.[20]

Passive Range of Motion

The amount of joint motion available when an examiner moves a joint through its anatomical or physiological range, without assistance from the client, while the client is relaxed.[20,71]

Active Range of Motion

The amount of joint motion that can be achieved by the client during the performance of unassisted voluntary joint motion.[72]

Accessory Joint Motion

The range of motion within synovial and secondary cartilaginous joints that is not under voluntary control and, therefore, can only be obtained passively.[20]

These motions, also known as joint play movements, are essential for full and pain-free active range of motion.

End Feel

The quality of motion or sensation that the clinician palpates or "feels" in the joint during overpressure at the end of passive range of motion.[20]

Impaired joint mobility can be the result of numerous primary impairments, such as impaired muscle extensibility, altered muscle tone, capsular restriction or inflammation, tendinopathy, neurological deficit, pain, or bony deformity. For the sake of clarity, relevant impairments are defined in separate sections, although examination techniques for general range-of-motion testing are summarized here.

Overview of Examination Techniques

Goniometry is the established approach to measuring joint range of motion for peripheral joints, and the universal goniometer is accurate and efficient.[72,73] Numerous studies have documented high degrees of intrarater (ICCs = 0.88 to 0.93) and interrater reliability (ICCs = 0.85 and 0.80) for the universal goniometric measurements of a variety of upper and lower extremity joints for novice and experienced clinicians.[74,75] Less sophisticated techniques for range-of-motion testing include the use of visual estimation of range of motion, the findings of which can be more variable for many peripheral joints, regardless of the therapist's level of experience,[76] but may be more reliable in joints such as the forefoot that are more difficult to measure with goniometry.[77] A parallelogram goniometer[78] is under investigation and shows good reliability (r = 0.85 and 0.87) for the knee joint. Other techniques for assessing range of motion of peripheral joints include wire tracing for joints of the hand[79] and a gravitational protractor.[73] Two-dimensional and three-dimensional computer-aided motion analyses can provide information on the range of motion of multiple joints in static and dynamic postures[80–82] that can be more reliable than that from goniometry, particularly in complex joints.[83] Although the measurement of joint range of motion has traditionally been conducted with the client's joints uncovered, recent studies have explored measurement of clothed range of motion. In this situation, a computerized six-degrees-of-freedom electromagnetic tracker may be more accurate than goniometry.[84] Finally, standardized measures of self-reported range of motion, such as the Single Assessment Numeric Evaluation method, which asks clients to rate their range of motion as a percentage of normal,[85] are now being used as outcome measures.

Clinicians have used a variety of tools for the measurement of the range of motion of the spine and pelvis. Measures of spinal range of motion include the Cervical Range of Motion (CROM) instrument,[86] three-dimensional electromagnetic tracking systems,[87] the double inclinometer,[73] electrogoniometers[88] (which can be precise but limited in accuracy,[89] and computer-assisted motion analysis.[80–82] There are more-simplistic measures of spinal range of motion that involve the measurement of various distances using a tape measure. The use of measured distances of the client's fingers to the floor in the testing of spinal range of motion may be the least reproducible approach and also reflects the range of motion of joints other than the spine.[73] Another approach, the Schoeber method of using a tape measure placed on spinal landmarks to evaluate the motion of the spine, may be associated with considerable error.[73] Pelvic range of motion can be difficult to measure; consequently devices such as the Palpation Meter, a caliper-inclinometer combination,[90,91] and basic inclinometry, can be used to facilitate accurate measurement.[73]

Accessory, or joint play, movements are measured with the joint in the loose-packed position.[20] One technique described by Kaltenborn involves the palpation of glide and traction/compression ranges of motion during passive movements and the use of a six-point grading system: hypomobile (0–2), normal (3), or hypermobile (4–6).[92] Accessory movement testing has shown poor-to-fair intrarater (r = 0.75) and interrater (r = 0.45) reliability.[14,93–95] Laboratory or instrumented measures of accessory joint motion are now available; for

example, arthrometers are used to measure anterior-posterior translation (glide) in the knee joint.[96]

The quality of movement is as important as the quantity of range that is available. Clinicians should, therefore, assess the quality of the movement throughout the range and at the end of range as they perform passive range of motion. In doing so, they should apply over-pressure at the end of the range and note whether the end feel is normal (bone-to-bone, soft-tissue approximation, or tissue stretch) or abnormal for that joint (muscle spasm, hard capsular, soft capsular, bone-to-bone, empty, or springy block).[20]

IMPAIRED MUSCLE INTEGRITY
Definitions and Etiology
Muscle Integrity
The extent to which a muscle conforms to the expected anatomical and biomechanical norms.[50]

Muscle Extensibility
The ability of the muscle and its associated fascia to undergo lengthening deformation during the movement of a joint through its anatomical range.[97]

Contracture
A permanent muscular shortening due to a variety of physiological changes in muscle, such as fibrosis or loss of muscular balance.[24] Physiological contractures, as defined by Simons and Mense,[98] are permanent muscular contractions or shortening that does not involve motor activity. The shortening of involved muscles in Volkman's ischemic contracture, for example, involves prolonged ischemia, myonecrosis, proliferation of fibroblasts, scar contraction, and formation of myotendinous adhesions.[99] Muscle contractures may be associated with muscle imbalances that result from neurological disorders, such as the presence of hypertonia in cerebellar lesions.[100] They can also be associated with atrophy and fibrosis, as is the case in Duchenne's muscular dystrophy, in which biopsies of contractures in selected muscles showed a combination of muscle fiber atrophy with peri- and endomysial fibrosis.[101]

Muscle Strain or Tear
Lesion or inflammation of muscle fibers that can occur in response to trauma.[102]

Tendinitis
Inflammation of the peritendinous tissues that can occur in response to repetitive mechanical trauma.[103]

Tendinosis
Unlike tendinitis, which is an inflammatory condition, tendinosis refers to common overuse tendon conditions

with a histopathology that is consistent with a noninflammatory, degenerative condition of unknown etiology.[104]

Myofascial Trigger Point

A hyperirritable spot in skeletal muscle that is associated with a hypersensitive palpable nodule in a taut band.[16] The area is painful on compression and can give rise to a variety of symptoms, such as referred pain, tenderness, motor dysfunction, and autonomic phenomena.

ACTIVE TRIGGER POINTS

Refer pain in a characteristic pattern when the muscle in which they are located are working or at rest.

LATENT TRIGGER POINTS

Are not painful in and of themselves unless they are being palpated.

Overview of Examination Techniques

Impaired muscle extensibility is measured clinically using stretch tests (i.e., passive range-of-motion tests in which the muscle in question is placed in a stretched position) that have been defined for the given muscle group.[20] Extensibility of the hamstring muscles, for example, can be measured using goniometric measures of passive knee extension with the pelvis stabilized, a test that can be reliable (r = 0.99) and performed with little associated pelvic motion.[105] The Sit-and-Reach Test is another commonly used measure of hamstring extensibility; it is less accurate than the measurement of hip joint angle in this test position, since the Sit-and-Reach Test also appears to reflect spinal mobility and anthropometric factors.[106] Laboratory or instrumented measures of muscle extensibility include the use of force/angle data from isokinetic dynamometers, such as the KinCom, to measure muscle extensibility with high levels of reliability (ICC = 0.95 and 0.81) for selected muscle groups,[107] and dynamic ultrasonography.[108]

Tendinopathies and muscle strains or tears are assessed using the methods of selective tissue tension testing outlined above.[102,103] In this case, the clinician is looking for a relatively strong contraction of the muscle, with pain on contraction of the muscle (active movement in one direction), pain on stretch of the muscle (passive movement in the opposite direction), pain on isometric movement, and a possible decrease in range of motion if there is a gross hematoma.[20] The distinction between tendinous and muscular lesions is based on the location of pain during testing and the results of palpation of tenderness. Magnetic resonance imaging can be used when additional diagnostic information is required.[102]

Impaired muscle integrity will also be associated with impaired muscle performance and pain that are described in detail in other sections.

IMPAIRED MUSCLE PERFORMANCE

Definitions and Etiology

Muscle Performance

The muscle's capacity to do work based on its length, tension, and velocity.[50] Neurological stimulus, fuel storage, fuel delivery, balance, and timing and sequencing of muscle contraction influence integrated muscle performance.

Muscle Strength

The force or torque produced by a muscle or group of muscles to overcome a resistance during a maximum voluntary contraction.[50,109]

Muscle Power

Work produced by a muscle per unit of time (strength × speed).[50,109]

Muscle Endurance

The muscle's ability to contract, or maintain torque, over a number of contractions or a period of time.[50,109] Conversely, fatigue is inability to maintain torque or the loss of power over time.

Because of the multiple inputs required for integrated muscle performance, impaired muscle performance can be the result of adhesions, impaired muscle integrity, abnormal neuromuscular tone, impaired joint mobility, impaired joint integrity, swelling, impaired connective tissue integrity, pain, and postural malalignment, which are described in detail in other sections of this chapter. Muscle weakness, a primary cause of impaired muscular performance, is not described in this chapter, since massage techniques do not have a direct effect on increasing muscle strength.

Overview of Examination Techniques

Muscle strength can be measured isometrically, isotonically, and isokinetically. The graded manual muscle test is a long-standing clinical approach to isotonic strength testing that has questionable interrater reliability[110] but good intrarater reliability (r = 0.88).[111] Handheld dynamometers are an accurate and reliable means of measuring isometric muscle strength that have become the mainstay of clinical practice.[112,113] Hand strength testing is performed primarily with the grip strength dynamometer, the modified sphygmomanometer, and the pinch meter.[109] Isokinetic strength can be measured in a variety of ways using isokinetic dynamometers, such as peak torque, mean peak torque, and force-frequency relationship.[109,114-117] Muscle power is described in terms of peak power, mean power, instantaneous power, and torque-velocity relationships achieved through isokinetic testing.[113-117] Isoinertial devices produce constant resistance to a movement, which enables clinicians to measure isoinertial performance, particularly in trunk muscle testing.[109,118]

Muscle endurance can be assessed using simple clinical measures, such as the number of repetitions performed, or more complex tests that include endurance time to limit of endurance and mean power frequency derived from an electromyogram.[119] The client's perceived rate of exertion can be measured using rate of perceived effort tests, such as the Borg Perceived Effort Test, and correlated with objective measures of fatigue.

Clients with certain clinical conditions may require modifications to the usual muscle performance testing measures. The modified sphygmomanometer is a reliable (ICCs for interrater reliability of up to 0.85) means of assessing isometric strength, particularly in geriatric clients and those with rheumatoid arthritis.[120] Pedaling activities have been used to measure mechanical work and joint power generation patterns in clients who have had cerebrovascular accidents.[121,122]

The clinician can also assess the impact of an individual's muscle performance on his ability to perform functional tasks. The Sit-to-Stand Test, for example, shows the impact of lower extremity strength on the client's ability to perform a functional transfer.[123] The functional capacity evaluations used in occupational medicine measure a client's ability to perform work-related tasks, such as pulling, lifting, carrying, and handling weights, which reflect muscle performance.[124,125] Kinematic and kinetic gait analysis using two- or three-dimensional computer-assisted motion analysis and force analysis shows the impact of muscle performance on gait.[80,82]

ABNORMAL MUSCLE RESTING TENSION
Definitions and Etiology
Muscle Resting Tension
The firmness to palpation at rest observed in muscles with normal innervation.[126] Traditionally, resting muscle tension has been described as being the result of the physiological properties of muscle, such as viscosity, elasticity, and plasticity, rather than motor unit firing. For example, connectin is a giant elastic protein of striated muscle that may contribute to resting tension generation.[127] Animal studies suggest, however, that the resting tension of a relaxed muscle fiber is not entirely due to passive elasticity.[128] Instead, a portion of the resting tension—the filamentary resting tension—may be produced by a low level of active force generation.

Muscle Tone
Muscle resting tension and responsiveness of muscles to passive elongation or stretch.[129]

Hypertonia
A general term used to refer to muscle tone that is above normal resting levels, regardless of the mechanism for the increase in tone.[129]

Muscle Spasm
Involuntary contraction of a muscle that results in increased muscular tension and shortness that cannot be released voluntarily.[98] Research suggests that increased excitability of alpha-motor neuron pools contributes to the occurrence of muscle spasm.[130,131]

Overview of Examination Techniques
Muscle resting tension and muscle spasm can be assessed using a variety of tests, although research suggests that palpation is still the most important and exact method for measuring spasm.[132] The other tests for muscle spasm include the Tissue-Compliance Meter, which measures the consistency of soft tissue; badismography; the continuous electromyogram; and thermography.

PAIN
Definitions and Etiology
Pain
An unpleasant sensation associated with actual or potential tissue damage, which is mediated by specific nerve fibers to the brain where its conscious appreciation may be modified by various factors.[24]

Acute
Pain provoked by noxious stimulation produced by injury and/or disease, with unpleasant sensory and emotional experiences.[24]

Chronic
Pain that persists beyond the usual course of healing of an acute disease or beyond the reasonable time in which the injury is expected to heal.[25] There is some ambiguity in the definition of chronic pain. Some authors define it in terms of duration of pain, with a lower range of 6 weeks to 6 months,[133,134] while others define chronic pain in terms of an increasing dissociation from the physical cause and increasing affective and cognitive dimensions of pain[135] (see the definition of chronic pain syndrome).

Chronic Pain Syndrome
A clinical syndrome in which clients present with high levels of chronic pain, functional impairment, and depression.[136] This clinical pattern is seen more often in younger and middle-aged clients than in geriatric clients.[137]

Nociceptive Pain

Sensitization of peripheral nociceptors as a result of injury to a muscle or a joint that causes an increased release of neurotransmitters in the dorsal horn of the spinal cord.[138–140] The sensitized dorsal horn neurons demonstrate an increased background activity, an increased receptive field size, and increased responses to peripherally applied stimuli. Nociceptive pain may be implicated in most clients seen in clinical practice.[141]

Neurogenic Pain

Pain that occurs as a result of noninflammatory dysfunction of the peripheral or central nervous system that does not involve nociceptor stimulation or trauma.[139,142]

Referred Pain

Pain that is felt at another part of the body that is at a distance from the tissues that have caused it, because the referred site is supplied by the same or adjacent neural segments.[20] Referred pain can be distinguished from localized pain when clients report pain in a generalized area that is felt deeply, that radiates segmentally without crossing the midline, and that has indistinct boundaries.[20]

RADICULAR PAIN

Pain that is felt in a dermatome, myotome, or sclerotome because of direct involvement of a spinal nerve or nerve root;[20] also known as radicular, or nerve root, pain.

DERMATOMAL PAIN

A dermatome is an area of skin supplied by one dorsal nerve root. Injury of a dorsal root can result in sensory loss in the skin or be felt as a burning or electric pain.[6] For example, irritation of the C7 nerve root can lead to sensory changes in the C7 dermatome: lateral arm and forearm to the index, long, and ring fingers on the palmar and dorsal aspect.

SCLEROTOMAL PAIN

Pain in a sclerotome, an area of bone or fascia innervated by one segmental nerve root.[20,24] For example, hip pain can be referred to the groin, sacroiliac joints, lumbar spine, knee, or ankle.

MYOTOMAL PAIN

Pain in a myotome, or a group of muscles that are supplied by one nerve root.[20] For example, injury to the teres minor can result in referred pain near the insertion of the deltoid.

VISCERAL PAIN

Pain in areas of the viscera that are supplied by a nerve root.[65] For example, injury to the small intestine can refer pain to the same area supplied by the T9-10 dermatome: an area encircling the trunk, reaching the level of the umbilicus.

Trigger Point Pain

Referred trigger point pain arises in a trigger point but is felt at a distance, often entirely remote from its source.[5] The pattern of referred pain is diagnostic of its site of origin. The distribution of referred trigger point pain rarely coincides entirely with the distribution of a peripheral nerve or dermatomal segment. Untreated trigger points can be associated with pain syndromes that include, but are not limited to, radiculopathy, tennis elbow, tension headache, occipital headache, and frozen shoulder.[16]

Overview of Examination Techniques

The client's general experience of pain can be elicited through pain interviews about the 24-hour pain behavior (see Appendix B, Selected Soft-Tissue Examination Techniques). This interview can be augmented with the use of body diagrams that the client can use to map the locations and quality of pain.[143] Pain intensity can be assessed using the Visual Analog Scale, the Verbal Rating Scale, the Numerical Rating Scale, and the Descriptor Differential Scale.[143] The affective component of pain, how the client behaves in response to pain, can be assessed using the Verbal Rating Scale, the Visual Analog Scale, the Pain Discomfort Scale, the McGill Pain Questionnaire, and the Descriptor Differential Scale. The impact of the client's pain on his level of function can be evaluated using standardized self-report measures, such as the Oswestry Back Pain Questionnaire, the Sickness Impact Profile, the Dallas Pain Questionnaire, and the Millon Visual Analog Scale.[124] Pain that the client reports remains constant, regardless of activity, rest, or sleep, may be from a nonmusculoskeletal cause, such as cancer, that warrants a referral to the client's physician for further assessment.[144]

Physical tests that are used in the identification of pain syndromes include neural tissue tension or provocation tests,[139,142,145,146] active and passive movement analysis, and nerve or tissue palpation.[145] The client's sensitivity to the pressure of palpation can be quantified accurately[147] and reliably (interrater reliability ICCs ranging from 0.75 to 0.84, intrarater reliability ICCs ranging from 0.64 to 0.96) using a pain threshold meter or pressure algometer.[148–151] The combination of client history and palpation is the primary clinical means of identifying trigger points[16] (see Appendix B, Selected Soft-Tissue Examination Techniques), although the palpation of latent trigger points may be less reliable than that of active trigger points.[152] Electrophysiological studies (nerve conduction), electromyography, and thermography are among the laboratory or instrumented tests used in the diagnosis of pain syndromes.[133,153,154]

POSTURAL MALALIGNMENT
Definitions and Etiology
Posture

The positioning and alignment of the skeleton and associated soft tissues in relation to gravity, the center of mass, and the base of support of the body.[50]

Postural Malalignment

Abnormal joint alignment caused by soft tissue or deformity within a bone.[155] Since all tissue growth and repair can be influenced by mechanical loading and body posture, postural malalignment can contribute to the development of neurovascular and musculoskeletal dysfunction directly or as a result of the compensatory motions or postures that can accompany postural malalignment.[155,156] For example, chronic placement of the head anterior to the body's center of gravity is a common postural malalignment that is associated with neurological and musculoskeletal dysfunction.

Overview of Examination Techniques

Visual inspection of the symmetry of bony landmarks, muscle contours, and other tissues with the client in static postures, such as sitting, standing, or lying, is the common clinical approach to assessing postural alignment (see the Appendix B, Selected Soft-Tissue Examination Techniques).[20,71] Visual inspection of dynamic posture is of greater importance in the assessment of fascial restrictions.[28] The technique of visual inspection can be refined through the use of postural grids, photography, and various posture analysis forms, such as the Portland State University Posture Analysis Form.[157] In addition, the client's postural awareness can be elicited during the client interview.

Goniometry, plumb lines, inclinometers, tape measures, and video image and frame analysis are among the tools that can be used to quantify postural malalignment.[158,159] For example, sagittal-plane postural alignment of the head and shoulder in relationship to the lateral malleolus can be measured using a carpenter's tri-square with a line level attached to the horizontal arm and a goniometer with a line level attached to the horizontal arm.[160]

More-sophisticated measures of postural alignment include three-dimensional electrogoniometers, such as the Metrecom Skeletal Analysis System,[161] a force platform,[157] x-ray line-drawing analysis for sagittal-plane spinal displacement,[160,162] and visual estimation of lumbar lordosis from radiographs (which can be inaccurate and unreliable[163]). Dynamic postural analysis can be performed using three-dimensional computer-assisted motion analysis, with or without electromyography.[164] Finally, postural alignment during functional activity can be assessed using measures such as the Ovako Working Analysis System.[165]

IMPAIRED SENSATION SECONDARY TO ENTRAPMENT NEUROPATHY
Definitions and Etiology
Entrapment Neuropathy

Nerve compression can result from muscle and connective tissue shortening and inflammation associated with trigger point activity, fascial restrictions, overuse syndromes, and other clinical conditions.[166–168] The client with an entrapment neuropathy will present with pain, paresthesia, numbness, or loss of range of motion. Common peripheral entrapment neuropathies include carpal tunnel syndrome, cubital tunnel syndrome, and tarsal tunnel syndrome.[169,170] Less common entrapment neuropathies include posterior interosseous nerve syndrome and anterior interosseous nerve syndrome.[171,172]

Overview of Examination Techniques

Clinical evaluation of entrapment neuropathies includes dermatome testing, such as light touch, hot/cold, pinprick, and filament testing; myotome testing through isometric movements and reflexes; palpation of the nerve in the area of possible compression; and neural tension testing.[20]

Electrophysiological testing (nerve conduction studies) evaluates late responses (F waves and H reflexes) and long latency reflexes.[154] These studies enable the clinician to identify the location and severity of the neuropathy.[173,174] Electroneurometry (skin-surface electrical stimulation of the motor nerve), single-frequency (120 Hz) vibrometry tests, and magnetic resonance imaging are also of value in the diagnosis of entrapment neuropathies.[175,176]

SWELLING
Definitions and Etiology
Swelling

An abnormal enlargement of a segment of the body.[20]

Edema

An accumulation of fluid in cells, tissues, or serous cavities.[177] Edema has four main causes: increased permeability of capillaries, decreased plasma protein osmotic pressure, increased pressure in capillaries and venules, and lymphatic flow obstruction.

Effusion

Excessive fluid in the joint capsule, indicating irritation or inflammation of the synovium.[177]

Lymphedema

Accumulation of abnormal amounts of lymph fluid and associated swelling of subcutaneous tissues that results from the obstruction, destruction, or hypoplasia of lymph vessels.[178,179]

Dependent Edema

An increase in extracellular fluid volume that is localized in a dependent area, such as a limb.[24] Dependent edema can be associated with swelling or pitting.

Pitting Edema

Edema that retains the indentation produced by the pressure of palpation.[24]

Overview of Examination Techniques

The client's description of his swelling and related symptoms can be obtained through the client interview in conjunction with the use of a body diagram.[20] Visual inspection of swelling can assist the clinician in determining how best to measure the client's swelling.[20] Palpation of swelling provides data on the quality of the swelling and the degree of edema that is present.[20] Girth measurements of swollen body segments can be taken using a flexible tape measure, jeweler's ring, or wire.[180,181] Volumetric analysis, in which the amount of fluid displaced by the limb is measured, provides a simple means of quantifying the extent of swelling, which is more appropriate for swelling of the extremities.[177] Comparison of volumetric analysis and estimation of limb volume using measurements of the limb perimeter showed that there was no significant difference between the two measures of limb volume for the arm, but volumetric analysis was more reliable and accurate for the hand.[182] See Appendix B, Selected Soft-Tissue Examination Techniques for further information on the measurement of swelling.

Laboratory or instrumented measures of swelling include multiple-frequency bioelectrical impedance analysis, magnetic resonance imaging, and laser-Doppler flowmetry.[181,183]

NEUROLOGICAL IMPAIRMENTS

ABNORMAL NEUROMUSCULAR TONE

Definitions and Etiology

Muscle Tone

Resting tension and responsiveness of muscles to passive elongation or stretch.[129]

Postural Tone

The development of muscular tension in skeletal muscles that participate in maintaining the positions of different parts of the skeleton. The cerebellum regulates postural tone.[184] Unlike muscle resting tension, constant muscle activation is required for the maintenance of postural tone, and the self-sustained firing of motoneurons may reduce the need for prolonged synaptic input in this situation.[185]

Hypertonia

A general term used to refer to muscle tone that is above normal resting levels, regardless of the mechanism for the increase in tone.[129]

Hypotonia or Flaccidity

A general term used to refer to muscle tone that is below normal resting levels, regardless of the mechanism for the decrease in tone.[129]

Spasticity

Increased muscular tone that is a result of an upper motor neuron lesion that may or may not be associated with reflex hyperexcitability.[186,187] Spastic muscle exhibits a velocity-dependent increase in tonic stretch reflexes.[24,129] The quicker the stretch, the more pronounced the resistance of the spastic muscle.

Rigidity

Increased muscular tone that occurs as a result of brainstem or basal ganglia lesions. Rigidity involves a uniformly increased resistance in both agonist and antagonist muscles, resulting in stiff, immovable body parts, independent of the velocity of the stretch stimulus.[129] Patients exhibit two types of rigidity: *(a)* cogwheel rigidity, which is a ratchetlike response, alternating giving way and increased resistance to passive movement, and *(b)* lead-pipe rigidity, which is a constant response to passive movement.

DECORTICATE RIGIDITY

Occurs as a result of brainstem lesions.[129] It presents clinically as sustained contraction and posturing of the trunk and lower limbs in extension and the upper limbs in flexion.

DECEREBRATE RIGIDITY

Occurs as a result of brainstem lesions.[129] It presents clinically as sustained contraction and posturing of the trunk and lower limbs in extension.

PARKINSONIAN RIGIDITY

Occurs as a result of basal ganglia lesions.[129] It presents clinically as a tight contraction of both agonist and antagonist muscles throughout the movement (lead-pipe rigidity).

Clonus

A cyclical, spasmodic hyperactivity of antagonistic muscles that occurs at a regular frequency in response to a quick stretch stimulus.[129]

Overview of Examination Techniques

The measurement of abnormal muscular tone requires an understanding of neurological lesions. Manual passive motion testing and the use of tone grading scales, such as the Ashworth Scale, are central to the examination of abnormal tone.[129,188] The client examination for spasticity can also include the pendulum test (using isokinetic dynamometers or a goniometer); torque/electromyogram curves for ramp and hold or sinusoidal oscillation; or the use of handheld or isokinetic dynamometers to measure resistance to passive movement.[187,189]

Some standardized assessments of motor control, such as the Fugl-Meyer and the Montreal Assessment include sections on manual testing of muscle tone.[190] In addition to manual passive motion testing, spasticity can be evaluated using electrophysiological measures that measure the electrical and mechanical features of hypertonic muscle.[187] These measures include electromyographic testing of reflexes, such as the T-reflexes, H-reflexes, F-responses, long-latency stretch reflexes, the tonic vibration reflex, and flexor reflexes. Research suggests, however, that there is a stronger correlation between Ashworth Scale scores and spasticity than with laboratory or instrumented tests of reflex activity.[191] Testing for exaggerated or clonic deep tendon reflexes in hypertonic individuals and absent or decreased reflexes for hypotonic states is also possible.[129]

In light of the impact that neurological conditions can have on an individual's functional level, there are numerous functional measures that are used in the client examination.[190] These measures are similar in their emphasis on motor recovery and the functional tasks that are most often affected in individuals who have had strokes; however, they differ in the philosophical principles on which they are based. For example, the measures that reflect Neurodevelopmental therapy principles include the Rivermead Motor Assessment Protocol and the Montreal Assessment. The Fugl-Meyer uses Brunnstrom's sequence of motor recovery. The Functional Test for the Hemiparetic Upper Extremity is based on both Brunnstrom and Neurodevelopmental therapy principles. Other measures, such as the Motor Assessment Scale, the Physical Assessment for Stroke Patients, and the Arm Function Test are not structured on the basis of either the Brunnstromm or neurodevelopmental philosophy.

CARDIOPULMONARY IMPAIRMENTS

IMPAIRED AIRWAY CLEARANCE
Definitions and Etiology
Airway Clearance
Ability to move pulmonary secretions effectively through the use of normal mechanisms of cough and the mucociliary escalator.[192]

Chronic Obstructive Pulmonary Disease
Pulmonary disorders that are characterized by the presence of increased airway resistance.[192,193] These disorders are associated with increased sputum production and cough that can predispose the individual to recurrent bronchial infection. Examples of chronic obstructive pulmonary disease include emphysema, chronic bronchitis, and asthma.

Chronic Restrictive Pulmonary Disease
Pulmonary disorders that are characterized by the restriction of lung expansion, such as interstitial fibrosis.[192]

Overview of Examination Techniques
The clinical examination of impaired airway clearance is based on a number of clinical signs and symptoms, many of which are summarized in the Respiratory Nursing Diagnosis Scale (RNDS) that defines major and minor characteristics of impaired airway clearance.[194,195] According to this scale, the most important characteristic of impaired airway clearance is an ineffective cough. The minor characteristics included tenacious sputum; subjective complaints of inability to cough up secretions; increased or copious sputum; absent, decreased, or abnormal breath sounds; air hunger; abnormal respiratory pattern; nasal flaring; anxiety; dyspnea at rest; cyanosis or other change in color; and restlessness. Characteristics that were deemed less relevant to impaired airway clearance included asymmetrical chest excursion, abnormal inspiratory-to-expiratory ratio, dyspnea on exertion, diaphoresis, and pain.

A number of clinical tests can be used to collect the data on which to base the identification of impaired airway clearance.[196–197] Visual inspection of cough; visual inspection of the volume and quality of sputum, respiration rate, and pattern; color; and accessory muscle use are essential starting points.[192] Oxygen saturation—the degree to which arterial blood is oxygenated—is measured by pulse oximeters.[197] Auscultation is used to assess breath sounds and heart rate.[192] Clinicians can use self-report measures to elicit client's perception of breathlessness (measured on a visual analog scale), rating of dyspnea on a dyspnea rating scale, or perceived exertion on a perceived exertion rating scale.[197]

Laboratory tests of symptoms associated with impaired airway clearance include arterial blood gases, which show oxygenation, acidosis, alkalosis, compensatory mechanisms, and buffer systems;[192] pulmonary function tests, which show inspired volume, respiratory exchange ratio,[197] forced expiratory volumes,[197,198] inspiratory capacity, and vital capacity;[199] and measures of oxygen consumption.[196] Laboratory measures of actual particle clearance rates are not yet appropriate for use with humans, although they are commonly used in animal research.[200]

The client's perception of the impact of impaired airway clearance and chronic respiratory disease on his functional level and quality of life can be measured using a variety of self-report functional measures, such as the Nottingham Health Profile for quality of life[201] and the Self-Efficacy for Functional Activities questionnaire.[202]

DYSPNEA

Definitions and Etiology

Dyspnea

Shortness of breath, labored or difficult breathing, or uncomfortable awareness of one's breathing.[192,203] Dyspnea is usually an indication of inadequate ventilation or insufficient amounts of oxygen in the circulating blood. Dyspnea is a complex sensation that involves *(a)* the physiological and psychological events or stimuli preceding the development of dyspnea; *(b)* the characteristics of an individual or his environment, which mediates his response to the dyspnea; and *(c)* the outcomes that result once the individual has reacted to the dyspnea.[192,204]

Overview of Examination Techniques

Clinical examination of a client with dyspnea can include visual inspection for posture used during respiration; quality, rate, and pattern of breathing; accessory muscle use; color; and affect. Laboratory tests of decreased ventilation include arterial blood gases, which show oxygenation, acidosis, alkalosis, compensatory mechanisms, and buffer systems,[198] and capnography, which determines levels of carbon dioxide.[203]

A critical review of measures for dyspnea performed by Hutter and Wurtemberger[193] showed only a fair association between perceived dyspnea and actual physiological lung function (less than 30% of the common variance). This may occur because of the different components that are antecedents, mediators, and outcomes of dyspnea that are outlined above. Mancini and Body[204] organize the various standardized self-report measures of dyspnea according to those components. For example, they state that measures, such as the British Medical Research Council Questionnaire, the American Thoracic Questionnaire, and the Dyspnea Interview Schedule can assess the events or stimuli that precede the dyspnea. The American Thoracic Questionnaire, the Chronic Respiratory Questionnaire, the Dyspnea Interview Schedule, the Pulmonary Functional Status Scale, and the Therapy Impact Questionnaire may measure characteristics that mediate the dyspnea. The Dyspnea Visual Analogue Scale, the Therapy Impact Questionnaire, and the Borg Perceived Exertion Scale measure an individual's reactions to dyspnea. Finally, the consequences of an episode of dyspnea can be measured using the Therapy Impact Questionnaire, the Baseline Dyspnea Index, the Transition Dyspnea Index, the Chronic Respiratory Questionnaire, the Oxygen Cost Diagram, the Dyspnea Interview Schedule, and the Modified Medical Research Council Dyspnea Scale.

IMPAIRED RIB CAGE MOBILITY

Definitions and Etiology

Rib Cage Mobility

The capacity of the rib cage to move within the available anatomical range of motion during respiration, based upon the arthrokinematics of the joints of the rib cage and the thoracic spine and the ability of the periarticular connective tissue to deform.

Overview of Examination Techniques

Examination of rib cage mobility involves both visual inspection and palpation. The visual inspection performed by the clinician should include general posture, breathing pattern, chest wall shape, symmetry of chest wall movement, accessory muscle use, and muscle contours.[192,203] Palpation of chest wall excursion during respiration should address lateral costal and diaphragmatic excursion through palpation of the intercostal spaces, sternal motion, and apical motion. Clinicians can also use palpation to assess the mobility of the thoracic spine, the costovertebral joints, and the sternocostal joints.[20,192] Palpation of muscle tension in the accessory muscles of breathing, such as the sternocleidomastoid, and the intercostal muscles will complete the palpation process. Finally, clinicians can quantify rib cage mobility by measuring rib cage excursion during respiration with a tape measure, using a consistent measurement site and position.[205]

PSYCHONEUROIMMUNOLOGICAL IMPAIRMENTS

STRESS

Definitions and Etiology

Chronic Stress

A prolonged and heightened state of arousal that has negative physiological and psychological consequences.[206] Chronic stress responses occur over the cognitive, physiological, affective, or behavioral domains and may have consequences, such as impaired cognitive function, depression or anxiety, muscle tension, and impaired social functioning.

Stress Response

The individual's cognitive, physiological, affective, or behavioral response to the stressor, or stress-causing agent.[207]

Cognitive Transactional Model of Stress

Lazarus and Folkman[208] define stress as the condition that results when a person's interactions with his environment leads him to perceive a discrepancy—whether real or not—between the demands of the situation and the resources of the person's biological, psychological, or social systems.

Physiological Model of Stress

Hans Selye's model of stress is based on the finding that the adrenal cortex and the neuroendocrine and immune systems interact during stress.[209,210] Selye defined stress as the body's automatic response ("fight or flight") to a demand that is placed on it. Seyle also made a distinction between negative and positive stress: distress and eustress, respectively.

Life Events Model of Stress

Holmes and Rahe defined a model of stress that examined the nature and consequences of negative life events and proposed that interpersonal stressors are predictive of increases in disease activity.[211]

Chronic psychosocial stress has numerous pathophysiological effects that may be related to excessive sympathetic nervous system activation.[212] In particular, adrenal glucocorticoid hormones may play a major role in the stress response because of their profound effects on mood, behavior, neurochemical transmission, and neuroendocrine control.[213]

The pathophysiological effects of chronic stress include insulin resistance, hyperinsulinemia, coronary heart disease risk,[214] infertility in females,[215] therapy-resistant periodontitis,[216] and impaired hippocampus-mediated memory processes.[217] In children, chronic stress may be associated with impaired mental and affective stability, integrity, and development.[218] Because of the subjective nature of stress, clients' perceptions of their symptoms and stress levels are a critical component of the client examination. Client interviews can elicit clients' reports of physical, mental, emotional, and behavioral symptoms of stress and descriptions of the situations they perceive to be stress provoking. Clinicians can use a visual analog scale to obtain a basic rating of the client's perceived stress level. There are also numerous standardized self-report stress-rating questionnaires that clinicians can use to assess their clients' perceived level of stress and the factors contributing to the stress that their clients experience. These tests provide a well-defined set of information and are usually designed and validated for a specific population. A clinician who wishes to use a standardized measure of stress is advised to consult the measure's manual for details of the professional training required prior to administering the measure and to determine whether that form of examination falls within her scope of practice. Some of these

measures are based on the dominant models of stress. For example, the Schedule of Recent Experience,[219] Impact of Events Scale, and the Social Readjustment Ratings Scale[220] are classic measures based on Holmes and Rahe's Life Events Model of Stress. The Cognitive Transactional Model of Stress provides the basis for the Hassles and Uplifts[221] and the Ways of Coping Questionnaire from Folkman and Lazarus.[222] Buros Mental Measurement Yearbook[223] is a useful source of information on standardized stress questionnaires that includes the test population, test purpose, test details, and reviews. Some of the many tests described in Buros are described in Box 3-3. In addition, there are health-related stress questionnaires, such as the Cardiac Event Threat Questionnaire.[224]

Clinicians can also use any of the range of physiological measures of chronic stress that are available. Clinical measures include heart rate,[225,226] systolic and diastolic blood pressure,[227,228] finger pulse volume,[229] skin conductance levels,[229,230] and finger temperature.[230] Electromyography, especially lateral frontalis electromyogram responses, is an indicator of stress.[225,226] Laboratory measures of blood samples include levels of lipid peroxides in venous blood samples;[231] levels of stress-related hormones prolactin,

---

Box 3-3
Selected Standardized Measures of Stress from Buros Mental Measurement Yearbook[223]

- Adolescent Coping Scale
- Coping Inventory for Stressful Situations
- Coping With Stress
- Daily Stress Inventory
- Life Stressors and Social Resources Inventory–Youth Form
- Personal Stress Assessment Inventory
- Questionnaire on Resources and Stress
- Stokes-Gordon Stress Scale
- Stress Analysis System
- Stress Audit
- Stress Impact Scale
- Stress Indicator and Health Planner
- Stress Management Questionnaire
- Stress Resiliency Profile
- Stress Response Scale
- Understanding and Managing Stress

cortisol, and testosterone;[232] and glycated hemoglobin levels.[233] Finally, saliva can be analyzed to determine salivary cortisol levels, a common physiological indicator of stress.[226,227,234]

SELF-CARE ACTIVITIES

Self-care activities refer to those daily tasks that an individual needs to perform to be independent.[235] These tasks include dressing, feeding, grooming, hygiene, functional mobility, and functional communication. Since an inability to perform any of these tasks is considered a functional limitation, clinicians are more frequently using standardized measures of self-care to assess the client's progress on the identified functional outcomes of care. For example, the Barthel Index is a self-care measure that consists of 10 items that represent basic self-care activities including feeding, wheelchair transfer, grooming, bathing, walking on level surface, climbing stairs, dressing, bowel control, and bladder control.[236] Although it is one of the oldest self-care measures, ongoing studies are evaluating its validity and reliability.[237] The Barthel Index is still widely used for the examination of clients with strokes, hip fractures, liver transplants, Parkinson's disease, amputations, and other clinical conditions.[238–243] Other self-care measures are discussed in relevant sections on impairments.

HEALTH-RELATED QUALITY OF LIFE

Health-related quality of life can be an issue to be addressed in the client examination for massage, since the impairments described above can have an impact on

---

Box 3-4
Selected Health-Related Quality of Life Measures

- Medical Outcome Study Health Status Questionnaire[245]
- Duke-UNC Health Profile[255]
- The Sickness Impact Profile[256]
- McMaster Health Index Questionnaire[257]
- Functional Status Questionnaire [258]
- Nottingham Health Profile[201]

---

the client's functional level and disability. Measures of health-related quality of life have a broader focus thanself-care measures, and they typically cover the domains of physical, psychological/emotional, and social function.[244] The Medical Outcomes Survey–Short Form 36 (MOS SF-36) is a frequently used health-related quality of life measure that has been validated for several diseases, such as venous leg ulcers, kidney disease, HIV/AIDS, epilepsy, systemic lupus erythematosus, strokes, alcohol dependency, and schizophrenia, and translated into other languages, such as Chinese.[246–253] Other health-related quality of life measures are listed in Box 3-4. In addition, disease-specific quality of life measures, such as the Rheumatoid Arthritis Quality of Life Scale,[254] are being used more frequently in clinical examination and studies.

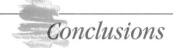

Conclusions

The client examination plays a critical role in outcome-based massage by providing the clinical findings on which the clinician can base the confirmation of her clinical hypothesis and her treatment planning. Consequently, clinicians who are conducting client examinations with a view to using massage as a primary or complementary treatment modality need to expand the focus of their standard approach to examination to include the assessment of soft-tissue dysfunction and the impairments that are relevant to the use of massage.

Palpation provides an important means of assessing a variety of aspects of soft-tissue function that can suggest the presence of impairments, such as temperature, tissue mobility, fluid status, tissue texture, and tissue consistency. In addition, the client's response to palpation can give the clinician other information about the client's presenting impairments. Yet palpation is not the only means of assessing a client's impairments; the clinician can also extend her interpretation of the findings from standard musculoskeletal, neurological, cardiopulmonary, or psychological tests and measures to include an analysis of the contribution of soft-tissue dysfunction. Finally, the client examination conducted by the clinician should also address the client's functional limitations, disability, and quality of life so that the clinician has data on which to base the identification of appropriate functional outcomes of care.

References

1. National Institute of Child Health and Human Development. Research plan for the National Center for Medical Rehabilitation Research. Public Health Service NIH Publication no. 93-3509. Bethesda, MD: National Institutes of Health, US Department of Health and Human Services, 1993.
2. Nagi S. Disability concepts revisited: implications for prevention. Executive summary. In: Pope A, Tarlov A, eds. Disability in America. Washington, DC: National Academy Press, 1991:1–4.
3. Chaitow L. Palpation skills. New York: Churchill-Livingstone, 1997.
4. Lewit K. Soft tissue and relaxation techniques in myofascial pain. In: Hammer WI. Functional soft tissue examination and treatment by manual methods. 2nd ed. Gaithersburg, MD: Aspen, 1999:479–532.
5. Greenman PE. Principles of manual medicine. 2nd ed. Baltimore: Williams & Wilkins, 1996.
6. Starkey C, Ryan J. Evaluation of orthopedic and athletic injuries. Philadelphia: FA Davis, 1996.
7. McKenzie AM, Taylor NF. Can physiotherapists locate lumbar spinal levels by palpation? Physiotherapy 1997; 83(5):235–239.
8. Keating J, Matyas TA, Bach TM. The effect of training on physical therapists' ability to apply specified forces of palpation. Phys Ther 1993;73(1):38–46.
9. Fritz S. Fundamentals of therapeutic massage. St Louis: Moseby-Lifeline, 1995.
10. Downey BJ, Taylor NF, Niere KR. Manipulative physiotherapists can reliably palpate nominated lumbar spinal levels. Manual Ther 1999;4(3):151–156.
11. Latimer J, Adams R, Lee M. Training with feedback improves judgements of non-biological linear elastic stiffness. Manual Ther 1998;3(2):85–89.
12. Maher CG, Simmonds M, Adams R. Therapists' conceptualization and characterization of the clinical concept of spinal stiffness. Phys Ther 1998;78(3):289–300.
13. Nicholson L, Adams R, Maher C. Reliability of a discrimination measure for judgements of non-biological stiffness. Manual Ther 1997;2(3):150–156.
14. Inscoe EL, Witt PL, Gross MT, Mitchell RU. Reliability in evaluating passive intervertebral motion of the lumbar spine. J Manual Manipulative Ther 1995;3(4):135–143.
15. Barral JP. Manual thermal diagnosis. Seattle, WA: Eastland Press, 1996.
16. Simons DG, Travell JG, Simons LS. Travell and Simons' myofascial pain and dysfunction: the trigger point manual, vol 1: upper half of body. 2nd ed. Baltimore: Williams & Wilkins, 1999.
17. DiGiovanna EL, Schiowitz S. An osteopathic approach to diagnosis and treatment. 2nd ed. Philadelphia: Lippincott-Raven, 1997:18.
18. Cantu R, Grodin A. Myofascial manipulation: theory and clinical application. Gaithersburg, MD: Aspen, 1992.
19. Thomson JS. Core textbook of anatomy. Philadelphia: JB Lippincott, 1977.
20. Magee DJ. Orthopedic physical assessment. Philadelphia: WB Saunders, 1997.
21. Hertling D, Kessler RM. Management of common musculoskeletal disorders. 3rd ed. Philadelphia: Lippincott-Raven, 1996.
22. Kisner C, Colby LA. Therapeutic exercise: foundations and techniques. 3rd ed. Philadelphia: FA Davis; 1996.
23. de Domenico G, Wood EC. Beard's massage. 4th ed. Philadelphia: WB Saunders, 1997.
24. Stedman TL. Stedman's medical dictionary. 25th ed. Baltimore: Williams & Wilkins, 1989.
25. Barnes JF. Myofascial release: the search for excellence. Paoli, PA: MFR Seminars, 1990.
26. Drape JL, Silbermann Hoffman O, Houvet P, et al. Complications of flexor tendon repair in the hand: MR imaging assessment. Radiology 1996;198(1):219–224.
27. Gerscovich EO, Maslen L, Cronan MS, et al. Spinal sonography and magnetic resonance imaging in patients with repaired myelomeningocele: comparison of modalities. J Ultrasound Med 1999;18(9):655–664.
28. Mannheim CJ, Lavett DK. The myofascial release manual. Thorofare, NJ: Slack (McGraw-Hill), 1989.
29. Scott J, Huskisson E. Vertical or horizontal visual analogue scales. Ann Rheum Dis 1979;38:560.
30. Chaitow L. Modern neuromuscular techniques. New York: Churchill-Livingstone, 1996.
31. Sucher BM, Heath DM. Thoracic outlet syndrome—a myofascial variant: part 3. Structural and postural considerations. J Am Osteopath Assoc 1993;93(3):334, 340–345.
32. Sucher BM. Thoracic outlet syndrome—a myofascial variant: part 2. Treatment. J Am Osteopath Assoc 1990;90(9):810–812, 817–823.
33. Sucher BM. Thoracic outlet syndrome—a myofascial variant: part 1. Pathology and diagnosis. J Am Osteopath Assoc 1990;90(8):686–696, 703–704.
34. Sucher BM. Myofascial manipulative release of carpal tunnel syndrome: documentation with magnetic resonance imaging. J Am Osteopath Assoc 1993;93(12):1273–1278.
35. Sucher BM. Myofascial release of carpal tunnel syndrome. J Am Osteopath Assoc 1993;93(1):92–94, 100–101.
36. Cisler TA. Whiplash as a total-body injury. J Am Osteopath Assoc 1994;94(2):145–148.

37. Hanten WP, Chandler SD. Effects of myofascial release leg pull and sagittal plane isometric contract-relax techniques on passive straight-leg raise angle. J Orthop Sports Phys Ther 1994;20(3):138–144.

38. Radjieski JM, Lumley MA, Cantieri MS. Effect of osteopathic manipulative treatment on length of stay for pancreatitis: a randomized pilot study. J Am Osteopath Assoc 1998;98(5):264–272.

39. Tillman LJ, Chasan NP. Properties of dense connective tissue and wound healing. In: Hertling D, Kessler RM, eds. Management of common musculoskeletal conditions. 3rd ed. Philadelphia: Lippincott-Raven, 1996:8–21.

40. Tillman LJ, Cummings GS. Biologic mechanisms of connective tissue mutability. In: Currier DP, Nelson RM, eds. Dynamics of human biologic tissues. Philadelphia: FA Davis, 1992:1–44.

41. Kessler RM, Hertling D. Friction massage. In: Hertling D, Kessler RM, eds. Management of common musculoskeletal conditions. 3rd ed. Philadelphia: Lippincott-Raven, 1996:133–139.

42. Hammer WI. Friction massage. In: Hammer WI. Functional soft tissue examination and treatment by manual methods. 2nd ed. Gaithersburg, MD: Aspen, 1999:463–478.

43. Palastanga N. The use of transverse frictions for soft tissue lesions. In: Grieve GP, ed. Modern manual therapy for the vertebral column. New York: Churchill-Livingstone, 1986:819–825.

44. de Brujin R. Deep transverse friction; its analgesic effect. Int J Sports Med 1984;5(suppl):35–36.

45. Cyriax J, Coldham M. Textbook of orthopedic medicine, vol 2. Treatment by manipulation, massage and injection. 11th ed. London: Bailliere-Tindall, 1984.

46. Chamberlain GJ. Cyriax's friction massage: a review. J Orthop Sports Phys Ther 1982;4(1):16–22.

47. Cyriax J. Deep massage. Physiotherapy 1977;63:60–61.

48. Walker JM. Deep transverse frictions in ligament healing. J Orthop Sports Phys Ther 1984;62:89–94.

49. Bajuk S, Jelnikar T, Ortar M. Rehabilitation of patient with brachial plexus lesion and break in axillary artery. Case study. J Hand Ther 1996;9(4):399–403.

50. Hammer WI. The use of friction massage in the management of chronic bursitis of the hip or shoulder. J Manipulative Physiol Ther 1993;16(2):107–111.

51. American Physical Therapy Association. Guide to physical therapist practice. Phys Ther 1997(11):77.

52. Junger M, Steins A, Zuder D, Klyscz T. [Physical therapy of venous diseases] (German). Vasa 1998;27(2):73.9. (Abstract).

53. Ogilvie Harris DJ, Myerthall S. The diabetic frozen shoulder: arthroscopic release. Arthroscopy 1997;13(1):1–8.

54. Siegel LB, Cohen NJ, Gall EP. Adhesive capsulitis: a sticky issue. Am Fam Phys 1999;59(7):1843–1852.

55. Gam AN, Schydlowsky P, Rossel I, et al. Treatment of "frozen shoulder" with distension and glucorticoid compared with glucocorticoid alone. A randomised controlled trial. Scand J Rheumatol 1998;27(6):425–430.

56. Schenk TJ, Brems JJ. Multidirectional instability of the shoulder: pathophysiology, diagnosis, and management. J Am Acad Orthop Surg 1998;6(1):65–72.

57. Cornelissen BP, Rijkenhuizen AB, van den Hoogen BM, et al. Experimental model of synovitis/capsulitis in the equine metacarpophalangeal joint. Am J Vet Res 1998;59(8):978–985.

58. Barozzi L, Olivieri I, De Matteis M, et al. Seronegative spondylarthropathies: imaging of spondylitis, enthesitis and dactylitis. Eur J Radiol 1998;27(Suppl 1):S12–17.

59. Coari G, Paoletti F, Iagnocco A. Shoulder involvement in rheumatic diseases. Sonographic findings. J Rheumatol 1999;26(3):668–673.

60. Hjelm R, Draper C, Spencer S. Anterior-inferior capsular length insufficiency in the painful shoulder. J Orthop Sports Phys Ther 1996;Mar;23(3):21–22.

61. Rozzi SL, Lephart SM, Gear WS, Fu FH. Knee joint laxity and neuromuscular characteristics of male and female soccer and basketball players. Am J Sports Med 1999;27(3):312–319.

62. Messina DF, Farney WC, DeLee JC. The incidence of injury in Texas high school basketball: a prospective study among male and female athletes. Am J Sports Med 1999;27(3):294–299.

63. Heitz NA, Eisenman PA, Beck CL, Walker JA. Hormonal changes throughout the menstrual cycle and increased anterior cruciate ligament laxity in females. J Athletic Train 1999;34(2):144–149.

64. Harris NL. Physical diagnosis of collateral ligament and combined ligament injuries. Oper Techniq Sports Med 1996;4(3):148–157.

65. Cyriax J. Textbook of orthopedic medicine, vol 1. Diagnosis of soft tissue lesions. 7th ed. London: Bailliere-Tindall; 1978.

66. Fritz JM, Delitto A, Erhard RE, Roman M. An examination of the selective tissue tension scheme, with evidence for the concept of a capsular pattern of the knee. Phys Ther 1998;78(10):1046–1056; discussion 1057–1061.

67. Pellecchia GL, Paolino J, Connell J. Intertester reliability of the Cyriax evaluation in assessing patients with shoulder pain. J Orthop Sports Phys Ther 1996;23(1):34–38.

68. Wilk KE, Andrews JR, Arrigo CA. The physical examination of the glenohumeral joint: emphasis on the stabilizing structures. J Orthop Sports Phys Ther 1997;25(6):380–389.

69. Blevins FT. Rotator cuff pathology in athletes. Sports Med 1997;24(3):205–220.

70. van Dijk CN, Mol BW, Lim LS, et al. Diagnosis of ligament rupture of the ankle joint. Physical examination, arthrography, stress radiography and sonography compared in 160 patients after inversion trauma. Acta Orthop Scand 1996;67(6):566–70.

71. Dyrek D. Assessment and treatment strategies for musculoskeletal deficits. In: O'Sullivan SB, Schmitz TJ, eds. Physical rehabilitation assessment and treatment. Philadelphia: FA Davis, 1994.

72. Norkin CC, White JD. Measurement of joint motion: a guide to goniometry. Philadelphia: FA Davis, 1985.

73. Gilliam J, Barstow IK. Joint range of motion. In: Van Deusen J, Brunt D, eds. Assessment in occupational therapy and physical therapy. Philadelphia: WB Saunders, 1997:49–77.

74. MacDermid JC, Chesworth BM, Patterson S, Roth JH. Intratester and intertester reliability of goniometric measurement of passive lateral shoulder rotation. J Hand Ther 1999;12(3):187–192.

75. Thoms V, Rome K. Effect of subject position on the reliability of measurement of active ankle joint dorsiflexion. Foot: Int J Clin Foot Sci 1997;7(3):153–158.

76. Bruton A, Ellis B, Goddard J. Comparison of visual estimation and goniometry for assessment of metacarpophalangeal joint angle. Physiotherapy 1999;85(4):201–208 (23 refs).

77. Somers DL, Hanson JA, Kedzierski CM, et al. The influence of experience on the reliability of goniometric and visual measurement of forefoot position. J Orthop Sports Phys Ther 1997;25(3):192–202.

78. Brosseau L, Tousignant M, Budd J, et al. Intratester and intertester reliability and criterion validity of the parallelogram and universal goniometers for active knee flexion in healthy subjects. Physiother Res Int 1997;2(3):150–166.

79. Ellis B, Bruton A, Goddard JR. Joint angle measurement: a comparative study of the reliability of goniometry and wire tracing for the hand. Clin Rehabil 1997;11(4):314–320.

80. Chiu HY, Su FC. The motion analysis system and the maximal area of fingertip motion. A preliminary report. J Hand Surg Br 1996;21(5):604–608.

81. Klein PJ, DeHaven JJ. Accuracy of three-dimensional linear and angular estimates obtained with the Ariel Performance Analysis System. Arch Phys Med Rehabil 1995;76(2):183–189.

82. Friedrichsen K. The validity and reliability of a two-dimensional computer-assisted video gait analysis system. Diss Abstr Int 1995;33-06:1863.

83. Mueller MJ, Norton BJ. Reliability of kinematic measurements of rear-foot motion. Phys Ther 1992;72(10):731–737.

84. Maulucci RA, Eckhouse RH. A technique for measuring clothed range of joint motion. J Appl Biomech 1997;13(3):316–333.

85. Williams GN, Gangel TJ, Arciero RA, et al. Comparison of the Single Assessment Numeric Evaluation method and two shoulder rating scales: outcomes measures after shoulder surgery. Am J Sports Med 1999;27(2):214–221.

86. Love S, Gringmuth RH, Kazemi M, et al. Interexaminer and intraexaminer reliability of cervical passive range of motion using the CROM and Cybex 320 EDI. J Can Chiropract Assoc 1998;42(4):222–228.

87. Barrett CJ, Singer KP, Day R. Assessment of combined movements of the lumbar spine in asymptomatic and low back pain subjects using a three-dimensional electromagnetic tracking system. Manual Ther 1999;4(2):94–99 (29 refs).

88. Troke M, Moore AP, Cheek E. Reliability of the OSI CA 6000 Spine Motion Analyzer with a new skin fixation system when used on the thoracic spine. Manual Ther 1998;3(1):27–33.

89. Christensen HW. Precision and accuracy of an electrogoniometer. J Manipulative Physiol Ther 1999;22(1):10–14.

90. Hagins M, Brown M, Cook C. Intratester and intertester reliability of the Palpation Meter (PALM) in measuring pelvic position. J Manual Manipulative Ther 1998;6(3):130–136.

91. Fischer P. The Palpation Meter (PALM). J Manual Manipulative Ther 1997;5(2):61–62.

92. Exelby L. Mobilisations with movement: a personal view. Physiotherapy 1995;81(12):724–729.

93. Fjellner A, Bexander C, Feleij R, Strender L. Interexaminer reliability in physical examination of the cervical spine. J Manipulative Physiol Ther 1999;22(8):511–516.

94. Ellem D. Assessment of the wrist, hand and finger complex. J Manual Manipulative Ther 1995;3(1):9.

95. Olson KA, Paris SV, Spohr C, Gorniak G. Radiographic assessment and reliability study of the craniovertebral side-bending test. J Manual Manipulative Ther 1998;6(2):87–96.

96. Huber FE, Irrgang JJ, Harner C, Lephart S. Intratester and intertester reliability of the KT-1000 arthrometer in the assessment of posterior laxity of the knee. Am J Sports Med 1997;25(4):479–485.

97. Zchezewski JE. Improving flexibility. In: Scully RM, Barnes MR, eds. Physical therapy. Philadelphia: JB Lippincott, 1989.

98. Simons DG, Mense S. Understanding and measurement of muscle tone as related to clinical muscle pain. Pain 1998;75(1):1–17.

99. Santi MD, Botte MJ. Volkmann's ischemic contracture of the foot and ankle: evaluation and treatment of established deformity. Foot Ankle Int 1995;16(6):368–377.

100. O'Dwyer NJ, Ada L, Neilson PD. Spasticity and muscle contracture following stroke. Brain 1996;119(pt 5):1737–1749.

101. Niamane R, Birouk N, Benomar A, et al. Rigid spine syndrome. Two case-reports. Rev Rhum Engl Ed 1999;66(6):347–350.

102. Noonan TJ, Garrett WE Jr. Muscle strain injury: diagnosis and treatment. J Am Acad Orthop Surg 1999;7(4):262–269.

103. Almekinders LC. Tendinitis and other chronic tendinopathies. J Am Acad Orthop Surg 1998;6(3):157–164.

104. Khan KM, Cook JL, Bonar F, et al. Histopathology of common tendinopathies. Update and implications for clinical management. Sports Med 1999;27(6):393–408.

105. Fredriksen H, Dagfinrud H, Jacobsen V, Maehlum S. Passive knee extension test to measure hamstring muscle tightness. Scand J Med Sci Sports 1997;7(5):279–282.

106. Cornbleet SL, Woolsey NB. Assessment of hamstring muscle length in school-aged children using the sit-and-reach test and the inclinometer measure of hip joint angle. Phys Ther 1996;76(8):850–855.

107. Allison GT, Weston R, Shaw R, et al. The reliability of quadriceps muscle stiffness in individuals with Osgood-Schlatter disease. J Sport Rehabil 1998;7(4): 258–266.

108. Siems JJ, Breur GJ, Blevins WE, Cornell KK. Use of two-dimensional real-time ultrasonography for diagnosing contracture and strain of the infraspinatus muscle in a dog. J Am Vet Med Assoc 1998;212(1): 77–80.

109. Simmonds M. Muscle strength. In: Van Deusen J, Brunt D, eds. Assessment in occupational therapy and physical therapy. Philadelphia: WB Saunders, 1997:27–48.

110. Knepler C, Bohannon RW. Subjectivity of forces associated with manual-muscle test grades of 3+, 4–, and 4. Percept Mot Skills 1998;87(3 pt 2):1123–1128.

111. Bohannon RW. Internal consistency of manual muscle testing scores. Percept Mot Skills 1997;85(2):736–738.

112. Bohannon RW. Research incorporating hand-held dynamometry: publication trends since 1948. Percept Mot Skills 1998;86(3 pt 2):1177–1178.

113. Reinking MF, Bockrath Pugliese K, Worrell T, et al. Assessment of quadriceps muscle performance by hand-held, isometric, and isokinetic dynamometry in patients with knee dysfunction. J Orthop Sports Phys Ther 1996;24(3):154–159.

114. Risberg MA, Holm I, Tjomsland O, et al. Prospective study of changes in impairments and disabilities after anterior cruciate ligament reconstruction. J Orthop Sports Phys Ther 1999;29(7):400–412.

115. Binder-Macleod SA, Lee SCK, Fritz AD, Kucharski LJ. New look at force-frequency relationship of human skeletal muscle: effects of fatigue. J Neurophysiol 1998;79(4): 1858–1868.

116. Wilkerson GB, Pinerola JJ, Caturano RW. Invertor vs. evertor peak torque and power deficiencies associated with lateral ankle ligament injury. J Orthop Sports Phys Ther 1997;26(2):78–86.

117. Whitcomb LJ, Kelley MJ, Leiper CI. A comparison of torque production during dynamic strength testing of shoulder abduction in the coronal plane and the plane of the scapula. J Orthop Sports Phys Ther 1995;21(4):227–232.

118. Bridgewater KJ, Sharpe MH. Trunk muscle performance in early Parkinson's disease. Phys Ther 1998;78(6): 566–576.

119. Fleming SL, Jansen CW, Hasson SM. Effect of work glove and type of muscle action on grip fatigue. Ergonomics 1997;40(6):601–612.

120. Kaegi C, Thibault M, Giroux F, Bourbonnais D. The interrater reliability of force measurements using a modified sphygmomanometer in elderly subjects. Phys Ther 1998;78(10):1095–1203.

121. Brown DA, Kautz SA. Speed-dependent reduction of force output in people with poststroke hemiparesis. Phys Ther 1999;79(10):919–930.

122. Perell KL, Gregor RJ, Scremin AME. Lower limb cycling mechanics in subjects with unilateral cerebrovascular accidents. J Appl Biomech 1998;14(2):158–179.

123. Bohannon RW. Alternatives for measuring knee extension strength of the elderly at home. Clin Rehabil 1998;12(5): 434–440.

124. Mueller BA, Adams ED, Isaac CA. Work activities. In: Van Deusen J, Brunt D, eds. Assessment in occupational therapy and physical therapy. Philadelphia: WB Saunders, 1997:477–521.

125. King PM, Tuckwell N, Barrett TE. A critical review of functional capacity evaluations. Phys Ther 1998;78(8): 852–866.

126. Smith LK, Weiss EL, Lehmkuhl LD. Brunnstrom's clinical kinesiology. 5th ed. Philadelphia: FA Davis, 1996.

127. Maruyama K: Connectin, an elastic protein of striated muscle. Biophys Chem 1994;50(1–2):73–85.

128. Campbell KS, Lakie M. A cross-bridge mechanism can explain the thixotropic short-range elastic component of relaxed frog skeletal muscle. J Physiol Lond 1998;510(pt 3):941–962.

129. O'Sullivan SB. Motor control assessment. In: O'Sullivan SB, Schmitz TJ, eds. Physical rehabilitation: assessment and treatment. Philadelphia: FA Davis, 1994.

130. Katavich L. Neural mechanisms underlying manual cervical traction. J Manual Manipulative Ther 1999;7(1): 20–25.

131. Katavich L. Differential effects of spinal manipulative therapy on acute and chronic muscle spasm: a proposal for mechanisms and efficacy. Manual Ther 1998;3(3): 132–139.

132. Kovac C, Krapf M, Ettlin T, et al. [Methods for detection of changes in muscle tones] (German). Z Rheumatol 1994;53(1):26–36. (Abstract).

133. Dvorak J. Epidemiology, physical examination, and neurodiagnostics. Spine 1998;23(24):2663–2673.

134. Song KM, Morton AA, Koch KD, et al. Chronic musculoskeletal pain in childhood. J Pediatr Orthop 1998;18(5):576–581.

135. Chaplin ER. Chronic pain and the injured worker: a sociobiological problem. In: Kasdan ML, ed. Occupational hand and upper extremity injuries and diseases. Philadelphia: Hanley and Belfus, 1991:13–45.

136. Simon JM. Chronic pain syndrome: nursing assessment and intervention. Rehabil Nurs 1996;21(1):13–19.

137. Corran TM, Farrell MJ, Helme RD, Gibson SJ. The classification of patients with chronic pain: age as a contributing factor. Clin J Pain 1997;13(3):207–214.

138. Sluka KA. Pain mechanisms involved in musculoskeletal disorders. J Orthop Sports Phys Ther 1996;24(4): 240–254.

139. Katavich L. Pain mechanisms underlying peripheral nerve injury—implications for mobilisation of the nervous system. NZ J Physiother 1999;27(1):24–27.

140. Khalsa PS. Muscle pain due to mechanical stimuli. J Neuromusculoskeletal Syst 1999;7(1):1–8.

141. Seaman DR, Cleveland C III. Spinal pain syndromes: nociceptive, neuropathic, and psychologic mechanisms. J Manipulative Physiological Ther 1999;22(7):458–472.

142. Hall TM, Elvey RL. Nerve trunk pain: physical diagnosis and treatment. Manual Ther 1999;4(2):63–73.

143. Ross RG, LaStayo PC. Clinical assessment of pain. In: Van Deusen J, Brunt D, eds. Assessment in occupational therapy and physical therapy. Philadelphia: WB Saunders, 1997:123–133.

144. Weinstein SM. Cancer pain. Phys Med Rehabil State Art Rev 1994;8(2):279–296.

145. Elvey RL. Physical evaluation of the peripheral nervous system in disorders of pain and dysfunction. J Hand Ther 1997;10(2):122–129.

146. Lewis J, Ramot R, Green A. Changes in mechanical tension in the median nerve: possible implications for the upper limb tension test. Physiotherapy 1998;84(6):254–261.

147. Marovino T, Blackmon CB, Sherman M, et al. Pain assessment. The accuracy and test-retest reliability of dolorimetry measurements in a healthy and chronic pain population. Am J Pain Manage 1995;5(3):94–97.

148. Delaney G, McKee A. Inter- and intra-rater reliability of the pressure threshold meter in measurement of myofascial trigger point sensitivity. Am J Phys Med Rehabil 1993;72:136–139.

149. Antonaci F, Sand T, Lucas GA. Pressure algometry in healthy subjects: inter-examiner variability. Scand J Rehabil Med 1998;30(1):3–8.

150. Hong C. Algometry in evaluation of trigger points and referred pain. J Musculoskeletal Pain 1998;6(1):47–59.

151. Nussbaum EL, Downes L. Reliability of clinical pressure-pain algometric measurements obtained on consecutive days. Phys Ther 1998;78(2):160–169.

152. Lew PC, Lewis J, Story I. Inter-therapist reliability in locating latent myofascial trigger points using palpation. Manual Ther 1997;2(2):87–90.

153. Ingber RS. Myofascial pain in lumbar dysfunction. Phys Med Rehabil State Art Rev 1999;13(3):473–498.

154. Hammond E. Electrodiagnosis of the neuromuscular system. In: Van Deusen J, Brunt D, eds. Assessment in occupational therapy and physical therapy. Philadelphia: WB Saunders, 1997:175–198.

155. Riegger-Krugh C, Keysor JJ. Skeletal malalignments of the lower quarter: correlated and compensatory motions and postures. J Orthop Sports Phys Ther 1996;23(2):164–170.

156. Troyanovich SJ, Harrison DE, Harrison DD. Structural rehabilitation of the spine and posture: rationale for treatment beyond the resolution of symptoms. J Manipulative Physiol Ther 1998;21(1):37–50.

157. Seegert EM, Shapiro R. From the field. Effects of alternative exercise on posture. Clin Kinesiol 1999;53(2):41–47.

158. Grimmer K. An investigation of poor cervical resting posture. Aust J Physiother 1997;43(1):7–16.

159. Villanueva MB, Jonai H, Sotoyama M, et al. Sitting posture and neck and shoulder muscle activities at different screen height settings of the visual display terminal. Ind Health 1997;35(3):330–336.

160. Harrison AL, Barry-Greb T, Wojtowicz G. Clinical measurement of head and shoulder posture variables. J Orthop Sports Phys Ther 1996;23(6):353–361.

161. Franklin ME, Chenier TC, Brauninger L, et al. Effect of positive heel inclination on posture. J Orthop Sports Phys Ther 1995;21(2):94–99.

162. Harrison DE, Harrison DD, Troyanovich SJ. Reliability of spinal displacement analysis on plain x-rays: a review of commonly accepted facts and fallacies with implications for chiropractic education and technique. J Manipulative Physiol Ther 1998;21(4):252–266.

163. Tuck AM, Peterson CK. Accuracy and reliability of chiropractors and Anglo-European College of Chiropractic students at visually estimating the lumbar lordosis from radiographs. Chiropract Techniq 1998;10(1):19–26.

164. Capodaglio EM, Capodaglio P, Panigazzi M, Bazzini G. [An ergonomic study of postures of toll collectors] (Italian). G Ital Med Lav Ergon (Italian) 1998;20(1):24–30. (Abstract).

165. Wright EJ, Haslam RA. Manual handling risks and controls in a soft drink distribution centre. Appl Ergonomics 1999;30(4):311–318.

166. Novak CB, Mackinnon SE. Repetitive use and static postures: a source of nerve compression and pain. J Hand Ther 1997;10(2):151–159.

167. Maigne JY, Doursounian L. Entrapment neuropathy of the medial superior cluneal nerve. Nineteen cases surgically treated, with a minimum of 2 years' follow-up. Spine 1997;22(10):1156–1159.

168. Berthelot JM, Delecrin J, Maugars Y, et al. A potentially underrecognized and treatable cause of chronic back pain: entrapment neuropathy of the cluneal nerves. J Rheumatol 1996;23(12):2179–2181.

169. Billi A, Catalucci A, Barile A, Masciocchi C. Joint impingement syndrome: clinical features. Eur J Radiol 1998;27(suppl 1):S39–41.

170. Idler RS. General principles of patient evaluation and nonoperative management of cubital syndrome. Hand Clin 1996;12(2):397–403.

171. Nakano KK. Nerve entrapment syndromes. Curr Opin Rheumatol 1997;9(2):165–173.

172. Huang KC, Chen YJ, Hsu RW. Anterior tarsal tunnel syndrome: case report. Chang Keng I Hsueh Tsa Chih 1999;22(3):503–507.

173. Preston DC. Distal median neuropathies. Neurol Clin 1999;17(3):407–424.

174. Lee CY. Lower limb entrapment neuropathies. Phys Med Rehabil State Art Rev 1999;13(2):231–249.

175. Cherniack MG, Moalli D, Viscolli C. A comparison of traditional electrodiagnostic studies, electroneurometry, and vibrometry in the diagnosis of carpal tunnel syndrome. J Hand Surg Am 1996;21(1):122–131.

176. Kleindienst A, Hamm B, Hildebrandt G, Klug N. Diagnosis and staging of carpal tunnel syndrome: comparison of magnetic resonance imaging and intra-operative findings. Acta Neurochir Wien 1996;138(2):228–233.

177. McCulloch J. Peripheral vascular disease. In: O'Sullivan SB, Schmitz TJ, eds. Physical rehabilitation assessment and treatment. Philadelphia: FA Davis, 1994:371–384.

178. Johansson K, Albertsson M, Ingvar C, Ekdahl C. Effects of compression bandaging with or without manual lymph drainage treatment in patients with postoperative arm lymphedema. Lymphology 1999;32(3): 103–110.

179. Todd JE. Symptom management. Lymphoedema—a challenge for all healthcare professionals. Int J Palliat Nurs 1998;4(5):230–239.

180. Ramadan A. Hand analysis. In: Van Deusen J, Brunt D, eds. Assessment in occupational therapy and physical therapy. Philadelphia: WB Saunders, 1997:78–122.

181. Palmada M, Shah S, O'Hare K. Issues in the measurement of hand oedema. Physiother Theory Pract 1998; 14(3):139–148.

182. Acebes O, Renau E, Sansegundo R, et al. [Evaluation of post-mastectomy lymphedema. Comparative study of two measurement methods] (Spanish). Rehabilitacion 1999; 33(3):190–194. (Abstract).

183. Cornish BH, Bunce IH, Ward LC, et al. Bioelectrical impedance for monitoring the efficacy of lymphoedema treatment programmes. Breast Cancer Res Treat 1996; 38(2):169–176.

184. Manni E, Petrosini L. Luciani's work on the cerebellum a century later. Trends Neurosci 1997;20(3):112–116.

185. Gorassini MA, Bennett DJ, Yang JF. Self-sustained firing of human motor units. Neurosci Lett 1998;247(1):13–16.

186. O'Dwyer NJ, Ada L. Reflex hyperexcitability and muscle contracture in relation to spastic hypertonia. Curr Opin Neurol 1996;9(6):451–455.

187. Agostinucci J. Upper motor neuron syndrome. In: Van Deusen J, Brunt D, eds. Assessment in occupational therapy and physical therapy. Philadelphia: WB Saunders, 1997:271–294.

188. Clarkson HM, Gilewich BG. Musculoskeletal assessment: joint range of motion and manual muscle strength. Baltimore: Williams & Wilkins, 1989.

189. Shaw J, Bially J, Deurvorst N, et al. Clinical and physiological measures of tone in chronic stroke. Neurol Rep 1999;23(1):19–24.

190. Sabari, J. Motor control. In: Van Deusen J, Brunt D, eds. Assessment in occupational therapy and physical therapy. Philadelphia: WB Saunders, 1997:249–270.

191. Vattanasilp W, Ada L. The relationship between clinical and laboratory measures of spasticity. Aust J Physiother 1999;45(2):135–139.

192. Frownfelter DL, Dean E. Principals and practice of cardiopulmonary physical therapy. 3rd ed. St. Louis: CV Mosby, 1996.

193. Hutter BO, Wurtemberger G. [Functional capacity (dyspnea) and quality of life in patients with chronic obstructive lung disease (COPD): instruments of assessment and methodological aspects] (German). Pneumologie 1999;53(3):133–142. (Abstract)

194. Parker L, Lunney M. Moving beyond content validation of nursing diagnosis. Nurs Diagn J Nurs Lang Classif 1998;9(4):144–150.

195. Carlson-Catalano J, Lunney M, Paradiso C, et al. Clinical validation of ineffective breathing pattern, ineffective airway clearance, and impaired gas exchange. Image: J Nurs Sch 1998;30(3):243–248.

196. Dallimore K, Jenkins S, Tucker B. Respiratory and cardiovascular responses to manual chest percussion in normal subjects. Aust J Physiother 1998;44(4):267–274.

197. Protas E. Cardiovascular and pulmonary function. In: Van Deusen J, Brunt D, eds. Assessment in occupational therapy and physical therapy. Philadelphia: WB Saunders, 1997:134–146.

198. Padman R, Geouque DM, Engelhardt MT. Effects of the flutter device on pulmonary function studies among pediatric cystic fibrosis patients. Del Med J 1999;71(1): 13–18.

199. Fujimoto K, Kubo K, Miyahara T, et al. Effects of muscle relaxation therapy using specially designed plates in patients with pulmonary emphysema. Intern Med 1996; 35(10):756–763.

200. Oberdorster G, Cox C, Gelein R. Intratracheal instillation versus intratracheal inhalation of tracer particles for measuring lung clearance function. Exp Lung Res 1997;23(1):17–34.

201. Fuchs-Climent D, Le Gallais D, Varray A, et al. Quality of life and exercise tolerance in chronic obstructive pulmonary disease: effects of a short and intensive inpatient rehabilitation program. Am J Phys Med Rehabil 1999;78(4):330–335.

202. Resnick B. Reliability and validity testing of the Self-Efficacy for Functional Activities scale: three studies. J Nurs Meas 1999;7(1):5–20.

203. Weinstock D, Andrews M, Cray J. Springhouse, professional guide to diseases. 6th ed. Springhouse, PA: Springhouse, 1998.

204. Mancini I, Body JJ. Assessment of dyspnea in advanced cancer patients. Support Care Cancer 1999;7(4):229–232.

205. Hill J, Johansen J, Pedersen S, LaPier TK. Site of measurement and subject position affect chest excursion measurements. Cardiopulmonary Phys Ther J 1997;8(4): 12–17.

206. Powell L, Eagleston J. The assessment of chronic stress in college students. In: Altmaier E, ed. Helping students manage stress: new directions for student services. San Francisco: Jossey-Bass, 1983.

207. Hackett G, Lonborg S. Models of stress. In Altmaier E, ed. Helping students manage stress: new directions for student services. San Francisco: Jossey-Bass, 1983.

208. Sarafino E. Health psychology: biopsychosocial interactions. New York: Wiley, 1990.

209. Berczi I. The stress concept and neuroimmunoregulation in modern biology. Ann NY Acad Sci 1998;851:3–12.

210. Szabo S. Hans Selye and the development of the stress concept. Special reference to gastroduodenal ulcerogenesis. Ann NY Acad Sci 1998;851:19–27.

211. Holmes T, Rahe R. The social readjustment rating scale. J Psychosomatic Research 1967;11:213–218.

212. Rozanski A, Blumenthal JA, Kaplan J. Impact of psychological factors on the pathogenesis of cardiovascular disease and implications for therapy. Circulation 1999;99(16):2192–2196.

213. Fuchs E, Flugge G. Stress, glucocorticoids and structural plasticity of the hippocampus. Neurosci Biobehav Rev 1998; 23(2):295–300.

214. Keltikangas-Jarvinen L, Ravaja N, Raikkonen K, et al. Relationships between the pituitary-adrenal hormones, insulin, and glucose in middle-aged men: moderating influence of psychosocial stress. Metabolism 1998;47(12): 1440–1449.

215. Sanders KA, Bruce NW. A prospective study of psychosocial stress and fertility in women. Hum Reprod 1997;12(10):2324–2329.

216. Axtelius B, Soderfeldt B, Edwardsson S, Attstrom R. Therapy-resistant periodontitis (I). Clinical and treatment characteristics. J Clin Periodontol 1997;24(9 pt 1):640–645.

217. Ohl F, Fuchs E. Differential effects of chronic stress on memory processes in the tree shrew. Brain Res Cogn Brain Res 1999;7(3):379–387.

218. Rothenberger A, Huther G. [The role of psychosocial stress in childhood for structural and functional brain development: neurobiological basis of developmental psychopathology] (German). Prax Kinderpsychol Kinderpsychiatr. 1997;46(9):623–644. (Abstract).

219. Amundson ME, Hart CA, Holmes TH. The schedule of recent experience. Seattle: University of Washington Press, 1986.

220. Holmes TH, Rahe RH. The Social Readjustment Rating Scale. J Psychosom Res 1967;11:213–218.

221. Lazarus RS, Folkman S. Hassles and Uplifts Scales research edition. Palo Alto, CA: Consulting Psychologists Press, 1989.

222. Folkman S, Lazarus RS. Ways of Coping Questionnaire research edition. Palo Alto, CA: Consulting Psychologists Press, 1988.

223. Impara J, Plake B, eds. The thirteenth mental measurements yearbook. Lincoln, NE: Buros Institute of Mental Measurements, 1998.

224. Bennett SJ, Puntenney PJ, Walker NL, Ashley ND. Development of an instrument to measure threat related to cardiac events. Nurs Res 1996;45(5):266–270.

225. Shalev AY, Bloch M, Peri T, Bonne O. Alprazolam reduces response to loud tones in panic disorder but not in posttraumatic stress disorder. Biol Psychiatry 1998;44(1): 64–68.

226. Rief W, Shaw R, Fichter MM. Elevated levels of psychophysiological arousal and cortisol in patients with somatization syndrome. Psychosom Med 1998;60(2): 198–203.

227. Stones A, Groome D, Perry D, et al. The effect of stress on salivary cortisol in panic disorder patients. J Affect Disord 1999;52(1–3):197–201.

228. Demaree HA, Harrison DW. Physiological and neuropsychological correlates of hostility. Neuropsychologia 1997; 35(10):1405–1411.

229. Davis PA, Holm JE, Myers TC, Suda KT. Stress, headache, and physiological disregulation: a time-series analysis of stress in the laboratory. Headache 1998; 38(2):116–121.

230. Wilhelm FH, Roth W. Acute and delayed effects of alprazolam on flight phobics during exposure. Behav Res Ther 1997;35(9):831–841.

231. Schneider RH, Nidich SI, Salerno JW, et al. Lower lipid peroxide levels in practitioners of the Transcendental Meditation program. Psychosom Med 1998;60(1): 38–41.

232. Anderzen I, Arnetz BB. Psychophysiological reactions to international adjustment. Results from a controlled, longitudinal study. Psychother Psychosom 1999;68(2): 67–75.

233. Schuck P. Glycated hemoglobin as a physiological measure of stress and its relations to some psychological stress indicators. Behav Med 1998;24(2):89–94.

234. Schmidt-Reinwald A, Pruessner JC, Hellhammer DH, et al. The cortisol response to awakening in relation to different challenge tests and a 12-hour cortisol rhythm. Life Sci 1999;64(18):1653–1660.

235. Law M. Self care. In: Van Deusen J, Brunt D, eds. Assessment in occupational therapy and physical therapy. Philadelphia: WB Saunders, 1997:421–434.

236. Mahoney F, Barthel D. Functional evaluation: The Barthel Index. Md State Med J 1965:61–65.

237. Engberg A, Bentzen L, Garde B. Rehabilitation after stroke: predictive power of Barthel Index versus a cognitive and a motor index. Acta Neurol Scand 1995; 91(1):28–36.

238. Levi SJ. Posthospital setting, resource utilization, and self-care outcome in older women with hip fracture. Arch Phys Med Rehabil 1997;78(9):973–979.

239. Kakurai S, Akai M. Clinical experiences with a convertible thermoplastic knee-ankle-foot orthosis for post-stroke hemiplegic patients. Prosthet Orthot Int 1996;20(3):191–194.

240. Hui E, Lum CM, Woo J, et al. Outcomes of elderly stroke patients. Day hospital versus conventional medical management. Stroke 1995;26(9):1616–1619.

241. Jonsson B, Overend T, Kramer J. Functional measures following liver transplantation. Physiother Can 1998; 50(2):141–146.

242. Patti F, Reggio A, Nicoletti F, et al. Effects of rehabilitation therapy on Parkinson's disability and functional independence. J Neurol Rehabil 1996;10(4):223–231.

243. Condie E, Treweek S, Jones D, Scott H. A one-year national survey of patients having a lower limb amputation. Physiotherapy 1996;82(1):14–20.

244. Jette AM. Using health-related quality of life measures in physical therapy outcomes research. Phys Ther 1993;73: 528–537.

245. Ware J, Sherbourne C. The MOS 36-item Short Form Health Survey (SF-36). Med Care 1992;30:473–483.

246. McHorney CA, Haley SM, Ware JE Jr. Evaluation of the MOS SF-36 Physical Functioning Scale (PF-10): II. Comparison of relative precision using Likert and Rasch scoring methods. J Clin Epidemiol 1997;50(4):451–461.

247. Thumboo J, Fong KY, Ng TP, et al. Validation of the MOS SF-36 for quality of life assessment of patients with systemic lupus erythematosus in Singapore. J Rheumatol 1999;26(1):97–102.

248. Daeppen JB, Krieg MA, Burnand B, Yersin B. MOS-SF-36 in evaluating health-related quality of life in alcohol-dependent patients. Am J Drug Alcohol Abuse 1998;24(4):685–694.

249. Lam CL, Gandek B, Ren XS, Chan MS. Tests of scaling assumptions and construct validity of the Chinese (HK) version of the SF-36 Health Survey. J Clin Epidemiol 1998;51(11):1139–1147.

250. Duncan PW, Samsa GP, Weinberger M, et al. Health status of individuals with mild stroke. Stroke 1997;28(4):740–745.

251. Russo J, Trujillo CA, Wingerson D, et al. The MOS 36-Item Short Form Health Survey: reliability, validity, and preliminary findings in schizophrenic outpatients. Med Care 1998;36(5):752–756.

252. Schlenk EA, Erlen JA, Dunbar-Jacob J, et al. Health-related quality of life in chronic disorders: a comparison across studies using the MOS SF-36. Qual Life Res 1998;7(1):57–65.

253. Wu AW, Hays RD, Kelly S, et al. Applications of the Medical Outcomes Study health-related quality of life measures in HIV/AIDS. Qual Life Res 1997;6(6):531–554.

254. de Jong Z, van der Heijde D, McKenna SP, Whalley D. The reliability and construct validity of the RAQoL: a rheumatoid arthritis-specific quality of life instrument. Br J Rheumatol 1997;36(8):878–883.

255. Parkerson G, Gehlbach S, Wagner E. The Duke UNIC Health Profile: an adult health status instrument for primary care. Med Care 1981;19:806–828.

256. Bergner MB, Bobbit R, Carter W, Gilson B. The SIP development and final revision of a health status measure. Med Care 1981;19:787–805.

257. Chambers LW, MacDonald LA, Tugwell P. The McMaster Health Index questionnaire as a measure of quality of life for patients with rheumatoid disease. J Rheumatol 1982;9:780–784.

258. Jette AM, Davies AR, Cleary PD. The Functional Status Questionnaire: reliability and validity when used in primary care. J Gen Intern Med 1986;1(3):143–149.

Suggested Readings

Field D. Anatomy, palpation, and surface markings. 2nd ed. Oxford, England: Butterworth-Heinemann, 1997.

Hoppenfeld S. Physical examination of the spine and extremities. New York: Appleton-Century-Crofts, 1976.

II

Treatment and Discharge

"Another common mistake is to suppose that anyone can 'do Massage', and that the whole art can be acquired in one or two easy lessons. Applicants for employment are anything but pleased when they are told that it takes nearly two years to learn, and that many people from lack of aptitude or defective general education never succeed in acquiring it ... Anyone can rub mechanically, but that is of no earthly use; a masseuse must work with her brain as well as her hands."

WILLIAM MURRELL, MD. MASSOTHERAPEUTICS OR MASSAGE AS A MODE OF TREATMENT. 4ᵀᴴ ED. LONDON: HK LEWIS, 1889:2, 65.

The chapters in this section cover the later phases of the clinical decision-making process: the Treatment Phase and the Discharge Phase. Chapter 4 describes the methods by which the clinician completes the psychological, physical, and material preparation for treatment, as well as the techniques for positioning and draping the client for treatment. Chapters 5 through 10 introduce categories of related massage techniques and detail the cognitive and psychomotor skills required to apply these techniques within a therapeutic treatment. These chapters also include discussions of the descriptive components (see Box P2-1) outcomes of care, indications, contraindications, cautions, and posttreatment care associated with each technique. Finally, Chapter 11 describes the principles and process that clinicians can use to design massage sequences and to progress treatment regimens that incorporate massage techniques from the initial intervention to discharge.

Section Objectives

After studying this section, the reader will be able to:

1. Discuss the components of the clinician's physical and psychological preparation for treatment.
2. Outline the materials used for massage interventions and the steps used in preparing these materials for treatment.
3. Outline and demonstrate how to position a client for the application of massage techniques to different regions of the body.
4. Describe and demonstrate how to perform appropriate draping techniques for different regions of the body.

5. Identify six basic categories of massage techniques and describe how each category of techniques affects different types of tissues.
6. Describe the impairment-level outcomes of care and clinical indications associated with each massage technique presented.
7. Define the seven components of massage techniques for each massage technique.
8. Recognize contraindications and cautions to the use of each massage technique.
9. Describe and demonstrate how to perform each massage technique and how to apply each technique in a practice sequence.
10. Identify appropriate posttreatment care and other appropriate techniques for each technique.
11. Outline methods of organizing massage techniques into regional and general sequences that address specific impairment-level outcomes of care.
12. Discuss the approach to the progression of treatment regimens for outcome-based massage.

General Guidelines for Practicing Massage

Novice clinicians are advised to consider the following guidelines when practicing the massage techniques outlined in this section.

1. Locate the tissues selected for treatment through palpation and be specific in your contact of these tissues.
2. Palpate continuously for the response of the client's tissues to the technique.
3. Frequently observe and elicit feedback on the client's response to the application of techniques.
4. First attempt to achieve penetration to deeper tissue layers through repetition of the technique rather than by increasing the pressure of application.
5. Decrease the rate of application when treating deeper tissue layers to provide a sufficient amount of time for the displacement of fluid and the intervening tissues.
6. Obtain feedback on the client's level of comfort after changes of position to eliminate positioning as a source of discomfort during the application of techniques.
7. Minimize client discomfort during treatment by modifying the application of techniques to ensure the client's comfort.
8. Adapt the application of each technique to the region of the body to which it is being applied.
9. Practice each technique individually to achieve competence in the execution of that technique before attempting to combine techniques into massage sequences. Unthinking repetition of anysort of routine may result in an inflexibility of treatment approach that may later impede the appropriate use of techniques in clinical situations.

Contact Surface: The portion of the clinician's hand or arm that is used to execute the stroke.

Pressure: The amount of force per unit area of contact surface that the clinician applies. We define categories of pressure as: "minimal" engages skin, "light" engages subcutaneous fascia and fat, "moderate" engages superficial muscle layers, and "heavy" engages deeper muscle layers.

Tissues Engaged: The target tissues or layers of tissue to which the clinician directs the pressure of the stroke and which are mechanically deformed by the application of the technique.

Direction: The direction of the applied force. The direction given in the description of techniques is the direction in which the greatest force is applied during the pressure phase of the stroke. Directions that are commonly specified include: centripetal (toward the heart), centrifugal (away from the heart), and transverse or parallel to the fibers of a reference structure.

Amplitude: An indication of the size of the area that is covered by a technique.

Rate: An indication of how fast the force is applied. This is a critical component since many desired effects occur only at certain rates of application. The rate may describe the speed of the movement of the clinician's hand over the client's skin (distance per second), the frequency of repetitions of a described technique (repetitions per second), or both rates.

Duration: An estimate of a reasonable length of time for which a single technique may have to be applied by a competent clinician in order to begin to achieve the specified impairment-level outcomes of care. This text provides a minimum duration that can be exceeded at the discretion of the clinician, for example "10 minutes or greater." If a longer duration of application of a technique can result in side effects or risks, this text provides a suggested upper limit, for example "1 to 10 minutes" and discusses how to determine an appropriate duration of treatment in the accompanying text.

Variations: Two common variations are presented in this text: "intergrades with" and "combines with." When one technique is said to "intergrade" with another, the two techniques can be performed consecutively and will merge gradually one into the other since there are intermediate hybrid forms of the technique that lie between and resemble both techniques. When one technique is said to "combine" with another, it means that the two techniques may be executed simultaneously.

Context: A brief description of how the technique is conventionally sequenced in relation to other techniques.

4

Preparation and Positioning for Treatment

*T*here is much preparation that must occur before the clinician applies a massage technique to the client's body. Most importantly, the clinician must prepare himself, both physically and mentally, before he initiates his interaction with the client. The clinician must also select and prepare a variety of treatment materials, such as tables, lubricants, and linen. During the intervention, there are other issues to which the clinician must attend. The clinician needs to ensure that the client is appropriately positioned and draped both prior to and during the application of techniques. In addition, the clinician also needs to ensure that he is appropriately positioned and uses correct body mechanics during the intervention. The importance of these activities cannot be overemphasized; appropriate implementation of these activities can enhance the quality of the clinician's execution of the manual technique for the massage techniques that are outlined in the chapters that follow.

Clinician's Physical Preparation for Treatment (Self-Care)

The practice of massage places considerable strain on the clinician's body. In particular, the soft tissues of the back and the upper kinetic chain are particularly prone to muscular fatigue, hypertonicity, trigger point syndromes, and repetitive strain injury. To maintain a trouble-free level of functioning and to prevent ongoing damage, any clinician who performs significant amounts of massage must develop a comprehensive exercise program that includes aerobic, flexibility, resistance, and balance training. Failure to pursue an exercise program can place the clinician at greater risk of injury and increases the likelihood that he will experience burnout. Comprehensive programs are beyond the scope of this book and are detailed elsewhere;[1–3] what follows is a selection of exercises that are of particular relevance for the clinicians who practice massage.

MOVEMENT

Different types of active exercises can be used for different purposes. Brisk active exercise increases heart rate, local blood flow, tissue temperature, and tissue extensibility. This can be used, prior to stretching exercises, to warm up at the beginning of the workday, and after breaks. Figures 4-1 to 4-4B show several shaking and "swinging" exercises for the whole body, which can be used to loosen the muscles of the shoulder girdle, back, and hips in preparation for performing massage.

Very slow, active movements are excellent for tension release and relaxation (Figs. 4-5 and 4-6). When performing these exercises, the clinician sits or reclines comfortably to promote relaxation throughout his body. A single isolated motion is then chosen (e.g., abduction of the shoulder) and is performed very slowly and at a consistent rate. The rate of movement should be sufficiently slow that it takes 60 to 90 seconds to complete movement through the available range. At the end of the movement, the clinician relaxes completely and rests for several seconds. He may then either repeat that movement or perform a movement for another joint. This procedure is most effective when it is used on several joints.

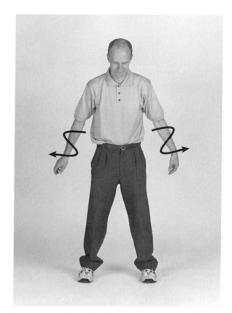

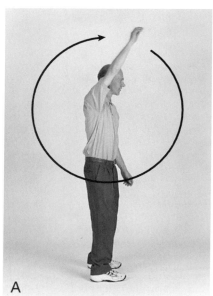

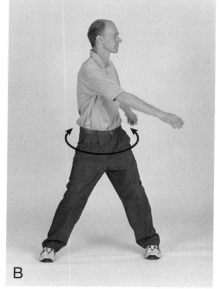

A

B

Figure 4-1. Shaking the hands, wrists, and forearms is a good way to relieve local neuromuscular tension immediately before or after massage. This can be done slowly and in a relaxed fashion or more briskly.

Figure 4-2. A. Each arm is circumducted vigorously 10 to 20 times. This movement opens the shoulder girdle and pushes blood in a centrifugal direction to the hand. **B.** The movement is done in both directions. The clinician coordinates bending of the knees as the arm descends, and straightening the knees as the arm ascends.

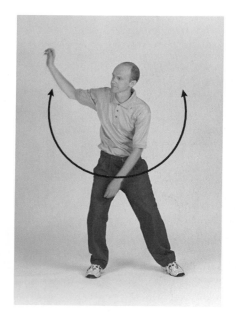

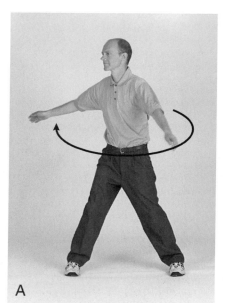

A

B

Figure 4-3. Swing the arms from side to side in the frontal plane; lift both arms up to one side, then relax and allow them to drop passively back down and in front of the body. Then swing them up to the other side, then relax down again to the center. Produce a continuous movement back and forth like a pendulum.

Figure 4-4. A. Swing the arms in the horizontal plane around the body in one direction and then back again. Allow the movement of the arms to be as loose as possible, so that the hands swing round to tap the opposite shoulder and hip at the end of each movement. **B.** You can power the movement of the arms by generating a forceful rotation of the trunk and pelvis in one direction and then back again (like a washing machine); the arms follow this movement.

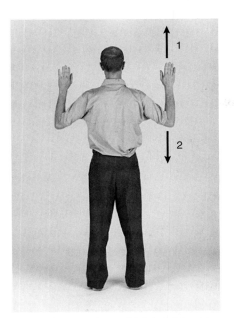

Figure 4-5. Lie supine on the floor in this position. Keep hands, arms, and shoulders as relaxed as possible and maintain maximum contact with the floor without forcing. Slide the arm(s) very slowly up as if reaching "over the head" and then back down. Pause occasionally to relax totally and take a full breath. Allow at least 2 min to go through the entire cycle up and down. Repeat the entire movement or concentrate on less fluid portions of the joint range of motion.

STRETCHING

Stretching techniques are an excellent method of maintaining and improving the flexibility of soft tissue, relieving neuromuscular tension, improving capacity for activity, and relieving pain and soreness related to activity.[4–7] While there are many different stretching techniques, the basic guidelines for effective static stretching are outlined below.[5,6]

1. Warm up first with slow active movement.
2. Move to the end of range to the point at which a comfortable stretch is experienced.
3. Breathe deeply throughout the stretch.
4. Hold the stretch position for 15 to 30 seconds.
5. Gently move farther into the range without bouncing.
6. Hold the stretch position for an additional 30 seconds.
7. Stretch both sides equally.
8. Never stretch to the point of experiencing pain.

The following stretches target areas that are frequently of concern to clinicians who perform massage. They can be assembled into short routines that the clinician can use at the beginning or end of the workday or even in the brief intervals that arise between clients (Figs. 4-7 to 4-25).

SELF-MASSAGE

Once the clinician acquires some expertise with performing the different massage techniques described later in this text, he can perform them on himself. Self-massage is particularly useful for relieving the tension that accumulates in the forearms and hands during treatment. These techniques can also be incorporated into the clinician's warm-up and warm-down routines (Figs. 4-26 to 4-33).

RECEIPT OF SKILLED MASSAGE

In recent years, as various forms of massage are receiving growing attention in scientific and public forums, there has been a trend toward allowing students to perform massage with little or no personal experience with massage or related forms of structured touch. This lack of on-the-table experience can make it difficult for students to acquire more than the most basic proficiency in massage. Students cannot rely on each other to

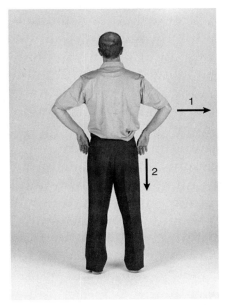

Figure 4-6. Lie supine on the floor in this position. Keep hands, arms, and shoulders as relaxed as possible, and maintain maximum contact with the floor without forcing. Slide the hands very slowly beside the body up toward the armpits (the elbows move out to the side) and then back down. Pause occasionally to relax totally and take a full breath. Allow at least 2 min to go through the entire cycle up and down. Repeat the entire movement, or concentrate on less fluid portions of the joint range of motion.

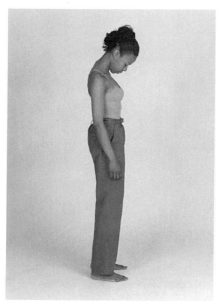

Figure 4-7. Active flexion of the neck—"chin to chest."

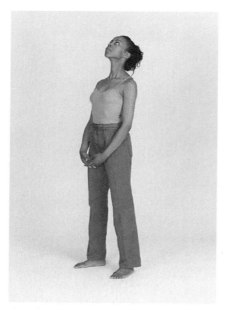

Figure 4-8. Active extension of the neck. Attempt to elongate the entire neck as cervical extension occurs, rather than just moving the occiput toward the first thoracic vertebra.

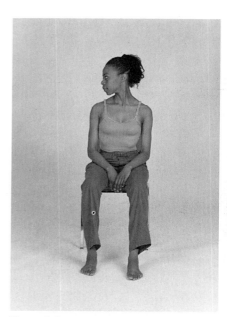

Figure 4-9. Active cervical rotation.

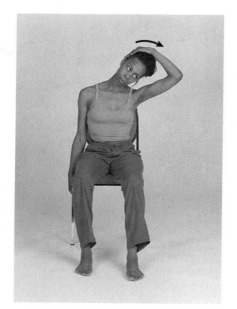

Figure 4-10. Cervical side-bending with gentle overpressure. The shoulder girdle can be stabilized by holding under the edge of the chair.

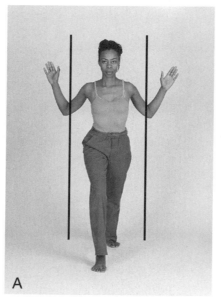

A

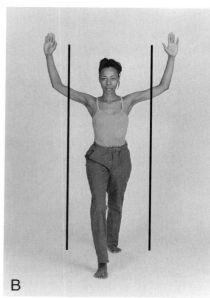

B

Figure 4-11. A. The "in doorway" stretch for pectoral muscles (the sides of the door frame are represented by the bars). The clinician pushes gently through the door frame toward the viewer, without arching the lower back. This position stretches the clavicular fibers of the pectoralis major. **B.** The "in doorway" stretch with the arms in the upper position stretches the sternal fibers of the pectoralis major.

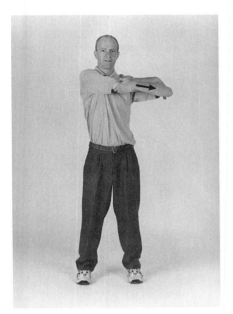

Figure 4-12. To stretch the posterior deltoid, the arm is drawn across the front of the body toward the opposite shoulder.

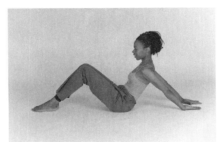

Figure 4-13. Biceps brachii can be stretched in several positions as long as the shoulder and elbow are extended and the forearm is pronated. In this position, extending the thoracic spine will intensify the stretch.

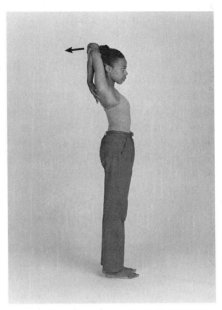

Figure 4-14. To stretch all of the triceps brachii both the shoulder and elbow need to be extended.

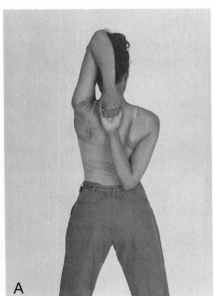

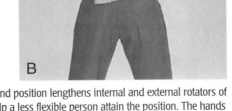

Figure 4-15. A. This behind-the-back clasped-hand position lengthens internal and external rotators of the shoulder on opposite sides. **B.** A towel can help a less flexible person attain the position. The hands can pull up or down to stretch the opposite shoulder.

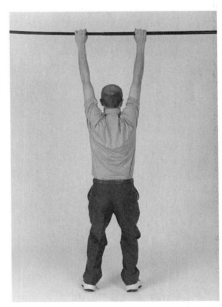

Figure 4-16. Hang from a bar of suitable height (or a door or door frame) to lengthen the entire torso. Maintain contact with ground. Perform a posterior pelvic tilt (tuck the pelvis) to stretch the latissimus dorsi.

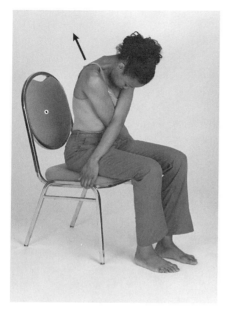

Figure 4-17. To stretch the interscapular area, assume this position, round the thoracic spine, and push through the sixth thoracic vertebra toward the ceiling.

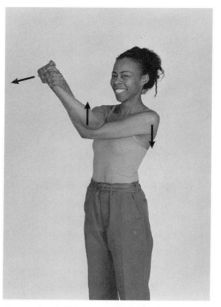

Figure 4-18. If done carefully, this yoga pose is an excellent stretch for the midtrapezius. Wrap the arms around each other, simultaneously depress the shoulder girdle, raise the elbows, and push the hands away from the face.

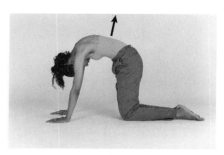

Figure 4-19. Arch upward to stretch the extensors of the spine. The weight can be shifted forward over the arms or back over the knees to focus the stretch more toward the thoracic or the lumbar extensors, respectively.

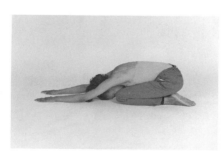

Figure 4-20. "Child's pose"—a most relaxing position for the back. The buttocks rest on the heels, or a less flexible person can place one or two pillows over the posterior calves for support.

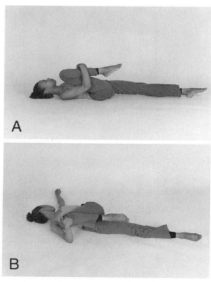

Figure 4-21. **A.** "Knee to chest" provides a unilateral stretch of the gluteus maximus in supine. **B.** "Knee to opposite chest" also stretches the gluteus maximus. To stretch the piriformis, bring the hip down from this position to exactly 90 degrees of flexion.

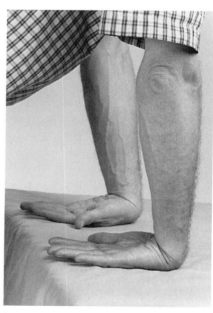

Figure 4-22. To stretch the wrist extensors, extend the elbows and use a gentle pressure of the dorsum of the hands against a vertical or horizontal surface to move the wrist into flexion. Do *not* lean on the wrists in this position.

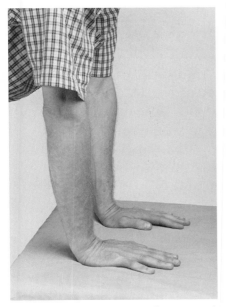

Figure 4-23. To stretch the wrist flexors, extend the elbows and use a gentle pressure of the palms against a vertical or horizontal surface to take the wrists into extension.

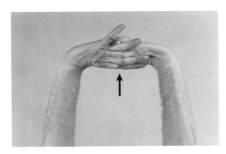

Figure 4-24. Another flexor stretch. Interlock the fingers and push the hands as far away as possible.

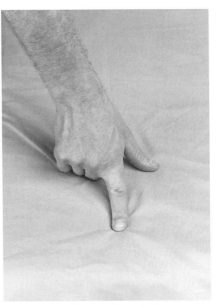

Figure 4-25. "Finger-splits" stretch the intrinsic muscles of the hand. A similar maneuver can be performed between each pair of adjacent digits.

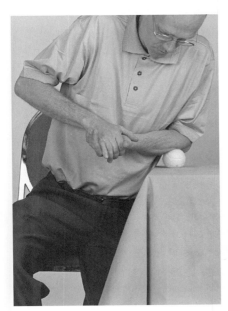

Figure 4-26. Compression administered to the extensors of the forearm with a tennis ball and body weight. See Chapter 7, Neuromuscular Techniques.

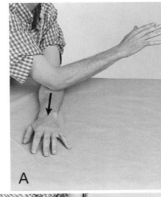

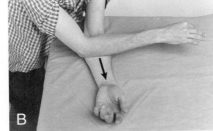

Figure 4-27. A. Self-administered direct fascial technique applied to the extensor surface of the forearm. See Chapter 8, Connective Tissue Techniques. **B.** Self-administered direct fascial technique applied to the flexor surface of the forearm. See Chapter 8, Connective Tissue Techniques.

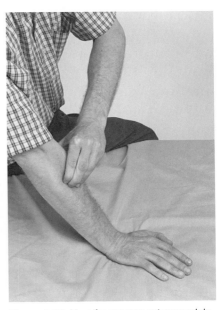

Figure 4-28. Near the common extensor origin, a frequent trouble spot for repetitive strain injuries. From this position, the clinician can apply stripping, direct fascial technique, or friction. See Chapter 7, Neuromuscular Techniques, and Chapter 8, Connective Tissue Techniques.

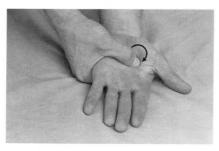

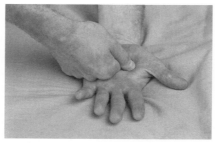

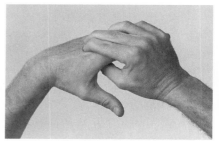

Figure 4-29. Thumb kneading applied to the muscles of the thenar eminence. This can be continued with good effects for 5 to 10 min or more per hand. See Chapter 7, Neuromuscular Techniques.

Figure 4-30. Specific digital compression applied with a reinforced thumb to the muscles of the thenar eminence. See Chapter 7, Neuromuscular Techniques.

Figure 4-31. The index finger and the thumb (hidden) work on opposite sides of the inter-metacarpal space to free the intrinsic muscles of the hand. Manipulations that can be applied in this position include specific compression, stripping, and direct fascial technique. See Chapter 7, Neuromuscular Techniques, and Chapter 8, Connective Tissue Techniques.

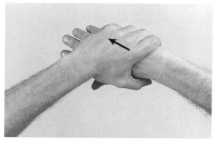

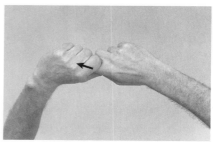

Figure 4-32. Performing massage exerts considerable compressive force on joints of the wrist and hand that can be countered with automobilization. Here, distraction of the wrist includes both proximal and distal joints.

Figure 4-33. Distraction can be performed at the metacarpophalangeal joints and all other joints of the hand.

demonstrate refined touch in classroom exchanges. In addition, the brief exposure to the touch of very qualified teachers in the classroom does not demonstrate overall flow, pacing, and rhythm to the students. Furthermore, while watching experienced clinicians work is extremely useful, it fails to convey the subtleties of touch. In addition, the authors have observed that students who have received touch from competent professionals prior to studying massage techniques may demonstrate much more rapid improvement in their manual skills. On this basis, the authors propose that few preparations will facilitate students' achievement of mastery of the craft of massage as much as the repeated receipt of massage or other manual techniques from competent, experienced professionals. This repeated exposure to "Intelligent Touch" can impart certain kinesthetic essentials that cannot be conveyed in words, ideas, or images.

Clinician's Psychological Preparation for Treatment

The clinician must ensure that adequate time is allocated to perform the types of treatment that are scheduled, to review clients' files, to check reference material, and to think about each client. Ideally, the clinician who performs massage should be able to manage his own treatment schedule. This will enable him to consider and reconcile clients' needs, the facility's policies, charting requirements, reimbursement issues, and his own capacity for performing treatments when scheduling clients. If another individual is responsible for booking, the clinician will need to clearly communicate his guidelines for booking to that person so that an unreasonable and rushed schedule is not imposed on him.

Once the clinician ensures that he has adequate time for treatment and other supporting activities, he can use some of the physical modalities previously described, such as gentle stretching, to facilitate his psychological preparation. In the same manner, conscious diaphragmatic breathing, correct body mechanics, and the use of controlled repetitive movement during the performance of massage techniques can actually deepen the clinician's level of relaxation.

Professions that use massage are usually service-oriented professions. For this reason, it is invaluable for the clinician to practice some routine of calming the mind throughout the workday, especially in the few minutes preceding sessions. Clinicians may draw upon a number of different resources for informing and deepening their ethical commitment to others and cultivating an attitude of peaceful, fulfilling service to others. These include a variety of forms of nonsectarian and sectarian spiritual practice, such as the use of autogenic or visualization exercises for relaxation or drawing upon an established faith. Spiritual practices of any sort are indispensable to the clinician who is in a "helping" profession. Since isolation contributes to the experience of "burnout" that is so common in service-oriented professions, the clinician is also wise to include in his clinical practice opportunities for interactions with colleagues, such as continuing education courses, review of clients, and professional meetings. Finally, service to others should not be at the expense of taking care of oneself.

Clinician's Preparations of Materials for Treatment

TABLES

The massage or treatment table is an essential tool in the practice of massage. Since massage tables come in a variety of makes and styles, the clinician should consider his anticipated needs carefully prior to purchasing a table. Any table that is used for massage must be solid, stable, easy to clean, at least 28 × 72 inches, and adjustable for height, to accommodate different clients and types of work. Ideally, the table will be padded with high-density foam on both the top and sides of the tabletop, since the clinician may frequently lean or brace himself against the sides of the table. A well-designed, adjustable face cradle or head support is a desirable addition to the basic massage table. This is an appropriate alternative to the use of face holes, since the latter rarely fit all clients equally well.

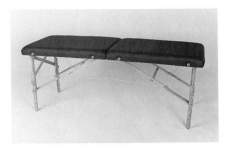

Figure 4-35. A portable table.

Stationary tables are preferable for the clinic or office setting, since they are extremely strong and stable, though heavy and not easily moved (Fig. 4-34). A hydraulic or electric height-adjustable table provides quick adjustment to the different heights that are required for the most efficient application of different techniques.

Clinicians who travel frequently have many styles of well-built portable tables from which to choose (Fig. 4-35). These tables weigh between 10 and 20 kg, are strong and attractive, are equipped with face cradles and arm shelves, and lack only the ability to be adjusted for height. As a result, some clinicians use portable tables for their primary place of practice.

If a clinician selects a table that lacks a mechanism for adjusting height quickly, he should choose a lower table height. The use of a lower table height requires the clinician to have training and practice in the correct use of his legs. Novice clinicians frequently set their tables

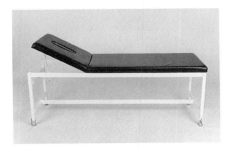

Figure 4-34. A metal-frame stationary table with face hole and adjustable legs, which can be partially tilted.

too high, which predisposes them to make many errors in body mechanics. When the clinician is performing work that requires use of a substantial amount of body weight, such as neuromuscular and connective tissue techniques, he may set the height of the table to the level of his extended fingertips or even lower (Fig. 4-36). For lighter work, such as superficial reflex and passive movement techniques, the clinician may set the table height to the level of his wrist or even higher.

Portable massage chairs are specifically designed for "on-site" or "mobile" practices of massage (Fig. 4-37A). These chairs offer comfort and ease of access to common problem areas for the office worker; however, they are not very versatile, and some clients may find the half-kneeling position difficult to assume (Fig. 4-37B).

Before and between clients, table, bed, or chair surfaces that come in contact with clients or draping should be cleaned with commercially available disinfectants or washed with soap and hot water and rinsed with a 10% bleach solution.[8]

SUPPORTS

The clinician can use either a commercially designed set of bolsters or a set of pillows to support clients who must be positioned on a bed or the floor. In addition, the clinician needs a large selection of pillows and bolsters of various sizes and shapes, including at least six standard-sized pillows (Fig. 4-38). If necessary, the clinician can place foam- or kapok-filled mats on the floor. The physical demands of working on the floor are extreme, however, and the repertoire of techniques that can be adapted for floor work is limited. Before and between clients, mat surfaces that come in contact with clients or draping should be cleaned with commercially available disinfectants or washed with soap and hot water and rinsed with a 10% bleach solution.[8]

LINEN

Sturdy, bleachable, opaque, cotton sheeting in white or pastels is recommended for clinical use. Although single (twin) flat sheets ensure ample coverage, a slightly narrower width of 50 to 54 inches is easier to handle and can reduce bunching of excess draping. Pillow cases, small and large towels, and blankets are among the basic linen supplies. Any linen that comes into contact with clients must be laundered after each use with detergent, bleach, and commercial degreaser. Whenever possible, professional laundering is recommended.

LUBRICANTS

Lubricants are used to control the amount of glide, friction, and drag that occurs between the clinician's moving hand and the client's skin. Although lubricants are applied to the skin, they affect the clinician's ability to palpate and effect changes in the client's subcutaneous tissues. Consequently, lubricant is absolutely required for some techniques, to be avoided for others, and of potential benefit for others only when carefully chosen and applied. Because of the different requirements for lubricants, the well-prepared clinician will have on hand a selection of lubricants to facilitate application of a range of techniques. Any lubricant that the clinician uses must be hypoallergenic and dispensed in a hygienic manner that does not contaminate the supply, such as a squeeze-bottle, pump, or shaker. Clients must give consent before the clinician adds scent to the lubricant as, for example, in aromatherapy.

OILS

Oils continue to be the lubricant of choice for classical neuromuscular techniques. Virtually any high-quality vegetable oil can be used, including olive, sunflower, safflower, almond, jojoba, and coconut oils. Mineral oil, on the other hand, is considered to be less nutritious for the skin.[9] Each oil has a slightly different density, stickiness, and rate of absorption. Oil has two drawbacks: it goes rancid and it stains. In addition, unabsorbed oil must be removed from the client's skin with disposable towels, which may be moistened with alcohol.

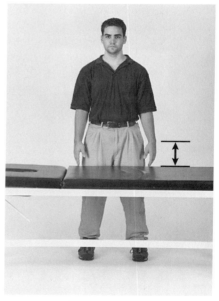

Figure 4-36. Correct table height varies with the technique that is being performed and the size of the client. Usually, the working height of the table lies between the height of the clinician's wrist and the tips of the extended fingers. Occasionally, the optimal height may be as low as the clinician's knees or as high as the waist.

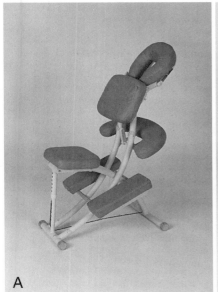
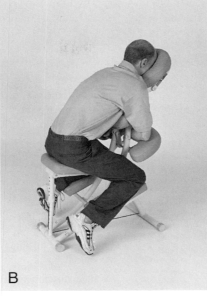

Figure 4-37. A. Portable massage chair with a strong, light, upholstered frame that folds into an easily carried unit. **B.** It offers good access to the back and neck.

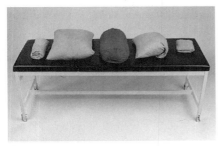

Figure 4-38. The clinician will require supports in a variety of shapes and sizes.

LOTIONS

Lotions are opaque, liquid suspensions of particles in either oil or water. Since they are readily absorbed into the skin, their lubricating qualities decline quickly with time. This rapid absorption can be an advantage when the clinician is preparing the client's tissues for deeper neuromuscular or connective tissue techniques.

CREAMS

Creams are thicker suspensions, often oil based, that fall midway between oils and lotions in terms of their rate of absorption. Creams can be quite oily and promote glide or they may contain sticky ingredients, such as lanolin and beeswax, that reduce glide and facilitate the clinician's ability to drag the client's skin. The ability of creams to reduce glide may be useful for connective tissue techniques.

POWDERS

Fine powder in the form of French chalk, cornstarch, or unscented baby powder can be used for techniques that require glide and when clients refuse oil. Furthermore, powder is the preferred lubricant for most lymph-drainage techniques.

Positioning and Draping the Client During Treatment

POSITIONING

In selecting the position for massage, the clinician will consider the aims of treatment, the areas to be accessed, the client's preferences, and the comfort of the client. Prone, supine, sidelying, seated, seated inclined, and long-sitting are common options, each of which has its own specific requirements for pillow placement and support. Box 4-1 summarizes which muscles, tissues, and regions are readily accessible in the common positions used for treatment.

Once the client is positioned correctly for massage on the treatment table, the clinician will adjust, add, or remove the pillows, bolsters, or rolled towels used for support as needed, to ensure that the client is comfortable. Figures 4-39A to 4-45 illustrate some common positions and how they can be supported with pillows. In practice, pillows are placed beneath the bottom sheet so that they can be reused without having to be recovered. Many other configurations are possible

---

Box 4-1
Treatment Positions for Various Muscles

Prone position is an excellent treatment position for
    Posterior cervical muscles
    Latissimus dorsi
    Rhomboids
    Mid- and lower trapezius
    Spinal extensors
    Gluteus maximus
    Hamstrings
    Triceps surae
    Foot intrinsics
Supine position is an excellent treatment position for
    All muscles of the head and neck
    Pectorals
    All muscles of the arm
    Abdominals
    Quadriceps
    Muscles of the anterior compartment
Sidelying position is an excellent treatment position for
(On uppermost side of the client's body)
    Scalenes
    Rotator cuff
    Pectoralis minor
    Serratus anterior
    Abdominals
    Quadratus lumborum
    Iliocostalis
    Gluteus medius and minimus
    Iliotibial tract
    Peronei
(On lower side of the client's body)
    Adductors of the hip
    Triceps surae
Seated upright position is an excellent treatment position for
    Upper trapezius
Seated inclined position is an excellent treatment position for
    All muscles of the posterior aspect of the head and neck
    All muscles of the upper back
    All muscles of the posterior aspect of the upper arms

---

and will be required if the clinician works in a hospital or rehabilitation setting.

DRAPING

Draping does more than place the client in a safe, warm, modest, and comfortable position in which to receive the intended massage. Appropriate draping can also serve to achieve and maintain appropriate client–clinician boundaries that are needed in all practice settings, including the classroom. Since draping sets a symbolic and an actual boundary between the clinician and the client during treatment, the clinician must make draping comfortable, yet precise and secured when exposing the client's body for treatment purposes.

The clinician's scope of practice, professional code of conduct, and local laws will dictate what is permissible in terms of exposing the client's body during treatment. When undraping the client, the clinician will adhere to the following rules.

1. Only one part is undraped at a time.
2. Only areas that are to be treated are undraped.
3. The gluteal cleft, perineum, genitals, and female breast are not undraped.

The following three exceptions[10,11] are generally considered to be legitimate exceptions to the rules noted above. In each case, the clinician must know whether local laws supersede the exception.

1. The female breasts may be exposed singly if breast massage is clinically indicated and, prior to treatment, the client has provided voluntary informed consent to this exposure.
2. The pelvis may be undraped if the client has provided voluntary informed consent to massage for the purposes of labor support and/or delivery. Clinicians for whom the treatment of pelvic floor dysfunction is within the professional scope of practice should consult their professional organization for guidelines on draping.
3. Infants under the age of 2 years may be treated undraped.

In a clinical setting, the clinician can use the following steps to introduce and carry out draping. Once the clinician has negotiated the plan of care with the client, he needs to identify the articles of clothing and jewelry to be removed and to explain the rationale for doing so. If the client chooses to remain clothed or partially clothed, the clinician must explain the technical consequences of this choice to the client. He then gives the client clear instructions on how to position herself on the table and how to arrange the draping and supports that have been provided. Once he is sure that he has answered the

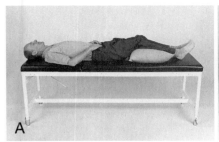
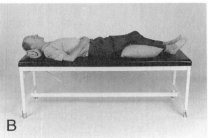

Figure 4-39. A. One or two pillows under the knees are commonly used when an individual is in supine, to reduce the strain on the lower back. **B.** An additional pillow or towel-roll may be needed under the cervical spine for the comfort of clients who have an anterior-head posture.

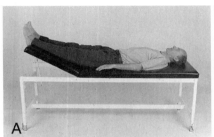
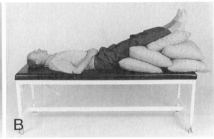

Figure 4-40. Legs can be elevated for drainage with (**A**) a treatment table that can be tilted or (**B**) a mound of pillows.

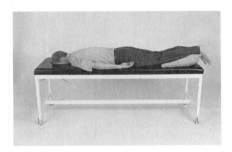

Figure 4-41. In prone, a single pillow under the ankles takes pressure off the knees.

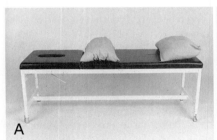
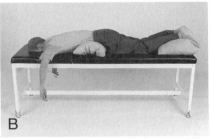

Figure 4-42. A, B. In prone, an additional small pillow can be placed under the abdomen to raise the lumbar spine into a less lordotic position. This may reduce the back pain of some clients with low back pain, such as those with acute facet derangement.

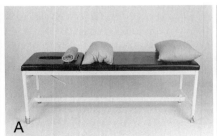
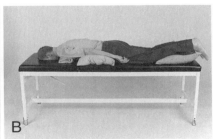

Figure 4-43. A, B. Another towel roll may be added under the upper chest to improve comfort for large-breasted women or to take the pressure off the thyroid cartilage.

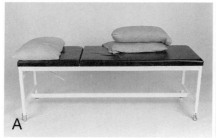
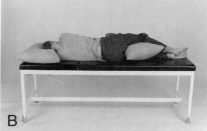
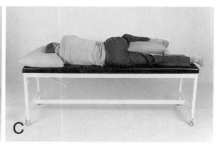

Figure 4-44. A. In sidelying, pillows are generally used for the head and legs. **B.** Usually one or two pillows are placed between the knees to enhance comfort. **C.** To access the medial tissues of the thigh and leg nearest the table, the hip and knee of the upper leg are flexed to 90 degrees, and pillows are used to support the upper leg so that the pelvis does not rotate.

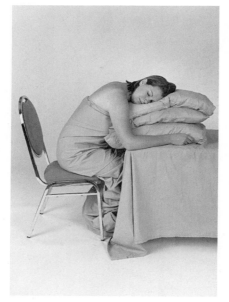
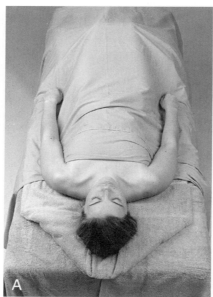
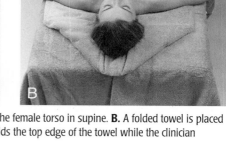

Figure 4-45. Several pillows support a relaxed seated position that offers good access to the upper back, shoulders, and posterior neck.

Figure 4-46. A. Starting position for undraping the female torso in supine. **B.** A folded towel is placed on top of the sheet over the breasts. The client holds the top edge of the towel while the clinician withdraws the sheet from under the towel.

client's questions, he leaves the room so that the client can undress in privacy.[10] If the client requires assistance undressing or getting onto the table, the clinician must clearly explain which items of the client's clothing—if any—he will be removing, where he will be touching or moving her, and obtain and record consent for this assistance before assisting the client.

Students must practice the process of appropriate draping repeatedly and extend appropriate respect to each other during classroom practice. In addition, it is useful for initial classroom practice to be done with the students clothed until students develop a reasonable level of skill in draping.

The following draping sequences (Figs. 4-46A to 4-59) all use two single (twin) flat sheets and a few towels. They can also be performed with sheets as

narrow as 4 feet. When these draping sequences are performed as described, they will be comfortable and secure and will ensure privacy for unclothed clients. The sequences for the legs can easily be modified should the client choose to wear her underwear. Certain clinical settings and client preference may require the use of a gown or modifications to the draping techniques presented in this text.

Following a clinical session, if there is sufficient time, the clinician can invite the client to rest before rising. He then instructs the client on how to get off the table safely, using statements such as "roll onto your side, let your legs drop off the table, and slowly come to a sitting position, using your arms to push up." If requested, he may also be required to give the client discreet assistance to sit up, to stand, or to dress after the session.

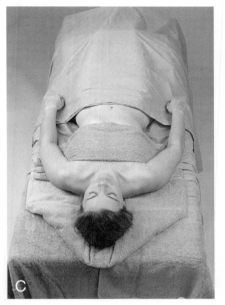

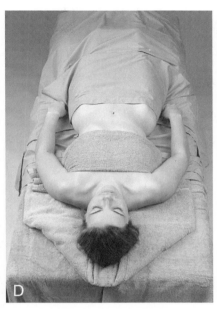

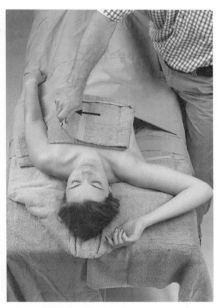

Figure 4-46 (continued). C. The towel is tucked under the torso or arms; then the abdomen is exposed. **D.** In the final position, the drape is securely tucked, and the abdomen is exposed from the xiphoid process to the anterior superior iliac spine.

Figure 4-47. For women, the chest towel can be folded back to undrape one breast at a time, if informed consent has been obtained and massage of breast tissue or the pectoral muscles is clinically indicated.

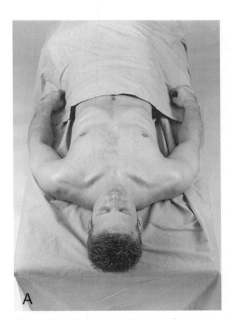

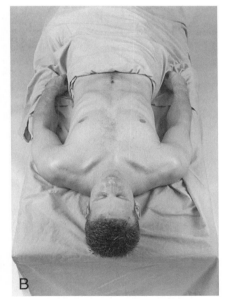

Figure 4-48. A. For men, the issue of consent to treat the anterior torso is less delicate. If extensive work is to be performed on the male client's torso, he can be undraped to the waist. If only abdominal massage is planned, he should still be offered a chest towel for warmth. **B.** The final drape tucked at the level of the anterior superior iliac spine.

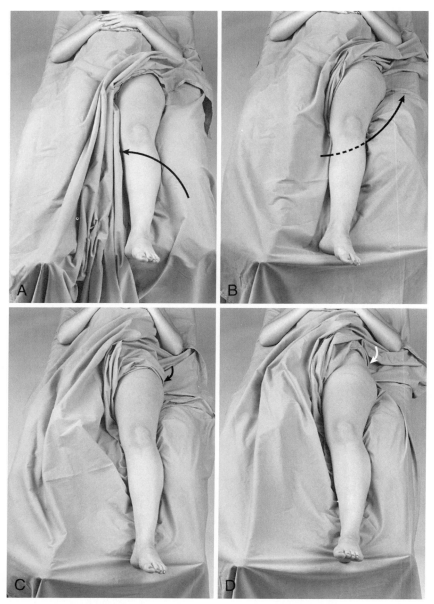

Figure 4-49. A. Undraping the anterior leg. The leg is exposed, and the extra sheet gathered between the legs. **B.** The extra sheet is then pulled underneath the exposed leg back toward the side of the table. Here, the sheet is securely anchored by the weight of the leg. **C.** The top edge of the drape can be tucked under the gluteal at the level of the greater trochanter. **D.** Or the edge can be rolled higher to expose the anterior superior iliac spine and tucked under the lower back.

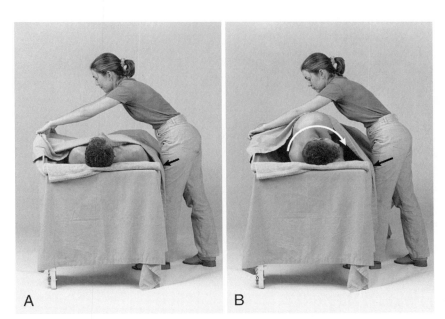

Figure 4-50. A. Turning to prone. The basic procedure is similar for turning from supine to prone, from prone to supine, or from either position to or from sidelying. The front of the thigh is used to pin the sheets against the near edge of the table, while the hands secure both sheets across the table. The client is instructed to turn. **B.** Throughout the turn, the clinician maintains control of both sheets at both sides of the table. Failure to do this will result in exposure of the client or a migrating bottom sheet that bunches uncomfortably under the client. The clinician must take care to minimize inadvertent touching of the client during the turn.

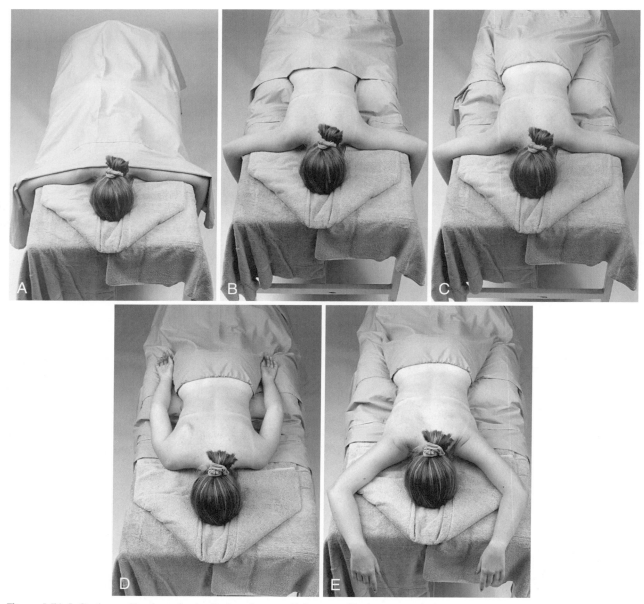

Figure 4-51. A. Starting position for undraping the torso in prone. **B.** For general back massage, the back is exposed to the level of the posterior superior iliac spine. **C.** The drape is securely tucked. **D.** The client may choose to position her arms at her sides. **E.** Or the client may position her arms overhead.

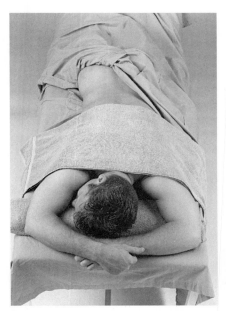

Figure 4-52. This angled draping unilaterally exposes the superior gluteal insertions. These must be worked on extensively when treating many lumbar conditions.

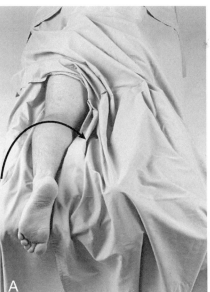

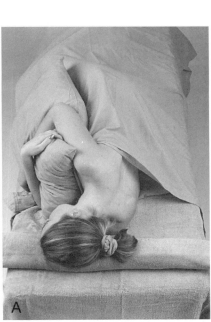

Figure 4-53. A. The procedure for undraping the posterior leg is similar to that for the anterior leg. The limb is exposed and the extra sheet is gathered between the legs. **B.** The extra sheet is then pulled underneath the exposed thigh back toward the side of the table. Here, the sheet is securely anchored by the weight of the leg.

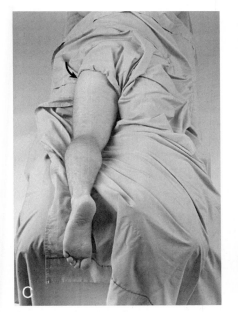

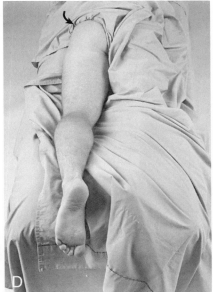

Figure 4-53 (continued). C. For a low drape, the upper edge of the sheet can be tucked under the anterior thigh at the level of the greater trochanter. **D.** A more common and much more useful technique is to roll the edge of the sheet toward the gluteal cleft and securely tuck it above the anterior superior iliac spine, thus exposing the bulk of the gluteals.

Figure 4-54. A. To expose the back and the flank of a sidelying female, the client is first instructed to clasp a standard-sized pillow in front.

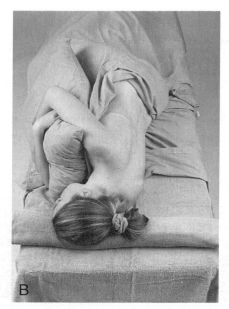

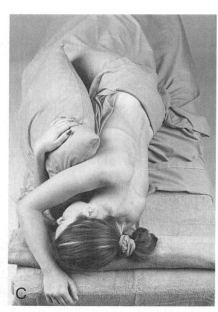

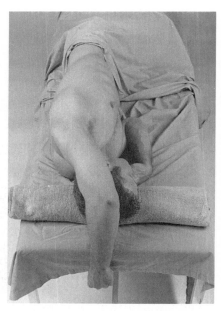

Figure 4-54 (continued). B. The back is undraped to the level desired. **C.** The drape is then securely tucked. The upper arm can be raised overhead, while the lower arm maintains the pillow in position.

Figure 4-55. The sidelying position potentially offers unparalleled access to the uppermost rotator cuff, serratus anterior, quadratus lumborum, and portions of the pectorals and spinal extensors.

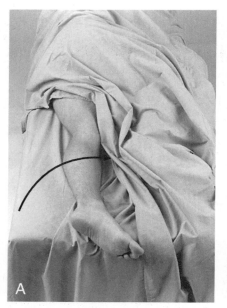

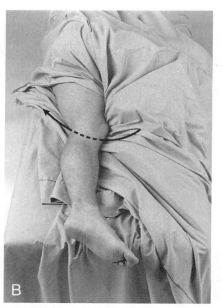

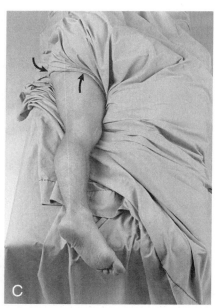

Figure 4-56. A. To undrape the bottom leg in sidelying (for work on the adductors, triceps surae, and tibialis posterior), first flex the knee and hip of the top leg to 90 degrees and use pillows to keep it forward and out of the way (see Fig. 4-44C). Then expose the bottom leg from behind and gather the extra sheet between the legs. **B.** The extra sheet is then pulled underneath the exposed leg back toward the posterior side of the table at the level of midthigh or slightly higher. Here, the sheet is securely anchored by the weight of the leg. At this point, a male client is instructed to move his genitals in a superior direction. **C.** The top edge of the drape is then rolled and pushed as close to the ischiopubic ramus as possible, and the posterior edge is tucked under the greater trochanter. Work performed on the adductor attachments onto the ramus may be best done through the sheet, for reasons of discretion.

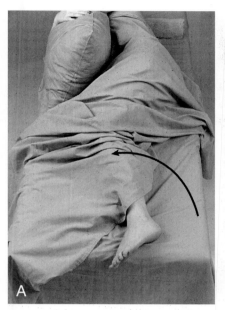
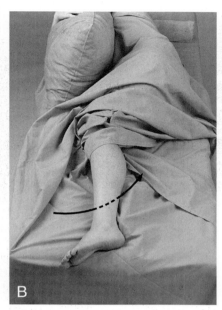
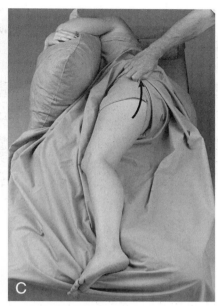

Figure 4-57. **A.** To expose the top leg in sidelying, fold the posterior portion of the sheet forward. Move as much of the extra sheet as possible out of the way in a superior direction. **B.** Pull the edge of the drape back under the leg. The leg to be exposed is now surrounded by the drape, as in a pant leg. The other leg is not exposed at any time during the procedure. Again, move as much of the extra sheet as possible out of the way in a superior direction. **C.** Keeping it tight to the leg, gradually work the "pant leg" drape up the thigh.

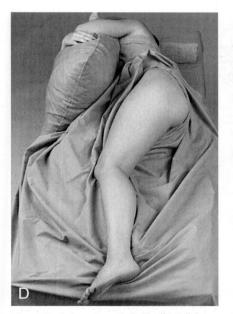
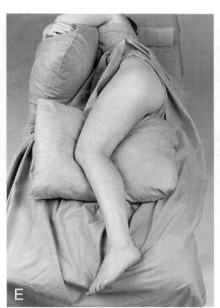
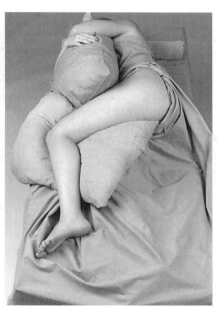

Figure 4-57 (continued). **D.** Finally, pull the superior edge of the drape toward the groin, toward the gluteal cleft, and roll it over the iliac crest. It takes practice to get this draping tight and secure. **E.** Gently lift the leg, and place a pillow under the knee for support.

Figure 4-58. The preferred position in which to work on the piriformis is with the knee and hip both flexed to 90 degrees. To achieve this draping, begin by placing the upper leg in the desired position under the sheet and then follow the steps described in Figure 4-57.

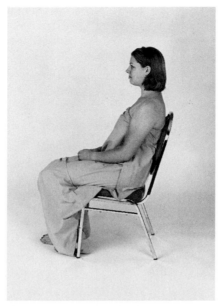

Figure 4-59. Wrap-around, or "toga-style," draping is useful for seated massage of the head, neck, and shoulders in a seated inclined position.

Clinician's Posture, Alignment, and Body Mechanics During Treatment

Efficient posture and movement constitute the physical foundation of effective execution of massage techniques. The outcomes and characteristic "feel" of well-performed massage techniques depend as much on the clinician's correct use of his feet, legs, pelvis, and respiratory apparatus as they do on the motion of his shoulder girdle. Students and clinicians who aspire to achieve expertise in performing massage strokes may have postural habits that must be systematically retrained. Furthermore, this retraining must start before instruction in manual technique begins, since the individual's attention to posture will diminish once he begins to learn manual technique. If the individual's habitually poor body mechanics are not corrected, then he will experience fatigue and pain when performing massage strokes; for many this unpleasant consequence can occur in as little as a few hours or weeks.

The following general principles of body mechanics apply during most clinical applications of the manual technique of massage.

1. Posture is aligned and as upright as possible, except during controlled transfer of body weight.
2. Both feet remain in contact with the floor.
3. The clinician reduces the vertical distance between himself and the client by bending his knees, rather than by bending over at the lumbosacral articulation.
4. The clinician reduces the horizontal distance between himself and the client by repositioning his legs or shifting his weight onto his forward leg, rather than by bending at the waist or reaching excessively.
5. The clinician orients his navel area toward the body segment of the client that he is treating.
6. Increases in pressure are achieved through the controlled use of body weight, rather than through muscle strength.
7. Controlled leaning toward the point of contact with the client is acceptable, but the clinician must control the amount of his body weight that is being transferred to the client, precisely and continuously.
8. The clinician's joints are positioned as close to neutral as possible, rather than being loaded while they are in a close-packed position.
9. The clinician changes his position (e.g., from sitting to kneeling) frequently, to vary the mechanical stress that is being placed on his body.

The use of the following postures[8,9,12,13] during the application of massage techniques will be discussed in the chapters on techniques. Ideally, before the clinician or student attempts to learn manual technique, he will practice the following posture and movement exercises often enough to use them automatically during practice. These exercises will assist the student or clinician in developing the relaxation, awareness, balance, coordination, flexibility, and strength that are required to perform massage techniques. A lack of familiarity with these or comparable exercises can compromise the quality of the individual's manual technique and increase his risk of injury. Furthermore, these exercises are worthwhile in their own right and can be incorporated into the clinician's daily warm-up or cool-down.

STANDING ALIGNED POSTURE

This deceptively simple posture can actually be quite difficult to maintain, since it often reveals and accentuates chronic patterns of tension in the body when the clinician first begins to use it. The steps for performing this posture are outlined below (Fig. 4-60A and B).

1. Stand with your feet positioned shoulder-width apart (glenoid fossa, not the lateral surface of the deltoid).
2. Breathe deeply and relax.
3. Let the weight settle down through your legs and into your feet.
4. Explore the manner in which your feet contact the ground by rocking from front to back, shifting from left to right, and shifting the inside to the outside.
5. Attempt to find the foot position in which the weight of your body is evenly distributed throughout your foot.
6. Let the top of your head rise up gently. You may want to have someone check whether you are incorrectly positioning your head by flexing or extending your neck.
7. Try to hold a standing aligned posture for 10 min, progressively refining both your foot contact with the ground and your sense of vertical alignment.

STANDING ALIGNED POSTURE WITH DIAPHRAGMATIC BREATHING

The steps for performing this posture are outlined below (Fig. 4-60C).

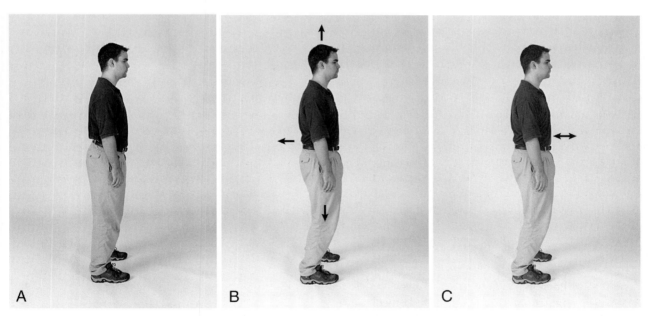

Figure 4-60. A. Lateral view of standing posture shows a forward lean; a shortening in this clinician's lumbar muscles, with an accompanying anterior pelvic tilt; and an anterior-head posture. These may be due to postural habit or chronic fascial shortening. **B.** His lumbar spine is in a more neutral position, and the whole posture is better aligned after he balanced the weight on his feet, softened his knees, let his sacrum drop, and let his head rise. Here, the clinician has overcompensated by bending his knees more than necessary. **C.** Using the diaphragm to breathe produces a passive rise of the abdomen on inhalation. Standing aligned posture is used for superficial reflex techniques that do not require application of pressure and need to be sustained for some time.

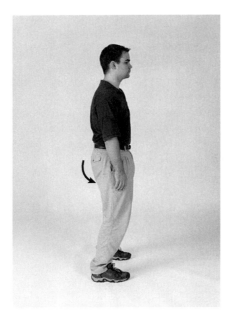

Figure 4-61. During a standing slow pelvic tilt, the pelvis is tucked under, while the thorax remains in the same position. This results in a lengthening of the lumbar region and a reduction of the normal lordosis. This movement is a prerequisite for later movements that involve bending the knees.

1. Assume a standing aligned posture until you feel very stable and relaxed.
2. Focus your attention on your breathing.
3. Let your upper chest remain still, and breathe using your diaphragm so that your abdomen passively rises during the inhalation and passively falls during the exhalation.
4. Remain in this position and continue to focus on the passive rise and fall of your abdomen. Gradually increase both the duration and depth of the inhalation.
5. Sustain focused breathing for 10 min, and periodically check the alignment of your body.

STANDING PELVIC TILT

The steps for performing this posture are outlined below (Fig. 4-61).

1. Assume a standing aligned posture until you feel very stable and relaxed.
2. Ensure that your knees are not hyperextended.
3. Focus your attention on your pelvis.
4. Keeping the legs and upper body motionless, perform a posterior pelvic tilt by letting your sacrum drop and rolling your anterior superior iliac spine in a posterior direction.

5. Place a hand on your lumbar spine and note whether you feel it flatten slightly; this indicates that the posterior pelvic tilt has occurred.
6. Hold the pelvic tilt and breathe deeply using your diaphragm in the manner outlined above.
7. Relax.
8. Perform this tilt and relax movement 10 to 20 times.
9. Vary your practice of this posture by making the movement larger or more subtle or by varying the amount you bend your knees.

Proper performance of a posterior pelvic tilt in standing requires some flexibility. If it is difficult to perform, practice this posture lying supine on a flat surface with your knees and hips flexed, progress to lying supine with your knees and hips extended, and then attempt to perform it standing with your back against a wall before reattempting the posture in unsupported standing.

SEATED ALIGNED POSTURE

The steps for performing this posture are outlined below (Fig. 4-62).

1. Sit upright on a level, firm, well-padded chair that allows your knees and hips to rest at 90 degrees of flexion. Place your feet on the floor, shoulder-width apart or slightly wider.

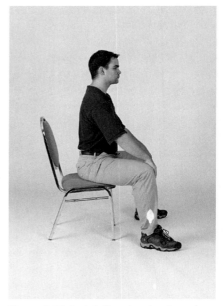

Figure 4-62. Seated aligned posture is used when applying many different techniques. Note the feet flat on the floor and the erect upper body supported by the ischiopubic rami.

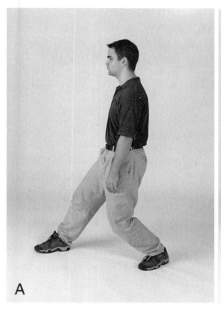
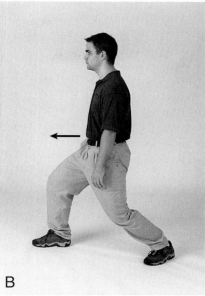

A　　　B

Figure 4-63. A. Lunge position with the weight over the back leg. **B.** Lunge position, shifting the weight toward the front leg (the rear leg can still be straightened some more). As the weight is shifted back and forth, the torso remains balanced and motionless in relation to the moving legs. This basic leg movement for many techniques requires some quadriceps strength.

2. First touch and then focus your attention on your ischial tuberosities.
3. Allow your spine to flex until you feel the weight of your upper body resting on your ischial tuberosities.
4. While maintaining your upper body in an upright position, slowly roll the contact point of your pelvis with the chair forward so that it shifts from being on the ischial tuberosities to being along the ischial rami in the direction of the symphysis pubis.
5. Since that movement should extend your lumbar spine, place your hand in the small of your back and note whether you feel the erector spinae muscles in your lumbar region.
6. Very slowly rock back and forward several times and locate the point on your pelvis, between your ischial tuberosities and symphysis pubis, at which your upper body feels upright and most comfortably balanced over the pelvis (somewhere around the perineum). The erector spinae muscles in your lumbar region should not be engaged in that position.
7. Breathe deeply using your diaphragm.
8. Let the top of your head rise up gently. You may want to have someone check whether you are incorrectly positioning your head by flexing or extending your neck.
9. Sit for 10 min, progressively refining both the contact of your pelvis with the chair and your sense of vertical alignment.

LUNGE

This position is also known as walk-standing, bow stance, or archer stance. The steps for performing this posture are outlined below (Fig. 4-63A and B).

1. Stand with your feet together.
2. Externally rotate your left hip to 20 to 45 degrees so that your left foot is turned out.
3. With your right foot, step forward and to the right of the left foot a comfortable distance.
4. Maintaining an upright torso, slowly straighten your left (back) leg without hyperextending your knee, and bend your right (forward) leg as you move your body over your forward foot.
5. Straighten your right (forward) leg and bend your left (back) knee as you shift your weight onto your back leg. Slowly shift your weight back and forth from your left to right foot, while keeping your torso perfectly poised and upright. Your head should remain equidistant from the floor throughout the movement.
6. You may also synchronize your breathing with the movement by inhaling as you shift your weight in the posterior direction and exhaling as you shift your weight in the anterior direction.
7. Continue for 5 min, and then repeat the exercise with the other foot forward.
8. Vary your practice of this posture and make it more challenging by gradually increasing the distance between your feet and the degree to which you flex your knees.

LUNGE AND REACH

The steps for performing this posture are outlined below (Fig. 4-64A and B).

1. Begin by performing the steps in the lunge movement previously described.
2. As you shift your weight onto your forward leg, extend both arms straight ahead at navel level without fully extending your elbows. As you shift your weight onto your back leg, flex your elbows and shoulders and bring your arms toward your body while keeping them at waist level.
3. Vary your practice of this posture by increasing the distance between your feet, by changing the degree to which you flex your knees, by varying the level of your arms, and by using different breathing patterns.

LUNGE AND LEAN

The steps for performing this posture are outlined below (Fig. 4-65).

1. Begin by performing the steps in the lunge movement previously described.
2. Rather than keeping the torso upright throughout the movement, incline the torso forward (lean) as you shift your weight onto the forward leg. At the forward portion of the motion, there should be a straight line from the top of your head, through your torso, to the heel of your back leg. The movement of this posture is from upright with your weight on your back leg to leaning with the weight on your front leg, and back again.

3. Once you have mastered the performance of the lean during the weight shift, add the arm movement previously described in the lunge and reach posture.

WIDE-STANCE KNEE BEND

This position is also known as the horse or warrior stance. The steps for performing this posture are outlined below (Figs. 4-66, 4-67A and B).

1. Stand with your feet placed more than shoulder-width apart and your feet pointed straight forward or in a small degree of external rotation.
2. While keeping your upper body upright, flex your hips and knees a few degrees. Hold this position. This is the "upper bent-knee position."
3. Adjust the distance (width) between your feet until you are in a position that you can comfortably hold for 2 to 3 min.
4. Slowly increase the degree of knee flexion so that you lower your body 6 to 8 inches. This is the "lower bent-knee position."
5. While keeping your torso upright, perform a posterior pelvic tilt (using the steps previously described) so that your lower spine lengthens as you lower your body. Place a hand on your lumbar spine to monitor its position during this movement.
6. Slowly extend your knees and return to the upper bent-knee position without hyperextending your lumbar spine or your knees.
7. Repeat.
8. Gradually work up to 100 repetitions of this sequence of movements from neutral to the upper and lower bent-knee positions.

Figure 4-64. **A, B.** Lunge and reach. Arms extend from an upright torso as the weight is shifted to the forward leg. This exact movement is used for superficial effleurage.

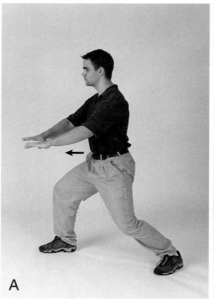
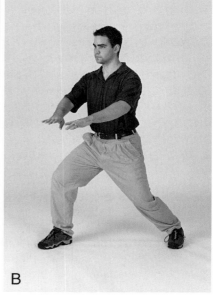

A   B

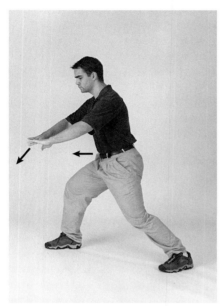

Figure 4-65. Lunge and lean. The clinician is shifting his weight over the front leg as he leans forward; extending his back knee slightly will complete the forward movement. Using exactly this movement, the clinician transfers pressure to the client during various neuromuscular and connective tissue techniques.

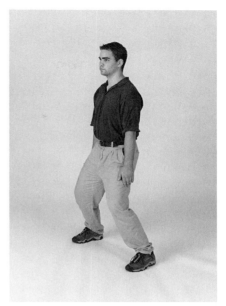

Figure 4-66. First, practice the wide stance (horse stance) without movement (the "upper bent-knee position").

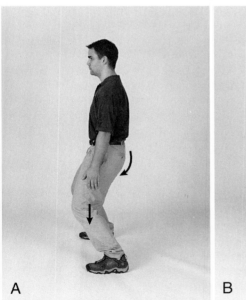

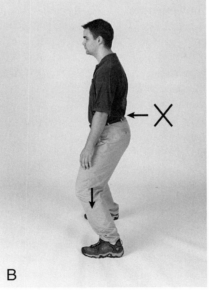

Figure 4-67. A. Knee bend in the wide stance. As the clinician bends his knees, he simultaneously executes a posterior pelvic tilt so that the lumbar region lengthens. This type of leg movement is used for some neuromuscular techniques like wringing. **B.** A common error of movement is to increase the lumbar lordosis as the knees are bending.

9. Vary your practice of this posture by changing the distance (width) between your feet, by flexing your knees more, by rotating your upright torso in one direction as you go down and rotating to the original position as you come up, and by performing the knee bend beside a massage table while transferring a portion of your upper body weight to the table through your bent arms.

STANDING CONTROLLED LEAN

The steps for performing this posture are outlined below (Fig. 4-68).

1. You need a massage table or other stable object against which you can lean to perform this posture. The table should be within reach of your partially extended arms.
2. Begin by performing the steps of the lunge and lean posture previously described.
3. As you shift weight onto your forward leg, lean forward and extend your arms. Allow your hands to contact the table and slowly transfer some of your weight to the table. As you do this, you should feel a shift of weight onto your extended back leg.
4. Slowly return your arms to their original position and shift your upper body back over your back leg.
5. Repeat this back-and-forth movement and transfer some of your body weight to the table at the appropriate point in each movement. The compression and release should be slow and controlled.

SEATED CONTROLLED LEAN

The steps for performing this posture are outlined below (Figs. 4-69A to 4-70).

1. Begin in the seated aligned posture facing a massage table or other stable object against which you can lean.
2. Place your hands on the supporting surface.
3. Gradually lean forward from your waist and apply pressure to the supporting surface so that you feel balanced as you do so.
4. Alternatively, sit upright on the edge of a firm bed or massage table and face one end of it. If you are on a massage table, the leg closest to the table will be off the ground and the other foot will have a secure contact with the floor.
5. Slowly lean forward to transfer your body weight in the manner described above.

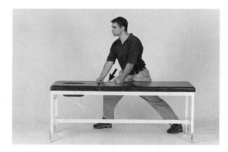

Figure 4-68. A standing controlled lean is used to apply pressure during many neuromuscular and connective tissue techniques.

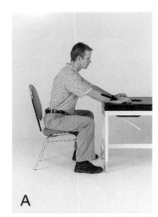

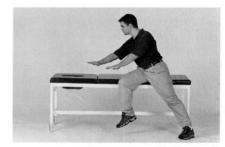

Figure 4-69. A. A seated controlled lean using a chair. This is often used when treating the client's shoulders. **B.** A seated controlled lean sitting on the edge of the table. When treating clients, it is acceptable to sit on the edge of the table as long as the clinician only contacts the client with his hands or forearms, not his thigh or pelvis.

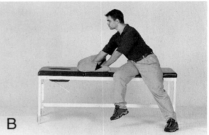

Figure 4-70. The clinician is obviously not using the client to support his body. He demonstrates flawless control of the amount of body weight that he could transfer to a client in this position.

6. Vary your practice of this posture by changing the amount of weight you transfer to the supporting surface, the height of contact, and the compression time (without losing continuous control and relaxed shoulders).

Conclusions

This chapter outlines many activities that a clinician must perform to prepare himself and his treatment materials prior to an intervention. It also discusses how the clinician should position himself and his client during the application of massage techniques. Knowledge of, and proper execution of, these activities are essential components of the appropriate application of the massage techniques that are outlined in the techniques chapters that follow. These strategies can also enhance the clinician's experience of providing interventions that incorporate massage techniques by minimizing the physical and psychological demands on the clinician.

References

1. Sharkey B. Fitness and health. 4th ed. Champaign, IL: Human Kinetics, 1997.
2. Jongsma D, Rice J. The active health and fitness book. Barrie, Ontario: Active Health and Fitness, 1998.
3. Moffat M, Vickery S. The American Physical Therapy Association book of body maintenance and repair. New York: Henry Holt & Co, 1999.
4. Alter MJ. Science of stretching. Champaign, IL: Human Kinetics, 1988.
5. Oswald C, Basco S. Stretching for fitness, health and performance: the complete handbook for all ages and fitness levels. New York: Sterling Publishing, 1998.
6. Anderson B. Stretching. Bolinas, CA: Shelter Publication, 1980.
7. Loving J. Massage therapy. Stamford, CT: Appleton & Lange, 1999.
8. Fritz, S. Fundamentals of therapeutic massage. St Louis: Moseby-Lifeline, 1995.
9. Salvo SG. Massage therapy. Philadelphia: WB Saunders, 1999.
10. Quality Assurance Committee of the College of Massage Therapists of Ontario. Code of ethics and standards of practice. Toronto: College of Massage Therapists of Ontario, 1999.
11. Curties D. Breast massage. New Brunswick, Canada: Curties-Overzet Publications, 1999.
12. Beck M. The theory and practice of therapeutic massage. Albany, NY: Milady, 1988.
13. Hollis M. Massage for therapists. 2nd ed. Oxford, England: Blackwell Science, 1998.

5

Superficial Reflex Techniques

Superficial reflex techniques are those massage techniques that palpate the skin and primarily affect level of arousal, autonomic balance, or the perception of pain. These techniques include static contact, superficial stroking, and fine vibration. This chapter describes each of these techniques, how to perform the technique, and how to apply it in a practice sequence. The chapter also includes a discussion of the indications, contraindications, cautions, outcomes of care, and postintervention care associated with each technique.

Table 5-1
Summary of Impairment-Level Outcomes of Care for Superficial Reflex Techniques

Impairment-Level Outcome of Care	Technique		
	Static Contact	*Superficial Stroking*	*Fine Vibration*
Increased sedation	✓	✓	✓
Decreased anxiety	✓	✓	P
Increased arousal	–	✓	–
Counterirritant analgesia	P	P	✓
Increased local resting muscle tension or neuromuscular tone	–	–	✓
Decreased local resting muscle tension or neuromuscular tone	–	✓	–
Stimulated peristalsis	P	P	P

✓, the outcome is supported by research summarized in this chapter; P, the outcome is probable; –, nonexistent, negligible, or improbable effects.

Static Contact

OTHER NAMES USED FOR THIS TECHNIQUE

"Resting position," "passive touch," "superficial touch," "light touch," "static touch," "maintained touch," "stationary holding."[1–7]

DEFINITION

Static contact: Motionless contact of the clinician's hands with the client's body, performed with minimal force.[1–7]

CLINICAL INDICATIONS AND IMPAIRMENT-LEVEL OUTCOMES OF CARE

Static contact is the least mechanically stimulating of the massage techniques. It can be used to enhance the flow of interventions, to achieve outcomes of care related to clients' psychological and physiological impairments, and to clarify client education. Static contact can be used to facilitate the flow and coherence of interventions in two ways: to establish a therapeutic rapport with the client[8–10] and to reduce anxiety and induce sedation at the beginning and end of massage interventions that incorporate other techniques.[1,3,4] The psychological effects of static contact are many: it can be used alone to decrease anxiety and the perception of pain in conditions in which the use of movement or force is contraindicated or poorly tolerated, for example, in situations of trauma, acute conditions, extreme or intractable pain, illness, dying, postsurgery, systemic weakness, convalescence, emotional distress, hypersensitivity, posttraumatic stress, and when there is a history of violence, sexual abuse, or poor physical self-image.[11–15] Research also suggests that static contact, superficial stroking, and gentle passive movement can have a positive effect on the physiological and psychological development of premature infants.[16–22] Static contact is indispensable when teaching a client breathing techniques (see Figs. 5-2 and 5-3) or when cueing a client to become aware of any part of the body,[23] and it can be used to facilitate movement. Finally, static contact is integrated into therapeutic approaches such as Therapeutic Touch, Reiki, and Polarity, in which the philosophy of treatment is conceptualized in terms of energy or life force.[24–31] The main impairment-level outcomes of care for static contact are summarized in Table 5-1.

CAUTIONS AND CONTRAINDICATIONS

Clinical training and supervised practice are critical for the proper application of static contact. Advanced training may be advisable in certain situations, particularly when dealing with pathological conditions. Static contact is a reflex technique; consequently, the contraindications for the use of mechanical techniques do not generally apply (see Chapter 2, "The Clinical Decision-Making Process").[1] The primary exception to this rule is that the use of static contact may be contraindicated locally in areas of acute inflammation because of pain. Furthermore, clients who are experiencing considerable pain or distress may not tolerate touch at all.

There are several cautions for the use of static contact.[1] Since it can be used with frail clients, high-risk infants, or terminally ill clients, the clinician needs to be sensitive to the emotional and physical needs of these clients. Although static contact looks deceptively simple and causes minimal mechanical effects, like all massage techniques it can give rise to very complex physical and emotional responses, including touch-triggered memory.[32] As with all massage techniques, informed consent from the client is therefore required for its use. When the client's condition results in an impairment of the client's cognitive function or level of consciousness, the clinician may have difficulty obtaining informed consent to treat. In addition, the clinician must maintain clear and consistent communication with the client throughout the intervention when the technique is applied for long periods or over large areas of the client's body.

Prerequisite Skills for Static Contact

Before practicing static contact, students should know how to

   Assess autonomic function

   Track autonomic function in a client

   Use standing aligned and seated aligned postures

   Perform diaphragmatic breath while standing and sitting

(See Chapter 3, Review of Client Examination Concepts for Massage, and Chapter 4, Preparation and Positioning for Treatment.)

Manual Technique begins on next page

MANUAL TECHNIQUE

Static Contact

In the following figures (Figs. 5-1 to 5-7), static contact is applied to the various regions of the body. Figures are ordered from head to foot in supine and then prone. Each figure illustrates most of the guidelines for manual technique outlined below.

1. Hands are relaxed and in full contact with the client's body in a position that allows them to conform evenly to the contours of the client's body.

2. Hands are commonly placed on the client's body in a symmetrical position. This enables the clinician to maintain contact with the left and right sides of the client's body simultaneously (Figs. 5-1A and B, 5-3, 5-6).

3. The clinician does not attempt to apply force or to physically manipulate the client's tissues in any way. The partial weight of the clinician's hands may rest on the client's body if the client reports that this is tolerable.

4. Hands make and break contact with the surface of the client's body gradually and gently. It is largely the manner with which contact is made and broken that establishes relaxation; however, making and breaking contact very frequently may decrease the sedative effect of this technique.

5. The clinician holds her hands steady while they are in contact with the client's body. The hands should not shake from fatigue, even during prolonged application.

6. The author's clinical observation suggests that the clinician is more likely to achieve the effect of deep relaxation when applying static contact for longer periods (5 minutes or longer) at the midsacrum and/or occiput[3] (Figs. 5-1B and 5-7). Contact with the hands, feet, and face may also be more likely to produce relaxation than that with other areas of the body,[3,10,13] possibly because of the density of nervous innervation in these areas (Figs. 5-5 and 5-6).

Components of Static Contact

Contact: Whole hand, fingertip(s), thumb

Pressure: Minimal

Engages: Skin

Direction: N/A

Amplitude/length: N/A

Rate: N/A

Duration: 60 sec to 15 min or more

Integrades[a] with: Compression, vibration

Context: May be used alone; it is commonly used as a "framing technique," performed at the beginning and end of regional or full-body sequences that use other techniques to engage deeper tissues

---

[a]To merge gradually one into the other.

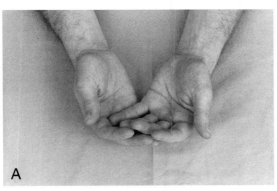

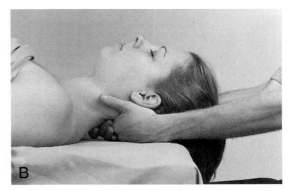

Figure 5-1. **A.** Hand position for applying static contact to the occiput with the client in supine. Note that the forearms are supported on the table. **B.** Static contact applied to the occiput. This nonthreatening approach to reducing spasm or hypertonicity in the client's neck can also produce sedative effects.[3]

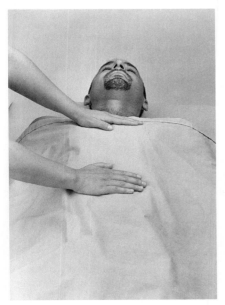

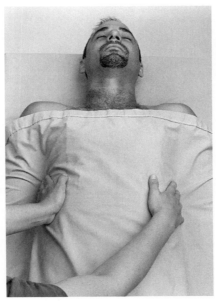

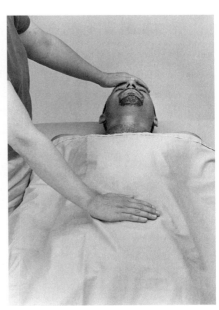

Figure 5-2. Static contact used to draw the client's awareness to the movement of the upper ribs and abdomen during breathing.

Figure 5-3. Static contact used to facilitate instruction of the client in lateral costal breathing.

Figure 5-4. Simultaneous contact to the forehead and abdomen.

Manual Technique Figures continue on next page

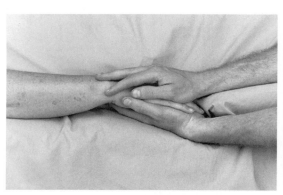

Figure 5-5. Appropriate contact to the hand(s) can be both intimate and comforting.[10]

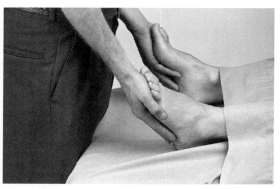

Figure 5-6. Bilateral static contact to the soles of the feet.

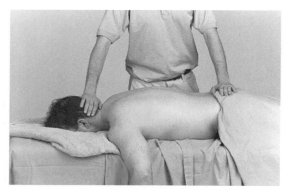

Figure 5-7. Prolonged simultaneous contact at occiput and sacrum can produce relaxation in the client.[3]

CLINICIAN'S POSITION AND MOVEMENT

1. The basic positions used by the clinician are described in Chapter 4, "Preparation and Positioning for Treatment," in the sections on standing aligned posture and seated aligned posture.
2. The clinician selects a posture that is comfortable and stable to minimize shaking when contact must be sustained for longer periods. This is necessary to avoid inadvertent shaking of the clinician's hands.
3. The clinician may prefer to sit when working on the client's feet and head or when working unilaterally. Sitting allows the clinician to support the forearms on the edge of the table, providing increased stability and reducing the likelihood of arm fatigue during the technique (Fig. 5-1A and B).

PALPATE

As she performs the technique, the clinician palpates the client's skin for the following:

1. Skin texture
2. Skin temperature
3. Presence of perspiration and moisture

OBSERVE

As she performs the technique, the clinician observes the client for changes in the level of arousal and autonomic balance that reflect increasing relaxation. The signs listed below may be indicative of increased relaxation:

1. Decrease in rate and depth of breathing
2. Deeper voice tone
3. Changes in skin color, such as flushing; pallor may indicate an undesirable sympathetic response
4. Systemic reduction of muscle resting tension, as evidenced by softening of the tissue contours or broadening and flattening of body segments
5. Muscle twitches and jerks
6. Increases in peristaltic noises
7. Decreases in heart rate as evidenced by change in pulses that are visible at the neck, wrist, and foot
8. Agitation or sweating, which may indicate an undesirable sympathetic response

COMMUNICATION WITH THE CLIENT

The clinician uses communication that may encourage general relaxation, guide the client's awareness of areas of the body, or facilitate the client's breathing pattern. Some examples of statements that the clinician can use are listed below.

1. "Let your . . . relax, as much as you're able."
2. "Feel the weight of your body" or "Let your body sink into the table."
3. "Notice what's occurring in your body. . . . It's not unusual to experience sensations some distance from the location of my hands."
4. "Let your awareness move to . . . "
5. "It's not unusual to have emotions or feelings arise in response to touch. Just observe them and express them if you need to."
6. "Deepen your breathing without forcing it in any way."
7. "Notice how your ribs move here when you inhale."
8. "What is happening with your pain?" This can be used when the technique is being applied to reduce pain, to periodically check how the client perceives that pain has been affected by the intervention.

OTHER APPROPRIATE TECHNIQUES

There are several modalities that the clinician can use in a complementary manner with static contact.

1. Progressive relaxation or diaphragmatic breathing[23] may be used prior to, or simultaneously with, static contact to enhance sedative effects. For example, the clinician can combine a prolonged occipital hold with the client in supine with instruction on diaphragmatic breathing.
2. Moist hot packs can enhance sedation and analgesia, if the use of heat is appropriate for the client's condition.[33]
3. Some craniosacral techniques may have a calming effect on the client.[34]

POSTINTERVENTION SELF-CARE

The clinician instructs the client to rest from 10 to 30 min and to resume activity slowly if experiencing the sedative effects of static contact.

A Practice Sequence for Static Contact

Practice time: 30 or 60 min per person.

Hold each position bilaterally about a minute for a half-hour session, or 2 min for a 1-hr session.

Clinicians who use static contact extensively often recommend a sequence that proceeds in a cephalocaudal direction, i.e., from head to toe, as is described here. We suggest that students try different orders and draw their own conclusions.

Supine	*Prone*
Vertex	Vertex
Occiput	Parietal bone
Eyes/frontal bone	Temporal bone
Cheeks/jaw	Occiput
Anterior neck	Posterior neck
Anterior shoulders	Upper trapezius
Upper ribs	Mid- and upper thorax
Lower ribs	Lower thorax
Elbows	Elbows
Dorsum of hands	Palms
Upper abdomen	Lumbar area
Lower abdomen	Sacrum
Hips	Gluteal area
Knees	Knees
Ankles	Ankles
Dorsum of feet	Plantar surface of feet

Home study: Devise comparable sequences that

1. Move in a caudocephalic direction
2. Incorporate more contact between joints
3. Spend half of the allotted time on a specified region, such as the legs

---

Superficial Stroking

OTHER NAMES USED FOR THIS TECHNIQUE

"Light stroking," "feather stroking," "nerve stroking."[2,3]

DEFINITION

Superficial stroking: Gliding over the client's skin with minimal deformation of subcutaneous tissues. This stroke is usually applied unidirectionally over large areas of the client's body.

NOTES

Some authors do not distinguish between stroking and effleurage or consider stroking to be similar to effleurage without the directional restriction.[1–7,35] This is discussed further in Chapter 6, "Superficial Fluid Techniques." This book uses Mennell's[36] definition, which considers superficial stroking to be a distinct reflex technique that is performed with a lighter pressure than that used with effleurage.

CLINICAL INDICATIONS AND IMPAIRMENT-LEVEL OUTCOMES OF CARE

Superficial stroking can be used to change the client's level of arousal, for pain reduction, and to facilitate changes in resting muscle tension and neuromuscular tone. Since superficial stroking can result in sedation or stimulation, depending on the contact, direction, and rate of application,[1,7,35] it is commonly used at the beginning or end of an intervention session to adjust the client's level of arousal. Like static contact, this technique is well suited to difficult situations in which the use of pressure is contraindicated.[37–41] Consequently, superficial stroking has been incorporated into interventions, such as the "slow-stroke back rub" described in the nursing literature, that are used to improve mood and relieve anxiety in the critically ill.[38–40] Forms of superficial stroking that can stimulate the client's level of arousal,[5,35] when judiciously applied, may temporarily ameliorate some symptoms of debility, convalescence, lethargy, and depression. Superficial stroking may have a role in treating pain when mechanical techniques are contraindicated. Pain relief may occur because light touch and vibration increase large-diameter afferent nerve input and may reduce the transmission of "slow" pain impulses through the spinal gate of the segment being touched.[5,7,42] Superficial stroking may minimally facilitate or inhibit local muscle tone via cutaneomuscular reflexes and may reduce spasm. It can be used locally and over the posterior primary rami to decrease limb spasticity.[5,43] The main impairment-level outcomes of care for superficial stroking are summarized in Table 5-1 at the beginning of this chapter.

CAUTIONS AND CONTRAINDICATIONS

Clinical training and supervised practice are critical for the proper application of superficial stroking. Advanced training may be advisable in certain situations, particularly when dealing with pathological conditions. Superficial stroking is a reflex technique; consequently, the contraindications for the use of mechanical techniques do not generally apply (see Chapter 2, "The Clinical Decision-Making Process").[1] The primary exception to this rule is that the use of superficial stroking may be contraindicated locally in areas of acute inflammation because of pain. In this situation, treat the client's pain by performing the technique on adjacent areas as tolerated by the client. Furthermore, clients who are experiencing considerable pain or distress may not tolerate touch at all.

There are several cautions for the use of superficial stroking.[1] When the client's condition results in an impairment of the client's cognitive function or level of consciousness, the clinician may have difficulty obtaining informed consent to treat. Since superficial stroking can be used with frail clients, high-risk infants, or terminally ill clients, the clinician needs to be sensitive to the emotional and physical needs of these clients. Although recent myocardial infarction was once considered to be a contraindication for massage, light massage is now considered to be permissible. A further cardiac-related caution is that a 48-hour wait is advisable after coronary artery bypass surgery.[44] Finally, if superficial stroking is being used for reflex stimulation, the clinician needs to ensure that the application of the technique does not become irritating. Ticklishness frequently occurs in areas where there is underlying muscular tension. If the application of superficial stroking tickles the client, the clinician should try the following strategies: Switch to a broader contact, add lubricant, check that the stroke direction doesn't run against the grain of the client's body hair, or change to a technique that uses more pressure.

Prerequisite Skills for Superficial Stroking

Before practicing superficial stroking, students should know how to

Assess autonomic function

Track autonomic function in a client

Hold standing aligned and seated aligned postures

Perform diaphragmatic breathing in standing

Use lunge, and lunge and reach movements

(See Chapter 3, Review of Client Examination Concepts for Massage, and Chapter 4, Preparation and Positioning for Treatment.)

Manual Technique begins on next page

MANUAL TECHNIQUE

Superficial Stroking

In the following figures (Figs. 5-8 to 5-15), superficial stroking is applied to the various regions of the body. Figures are ordered from head to foot in supine and then prone. Each figure illustrates most of the guidelines for manual technique outlined below.

1. Lubricant is not usually required to achieve glide without binding.

2. Hands are relaxed when the clinician is using the full palmar surface to perform the stroke. The clinician uses only the hand weight required to ensure good contact with the client's skin.

3. The clinician performs superficial stroking in one direction, unless the desired outcome of the intervention is stimulation, since the reflex effects of superficial stroking are direction dependent.

4. Hands are in the air for the return stroke to the starting position. The clinician uses the same speed for the return stroke as for the initiating stroke because this encourages a stable rhythm, which is necessary to achieve systemic sedation.

5. Though responses vary from person to person and with the context of treatment, the clinician can achieve different effects by adjusting the type of contact, rate, and direction of the stroke.[1,3–7,35] Palmar contact, slow steady rate, centrifugal direction on the limbs, and caudal direction on the back tend to produce sedation (Fig. 5-13A). Conversely, fingertip contact, fast or irregular rate, centripetal direction on the limbs, and cephalad direction on the back tend to produce arousal (Fig. 5-14). Fingertip stroking is usually stimulating and may sometimes be irritating (Figs. 5-9, 5-13B, and 5-14).

6. One hand remains in contact when the clinician substitutes a succession of overlapping short strokes for a single long stroke (Fig. 5-15). The technique of breaking up a long stroke into overlapping shorter ones is called "layering," "shingling,"[3] or "thousand hands."[7,35] This technique enables the clinician to cover a large area with less reaching for each stroke, and it creates a sensory experience that may help some clients to relax.

7. On the abdomen, the clinician may perform the stroke across the abdomen or in the direction of colonic flow (Figs. 5-10 and 5-11).[35]

8. Contact with the spinal column from occiput to sacrum, hands, feet, and face may produce stronger clinical effects than that with other areas of the body, possibly because of the density of nervous innervation in these areas (Figs. 5-8, 5-9, and 5-13A).

9. The clinician should use superficial stroking with caution on the plantar surface of the feet.

10. Superficial stroking can be applied effectively through the client's clothes or a sheet (Fig. 5-12). In this situation, the clinician must take steps to prevent bunching of the fabric over the skin, since this will detract from the regularity of the sensory input that the client receives during the stroke. The clinician may tuck the drape securely or use one hand to tighten the intervening fabric while the other hand performs the technique.

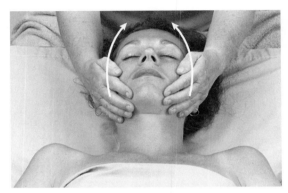

Figure 5-8. Slow, bilateral superficial stroking of the face with palmar contact can produce sedative effects.[1,3,35]

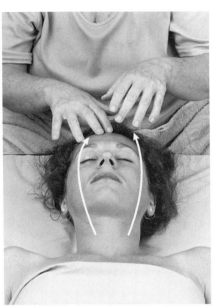

Figure 5-9. Fingertip superficial stroking of the face and scalp can provide a refreshing end to a massage sequence.

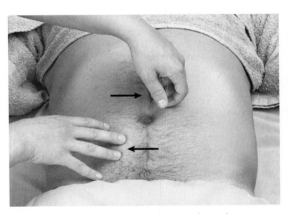

Figure 5-10. Dorsal and palmar contact surfaces alternate during transverse, bidirectional superficial stroking of the abdomen.

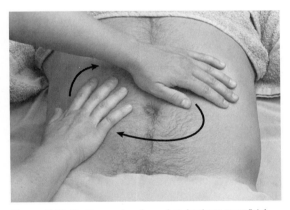

Figure 5-11. Continuous hand-over-hand palmar superficial stroking of the abdomen in the direction of colonic flow.

Manual Technique Figures continue on next page

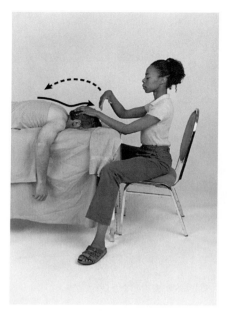

Figure 5-12. Superficial stroking can be applied through fabric, and the clinician may choose a seated aligned posture.

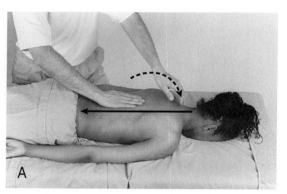

Figure 5-13. A. Slow, regular palmar stroking down the spine of produces sedative effects.[3] The return stroke in the air *(dotted line)* is made at the same rate as the stroke.

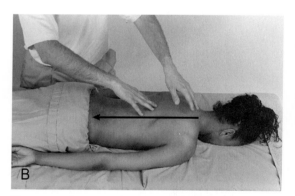

Figure 5-13 (continued). B. Fingertip contact can yield a more stimulating effect than palmar contact, with other components being the same.[1,3,35]

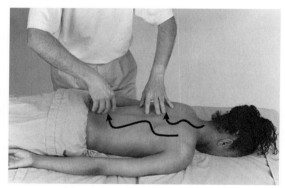

Figure 5-14. Fast, multidirectional, superficial fingertip stroking can be very stimulating and may be used judiciously to produce increased arousal in sedated clients.

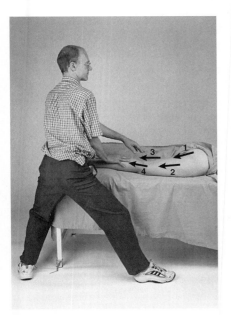

Figure 5-15. For long regions such as the posterior leg, the clinician may use overlapping short strokes instead of one long stroke.

Components of Superficial Stroking

Contact: Palmar surface of the hand, or fingertips

Pressure: Minimal

Engages: Skin only

Direction: Usually parallel to the long axis of the body part being stroked

Amplitude: The full length of the body part

Rate: 5 to 100 cm/sec

Duration: 10 sec to 10 min or more, depending on the clinician's intention

Integrades with: Superficial effleurage

Combines with: May be combined with fine vibration or shaking

Context: May be used alone; it is commonly used as a "framing technique," performed at the beginning and end of regional or full-body sequences that incorporate deeper techniques

CLINICIAN'S POSITION AND MOVEMENT

1. The basic positions used by the clinician are described in Chapter 4, Preparation and Positioning for Treatment, in the sections on standing aligned, seated aligned, lunge, and lunge and reach positions.
2. The clinician's shoulders and arms remain relaxed during the stroke, without straining to reach at the end of the stroke; the elbows are never fully extended.
3. The clinician can facilitate her ability to perform long strokes by using a relatively wide foot placement and by shifting the weight of an upright torso from one leg to the other as the stroke proceeds.

PALPATE

As she performs the technique, the clinician palpates the client's skin for the following:

1. Skin texture
2. Skin temperature
3. Presence of perspiration and moisture
4. Slight horizontal stretch of the skin, which occurs in the direction of movement; however, because of the light pressure and relatively fast rate, this stretch does not approach the elastic barrier of the skin.

OBSERVE

As she performs the technique, the clinician observes the client for increases or decreases in the client's level of arousal and autonomic balance. The signs listed below may be indicative of increased relaxation:

1. Change of rate and depth of breathing
2. Changes in voice tone
3. Changes in skin color, such as flushing or pallor
4. Systemic reduction of muscle resting tension, as evidenced by softening of the tissue contours or settling of body segments
5. Muscle twitches and jerks
6. Peristaltic noises
7. Change in heart rate as evidenced by change in pulses that are visible at the neck, wrist, and foot

8. Agitation or sweating may indicate an undesirable sympathetic response

COMMUNICATION WITH THE CLIENT:

The clinician uses communication that may encourage general relaxation or guide the client's awareness of areas of the body. Some examples of statements that the clinician can use are listed below.

1. "Let your . . . relax, as much as you're able."
2. "Feel the weight of your body" or "Let your body sink into the table."
3. "Notice what's occurring in your body. . . . It's not unusual to experience sensations some distance from the location of my hands."
4. "Let your awareness move to . . ."
5. "It's not unusual to have emotions or feelings arise in response to touch. Just observe them, and express them if you need to."
6. "What is happening with your pain?" This question can be used when the technique is being applied to reduce pain to periodically check how the client perceives that pain has been affected by the technique.

OTHER APPROPRIATE TECHNIQUES

There are several modalities that the clinician can use in a complementary manner to enhance sedation while using superficial stroking.

1. Progressive relaxation or diaphragmatic breathing[23,42] may be used prior to, or simultaneously with, superficial stroking, to enhance sedative effects.
2. Moist hot packs can enhance sedation and analgesia, if the use of heat is appropriate for the client's condition.[33]
3. Some craniosacral techniques may have a calming effect on the client.[34]

POSTINTERVENTION SELF-CARE

The clinician instructs the client to rest from 10 to 30 min and to resume activity slowly if experiencing the sedative effects of superficial stroking.

A Practice Sequence for Superficial Stroking

Practice time: 30 to 45 min per person.

Begin with palmar stroking down the spine from the crown to the sacrum; begin at a fast rate (100 cm/sec) and decrease the rate gradually over a period of 10 min until it is very slow (5–10 cm/sec). Follow with 5 min of static contact at both the sacrum and occiput.

After communicating changes in your intentions to your client, experiment with a variety of combinations of contact, rate, and direction that include different regions of the body in any orderly sequence. Examples of these combinations are

Moderate rate, palmar, layered from occiput to sacrum

Fast, palmar, across the back

Fast and irregular, fingertip, on the back

Slow, fingertip, down one limb

Fast, palmar, up the opposite limb

Moderate rate, palmar, across the abdomen

Slow, palmar or fingertip, up the face and scalp

Finish with palmar stroking down the spine and static contact at the sacrum and occiput. Ask the client for feedback.

Note: It takes time and repetition to produce sedative effects; it takes neither to achieve increased arousal.

Fine Vibration

OTHER NAMES USED FOR THIS TECHNIQUE

"Vibration," "mechanical vibration," "cutaneous vibration," "transcutaneous vibration," "vibratory stimulation."[45–70]

DEFINITION

Fine vibration: A fast, oscillating or trembling movement that is produced on the client's skin and that results in minimal deformation of subcutaneous tissues.[45–70]

NOTES

1. The term "vibration" has been used by some authors[3,5] to denote markedly differing techniques that involve shaking, compressing, or percussing the client's subcutaneous tissues with considerable force, as illustrated in Figure 5-21. In the current text, a distinction is made between fine vibration and the more vigorous forms of vibration that have mechanical effects and are described in Chapter 7, Neuromuscular Techniques, Chapter 9, Passive Movement Techniques, and Chapter 10, Percussive Techniques.

2. Recent research addresses fine vibration produced by small portable devices operating at frequencies varying from 40 to 200 Hz, with 100 Hz being the most commonly used.[45–70] The documented effects of machine-produced vibration, commonly referred to as mechanical vibration, cannot be extrapolated to manually produced fine vibration except with caution.

CLINICAL INDICATIONS AND IMPAIRMENT-LEVEL OUTCOMES OF CARE

Machine-produced vibration can be used to achieve pain relief and changes in neuromuscular tone. Machine-produced vibration can be an effective analgesic for acute and chronic pain of various causes, such as dental pain, phantom limb pain, myofascial pain, tendinous pain, neurogenic pain, and idiopathic pain.[45–65] Although the mechanism of analgesia is not well understood, researchers have noted that the reduction of pain and accompanying elevation of the pain threshold can persist for some time after intervention.[56,63,64] Analgesic effects are increased with sustained application of machine-produced vibration for 15 to 30 min or longer.[51,54] In addition, analgesic effects can be obtained when machine-produced vibration is applied to different regions of the client's body in relation to the site of pain, including direct application to the site of pain over a large area, distal to the site of pain, to the antagonist muscle group, to adjacent dermatomes, or even contralateral to the site of pain.[49,55,57,58,65] Combining the vibration with moderate pressure, if the client's condition permits, may enhance the analgesic effects of the vibration.[48,51,54,55]

Machine-produced vibration can result in an elevation of resting tone of the muscles under the site of application.[66–68] This effect may be used, when treating clients with neurological conditions, to promote more balanced movement and to prepare the client to perform functional activity.[67–68] Other effects ascribed to fine vibration are reflex relaxation, especially if it is applied to the feet,[69] and the healing of chronic peripheral nerve lesions.[70] The main impairment-level outcomes of care for fine vibration are summarized in Table 5-1 at the beginning of this chapter.

Effective application of manual fine vibration, using the technique described below, takes much practice. In addition, considerable skill on the part of the clinician is required to perform sustained application of manual fine vibration for more than a few minutes; hence the frequent use of machine vibration. The light touch of superficial stroking is a less-taxing manual alternative to manual fine vibration and also produces large-fiber afferent input.[42] Consequently, the clinician may alternate superficial stroking with, or substitute it for, fine vibration. In this situation, similar analgesic effects may be obtained if the duration of application is comparable.

CONTRAINDICATIONS AND CAUTIONS

Clinical training and supervised practice are critical for the proper application of fine vibration. Advanced training may be advisable in certain situations, particu-

larly when dealing with pathological conditions. Fine vibration is a reflex technique; consequently, the contraindications for the use of mechanical techniques do not generally apply (see Chapter 2, The Clinical Decision-Making Process). If, however, fine vibration is being used to treat pain in a client with an acute condition, the client may find the weight of the clinician's hand or a mechanical device intolerable. In this situation, the clinician should administer fine vibration in adjacent areas as tolerated by the client.

Prerequisite Skills for Fine Vibration

Before practicing fine vibration on a client, students should know how to

Assess pain

Assess and track autonomic function

Use standing aligned and seated aligned postures

Perform diaphragmatic breathing in standing

Generate a practice vibration in the air

(See Chapter 3, Review of Client Examination Concepts for Massage, and Chapter 4, Preparation and Positioning for Treatment.)

Manual Technique begins on page 136

MANUAL TECHNIQUE

Fine Vibration

In the following figures (see Figures 5-16 to 5-21), fine vibration is applied to the various regions of the body. Figures are ordered from head to foot in supine and then prone. Each figure illustrates most of the guidelines for manual technique outlined below.

1. The amplitude of fine vibration is scarcely visible and is generally less than 1 to 5 mm. Fine vibration exerts minimal mechanical effects beyond the surface of the client's skin.

2. The forearm and wrist are used to produce the motion, with as little recruitment of shoulder muscles as possible. One efficient method of generating fine vibration is to use a rapid, low-amplitude alternating pronation and supination of the forearm—a "flutter" (Fig. 5-16A and B). The clinician should avoid attempting to compress and release the client's tissues with the whole contact surface during the application of fine vibration. This action will usually recruit the clinician's shoulder muscles and result in a more vigorous and fatiguing manipulation that has mechanical effects on the client's subcutaneous tissues.

3. The two hands are rarely even in ability. The clinician can improve the ability of the less competent hand by practicing the application of fine vibration with both hands together in mirror image. Some clinicians choose to use only their dominant hand for fine vibration.

4. If the vibration is not being produced at an even rate, reduce the speed of application. It is preferable for the clinician to produce a slow, controlled vibration than a fast, uncontrolled one. Control and speed of application come with practice.

5. Fine vibration may be combined with superficial stroking to yield a "running" vibration whose reflex effects will also depend on the contact, rate, and direction of the stroking (Fig. 5-18).

Components of Fine Vibration

Contact: Palmar surface or fingertips are most common

Pressure: Minimal

Engages: Skin

Direction: N/A

Amplitude/length: Less than 1 to 5 mm

Rate: 4 to 10 Hz or more for manual vibration; 100 Hz is common for machine-produced vibration

Duration: 5 to 40 min for analgesia

Intergrades with: Shaking

Combines with: Can be combined with superficial stroking or compression

Context: Machine-produced vibration can be used alone; manual fine vibration is often alternated with superficial stroking and/or static contact in situations in which indications are similar

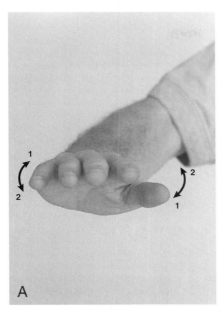

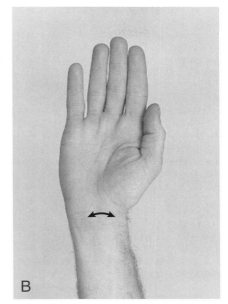

Figure 5-16. **A.** To create a fine vibration, the clinician may use low-amplitude alternating pronation and supination of the forearm. **B.** Or the clinician may use alternating radial and ulnar deviation of the wrist or forearm.

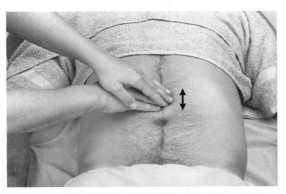

Figure 5-17. Fine vibration with stabilized fingertip contact applied to the abdomen.

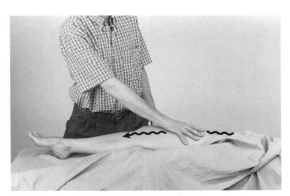

Figure 5-18. Fine vibration may be combined with stroking to produce a "running vibration," here shown on the quadriceps and anterior leg.

Manual Technique Figures continue on next page

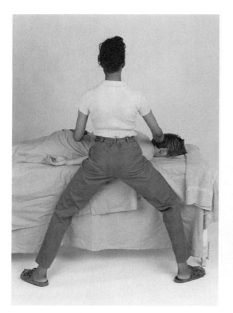

Figure 5-19. Whatever the manual method, posture must be aligned (standing or seated), and particular care must be taken to let the shoulders relax.

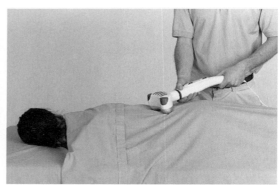

Figure 5-20. A handheld device for producing fine vibrations.

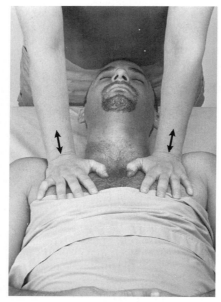

Figure 5-21. Coarser types of vibration that move subcutaneous tissue—such as the repeated rapid pumping of the ribcage shown here—have significant mechanical and proprioceptive effects and are discussed in later chapters.

CLINICIAN'S POSITION AND MOVEMENT

1. The basic positions used by the clinician are described in Chapter 4, Preparation and Positioning for Treatment, in the sections on basic standing aligned and seated aligned postures. See also Figure 5-19.
2. The shoulders are relaxed (down) and the elbows flexed. The clinician will experience less fatigue if the shoulder muscles are engaged as little as possible.
3. The clinician may find it helpful to sit, with the elbow or part of the forearm resting on the edge of the table.
4. The clinician's body position must be stable, since inadvertent postural shifts will detract from the intended effects of fine vibration.

PALPATE

As she performs the technique, the clinician palpates the client's skin for the following:

1. Skin texture
2. Skin temperature
3. Presence of perspiration and moisture

OBSERVE

As she performs the technique, the clinician observes the client for decreases in level of pain or general signs of relaxation. The signs listed below may signal this.

1. Decrease in rate and depth of breathing
2. Deeper voice tone
3. Changes in skin color, such as flushing; pallor may indicate an undesirable sympathetic response
4. Systemic reduction of muscle tension, as evidenced by softening of the tissue contours or broadening and flattening of body segments
5. Muscle twitches and jerks
6. Increases in peristaltic noises
7. Decreases in heart rate as evidenced by change in pulses that are visible at the neck, wrist, and foot

8. Agitation or sweating, which may indicate an undesirable sympathetic response

COMMUNICATION WITH THE CLIENT

The clinician uses communication that may encourage general relaxation or guide the client's awareness of areas of the body. Some examples of statements that the clinician can use are listed below.

1. "What is happening with your pain?" This question can be used when the technique is being applied to reduce pain, to periodically check how the client perceives that pain has been affected by the intervention.
2. "Deepen your breathing without forcing," "Let your body sink onto the table" can be used to facilitate relaxation; altered autonomic functioning may in turn affect the perception of pain.

OTHER APPROPRIATE TECHNIQUES

There are several modalities that the clinician can use in a complementary manner to enhance pain relief while using fine vibration.

1. Coapplication of transcutaneous electrical nerve stimulation (TENS) increases the analgesic effect of fine vibration.[61,62]
2. A variety of applications of heat, such as moist hot pack, fluidotherapy, and whirlpool, can enhance sedation and analgesia in the client.[33,71] Applications of cold, including cold packs, ice massage, and cold baths can enhance analgesia in the client.[33,71] The clinician must ensure that the selected modality is appropriate for the client's condition.

POSTINTERVENTION SELF-CARE

The clinician can instruct the client in the home use of a vibrating massage device and in appropriate hydrotherapy for analgesia.

Initial Practice of Manual Fine Vibration

Practice time: 15 min per day for several days.
No partner is required for initial practice of this technique. The steps in this practice sequence are listed below.

1. Stand with the shoulders down and elbows flexed to 90 degrees. Breathe deeply. Try to make an even vibration of the hand only of less than 1 cm in the air. The wrist and forearm will move slightly, too. Continue for 1 min, then rest for a minute.
2. Begin again. Try to generate an equal movement of the two hands. Continue for a minute, then rest again.
3. Begin again. Slightly flex and unflex the shoulders, then the elbows, then the wrists. Move through various combinations of shoulder, elbow and wrist flexion while continuing the vibration. Rest.
4. Place one hand on the opposite posterior deltoid. While vibrating with the free hand, can you tell if you are recruiting any shoulder girdle muscles to produce the vibration? Gradually increase the amplitude of the vibration to discover when the shoulder muscles begin to tense. Decrease the size again, and find the position and manual technique that recruits the shoulder muscles least. Switch arms. Practice this sequence once a day, gradually extending the time for which you can perform the fine vibration continuously without fatigue until you have reached 5 min. Then begin practice on clients, alternating periods of fine vibrations with superficial stroking.

Note: Remember to relax, breathe, and let the shoulders drop.

Clinical Example

Client profile

A 34-year-old male with late-stage AIDS who has been admitted to hospice from home for palliative care

Summary of clinical findings

Subjective
1. General complaints of pain and stiffness at rest and with activity
2. Complaints of pain during examinations of range of motion and functional activity
3. Complaints of anxiety and depression regarding terminal condition
4. Complaints of difficulty sleeping because of pain and anxiety

Objective
Impairments
1. Marked wasting of upper and lower extremity muscles
2. Strength: Range of motion—active and passive within normal limits in upper and lower extremities (pain throughout range)
3. Generalized weakness of upper and lower extremities, grade 2–3
4. Exercise tolerance: General debility, complains of fatigue and pain with less than 5 min of activity

Functional limitations
1. Bed mobility: Requires moderate assistance of one person
2. Activities of daily living: Requires moderate assistance of one person for dressing and feeding
3. Transfers: Requires maximal assistance of one person for lying to/from sitting, and sit to/from stand and side of bed
4. Mood: Appears anxious and depressed
5. Limited social interaction

(continued)

Treatment planning	*Treatment rationale* To provide relief of pain, stiffness, anxiety, and depression as the client's functional level declines

Impairment	Role of massage
Pain	Primary treatment; analgesia is a direct effect
Decreased muscle extensibility	Primary treatment; increased muscle extensibility is a direct effect
Muscle wasting	Improbable effect; wasting is due to disuse
Muscle weakness	Possible secondary effect; weakness is primarily due to disuse; pain reduction may facilitate willingness to perform movement through range
Poor exercise tolerance	Possible secondary effect; poor exercise tolerance is a result of debility; pain reduction may facilitate willingness to perform activities
Anxiety	Primary treatment; anxiety relief and systemic sedation are direct effects
Depression	Secondary effect; sensory arousal may ease some symptoms of depression and lethargy

Massage techniques	Static contact, soothing superficial stroking and manually produced fine vibration will almost certainly be tolerated and will all reduce pain, stiffness, and anxiety; machine-produced fine vibration, superficial effleurage, and gentle petrissage (see later chapters) may be tolerated depending on the client's sensitivity, level of debility, and previous familiarity with massage
Other appropriate techniques and interventions	Medical management, passive and active assisted range of motion, assisted activities of daily living, assisted bed mobility and transfers, counseling or pastoral care
Functional outcomes of care	1. Client will be able to perform feeding and dressing with assistance as required with decreased complaints of pain and stiffness 2. Client will be able to perform bed mobility and transfers with assistance as required with decreased complaints of pain and stiffness 3. Client will demonstrate increased social interaction with decreased complaints of depression 4. Client will demonstrate increased duration of sleep with decreased complaints of pain and anxiety interfering with sleep

References

1. Fritz S. Mosby's fundamentals of therapeutic massage. St Louis: Mosby-Lifeline, 2000.
2. American Physical Therapy Association. The guide to physical therapist practice. Phys Ther 1997;77(11):1155–1674.
3. Tappan FM, Benjamin P. Tappan's handbook of healing massage techniques. 3rd ed. Stamford, CT: Appleton & Lange, 1998.
4. Loving J. Massage therapy. Stamford, CT: Appleton & Lange, 1999.
5. de Domenico G, Wood EC. Beard's massage. 4th ed. Philadelphia: WB Saunders, 1997.
6. Salvo SG. Massage therapy. Philadelphia: WB Saunders, 1999.
7. Holey E, Cook E. Therapeutic massage. London, England: WB Saunders, 1997.
8. Knable J. Handholding: one means of transcending barriers of communication. Heart Lung 1981;10:1106.

9. Linn LS, Kahn KL. Physician attitudes toward the "laying on of hands" during the AIDS epidemic. Acad Med 1989;64(7):408–409.

10. McKorkle R. Effects of touch on seriously ill patients. Nurs Res 1974;3(2):125–132.

11. Lynch JJ, Thomas SA, Mills ME, et al. The effects of human contact on cardiac arrhythmia in coronary care patients. J Nerv Ment Dis 1974;158(2):88–89.

12. Lynch JJ, Flaherty L, Emrich C, et al. Effects of human contact on the heart activity of curarized patients in a shock-trauma unit. Am Heart J 1974;88(2):160–169.

13. Weiss SJ. Psychological effects of caregiver touch on incidence of cardiac dysrhythmia. Heart Lung 1986;15(5):496–503.

14. McCaffery M, Wolff M. Pain relief using cutaneous modalities, positioning, and movement. Hospice J 1992;8(1–2):121–153.

15. Werner R, Benjamin BE. A massage therapist's guide to pathology. Baltimore: Williams & Wilkins, 1998.

16. Solkoff N, Matuszak D. Tactile stimulation and behavioral development among low-birthweight infants. Child Psychiatry Hum Dev 1975;6(1):33–37.

17. Kattwinkel J, Nearman HS, Fanaroff AA, et al. Apnea of prematurity: comparative therapeutic effects of cutaneous stimulation and nasal continuous positive airway pressure. J Pediatr 1975;86(4):588–592.

18. Kramer M, Chamorro I, Green D, Knudtson F. Extra tactile stimulation of the premature infant. Nurs Res 1975;24(5):324–334.

19. White JL, Labarda RC. The effects of tactile and kinesthetic stimulation on neonatal development in the premature infant. Dev Psychol 1976;9(6):569–577.

20. Jay SS. The effect of gentle human touch on mechanically ventilated very short-term gestation infants. Matern Child Nurs J 1982;11(4):199–259.

21. Schanberg SM, Evoniuk G, Kuhn CM. Tactile and nutritional aspects of maternal care: specific regulators of neuroendocrine function and cellular development. Proc Soc Exp Biol Med 1984;175:135–146.

22. Field T, Schanberg SM, Scafidi F, et al. Tactile/kinesthetic stimulation effect on preterm neonates. Pediatrics 1986;77(5):654–658.

23. Kisner C, Colby LA. Therapeutic exercise: foundations and techniques. 3rd ed. Philadelphia: FA Davis, 1996.

24. Krieger D. The response of in-vivo human haemoglobin to an active healing therapy by direct laying on of hands. Hum Dimens 1972;1:12–15.

25. Krieger D. Healing by the laying on of hands as a facilitator of bioenergetic change: the response of in-vivo human haemoglobin. Psychoenerg Syst 1974;1:121–129.

26. Krieger D. Therapeutic Touch: the imprimatur of nursing. Am J Nurs 1975;75:784–787.

27. Krieger D, Peper E, Ancoli S. Physiologic indices of therapeutic touch. Am J Nurs 1979;14:660–662.

28. Krieger D. The Therapeutic Touch. New York: Prentice-Hall, 1979.

29. Siedman M. Like a hollow flute: a guide to polarity therapy. Santa Cruz, CA: Elan Press, 1982.

30. Gordon R. Your healing hands: the polarity experience. Santa Cruz, CA: Unity Press, 1979.

31. Stein D. Essential Reiki: a complete guide to an ancient healing art. Freedom, CA: Crossing Press, 1995.

32. Nathan B. Touch and emotion in manual therapy. Edinburgh: Churchill Livingstone, 1999.

33. Moor F, Peterson S, Manwell E, et al. Manual of hydrotherapy and massage. Oshawa, Canada: Pacific Press, 1964.

34. Upledger J, Vredevoogd JD. Craniosacral therapy. Seattle, WA: Eastland Press; 1983.

35. Hollis M. Massage for therapists. 2nd ed. Oxford, England: Blackwell Science, 1998.

36. Mennell JB. Physical treatment by movement, manipulation and massage. 5th ed. Philadelphia: Blakiston, 1945.

37. Longworth JCD. Psychophysiological effects of slow stroke back massage in normotensive females. Adv Nurs Sci 1982;6:44–61.

38. Sims S. Slow stroke back massage for cancer patients. Nurs Times 1986;82:47–50.

39. Fakouri C, Jones P. Relaxation treatment: slow stroke back rub. J Gerontol Nurs 1987;13(2):32–35.

40. Meek SS. Effects of slow stroke back massage on relaxation in hospice clients. Image J Nurs Scholar 1993;25(1):17–21.

41. Lewis P, Nichols E, Mackey G, et al. The effect of turning and backrub on mixed venous oxygen saturation in critically ill patients. Am J Crit Care 1997;6(2):132–140.

42. Hertling D, Kessler RM. Management of common musculoskeletal disorders. 3rd ed. Philadelphia: Lippincott-Raven, 1996.

43. Brouwer B, Sousa de Andrade V. The effects of slow stroking on spasticity in patients with multiple sclerosis: a pilot study. Physiother Theory Pract 1995;11:13–21.

44. Labyak SE, Metzger BL. The effects of effleurage backrub on the physiological components of relaxation: a meta-analysis. Nurs Res 1997;46(1):59–62.

45. Hansson P, Ekblom A. Acute pain relieved by vibratory stimulus. Br Dent J 1981;6:213.

46. Ottoson D, Ekblom A, Hansson P. Vibratory stimulation for the relief of pain of dental origin. Pain 1981;10:37–45.

47. Lundeberg T, Ottoson D, Hakansson S, Meyerson BA. 1983 Vibratory stimulation for the control of intractable chronic orofacial pain. Adv Pain Res Ther 1983;5:555–561.

48. Lundeberg TCM. Vibratory stimulation for the alleviation of chronic pain. Acta Physiol Scand Suppl 1983;523:1–51.

49. Bini G, Cruccu G. Hagbarth KE, et al. Analgesic effect of vibration and cooling on pain induced by intraneural electrical stimulation. Pain 1984;18(3):239–248.

50. Lundeberg T. The pain suppressive effect of vibratory stimulation and transcutaneous electrical nerve stimulation (TENS) as compared to aspirin. Brain Res 1984;294(2):201–209.

51. Lundeberg T. Vibratory stimulation for the alleviation of pain. Am J Chinese Med 1984;12(1–4):60–70.

52. Lundeberg T. A comparative study of the pain alleviating effect of vibratory stimulation, transcutaneous electrical nerve stimulation, electroacupuncture and placebo. Am J Chinese Med 1984;12(1–4):72–79.

53. Lundeberg T. Long-term results of vibratory stimulation as a pain relieving measure for chronic pain. Pain 1984;20: 13–23.

54. Lundeberg T, Nordemar R, Ottoson D. Pain alleviation by vibratory stimulation. Pain 1984;20:25–44.

55. Ekblom A, Hannson P. Extrasegmental transcutaneous electrical nerve stimulation and mechanical vibratory stimulation as compared to placebo for the relief of acute oro-facial pain. Pain 1985;23(3):223–229.

56. Lundeberg T. Naloxone does not reverse the pain-reducing effect of vibratory stimulation. Acta Anaesthesiol Scand 1985;29(2):212–216.

57. Lundeberg T. Relief of pain from a phantom limb by peripheral stimulation. J Neurol 1985;232(2):79–82.

58. Sherer CL, Clelland JA, O'Sullivan P, et al. The effect of two sites of high frequency vibration on cutaneous pain threshold. Pain 1986;25(1):133–138.

59. Lundberg T, Abrahamsson P, Bondesson L, Haber E. Effect of vibratory stimulation on experimental and clinical pain. Scand J Rehabil Med 1988;20(4):149–159.

60. Palmesamo TJ, Clelland JA, Sherer C, et al. Effect of high-frequency vibration on experimental pain threshold in young women when applied to areas of different size. Clin J Pain 1989;5(4):337–342.

61. Guieu R, Tardy-Gervet MF, Blin O, Pouget J. Pain relief achieved by transcutaneous electrical nerve stimulation and/or vibratory stimulation in a case of painful legs and moving toes. Pain 1990;42(1)43–48.

62. Guieu R, Tardy-Gervet MF, Roll JP. Analgesic effects of vibration and transcutaneous electrical nerve stimulation applied separately and simultaneously to patients with chronic pain. Can J Neurol Sci 1991;18(2):113–119.

63. Guieu R, Tardy-Gervet MF, Giraud P. Met-enkephalin and beta-endorphin are not involved in the analgesic action of transcutaneous vibratory stimulation. Pain 1992;48(1): 83–86.

64. Tardy-Gervet MF, Guieu R, Ribot-Ciscar E, Roll JP. [Transcutaneous mechanical vibrations: analgesic effect and antinociceptive mechanisms.] Rev Neurol (Paris) (French). 1993;149(3):177–185. (Abstract)

65. Yarnitsky D, Kunin M, Brik R, Sprecher E. Vibration reduces thermal pain in adjacent dermatomes. Pain 1997;69(1–2):75–77.

66. Cody FWJ, MacDermott N, Ferguson IT. Stretch and vibration reflexes of wrist flexor muscles in spasticity. Brain 1987;110:433–450.

67. Schmitt T, O'Sullivan S. Physical rehabilitation, assessment and treatment. 2nd ed. Philadelphia: FA Davis, 1988.

68. Hagbarth KE, Eklund G. The muscle vibrator: a useful tool in neurological therapeutic work. Scand J Rehabil Med 1969;1:26–34.

69. Matheson DW, Edelson R, Hiatrides D, et al. Relaxation measured by EMG as a function of vibrotactile stimulation. Biofeedback Self Regul 1976;1:285–292.

70. Spicher C, Kohut G. [A significant increase in superficial sensation, a number of years after a peripheral neurologic lesion, using transcutaneous vibratory stimulation.] Ann Chir Main Memb Super (French) 1997;16(2):124–129. (Abstract)

71. Michlovitz S. Thermal agents in rehabilitation. 3rd ed. Philadelphia: FA Davis, 1996.

Suggested Readings

Burke D, Hagbarth KE, Lofstedt L, Wallin BG. The responses of human muscle spindle endings to vibration of non-contracting muscles. J Physiol 1976;261(3):673–693.

Carter A. The use of touch in nursing practice. Nurs Stand 1995;9(16):31–35.

Cashar L, Dixon BK. The therapeutic use of touch. J Psychiatr Nurs 1967;5:442–451.

Ching M. The use of touch in nursing practice. Aust J Adv Nurs 1993;10(4):4–9.

Cochran-Fritz S. Physiological effects of massage on the nervous system. Int J Altern Complementary Med 1993;Sep: 21–25.

Cody FWJ, Plant T. Vibration-evoked reciprocal inhibition between human wrist muscles. Brain Res 1989;78: 613–623.

Doering TJ, Fieguth HG, Steuernagel B, Brix J, Konitzer M, Schneider B, Fischer GC. External stimuli in the form of vibratory massage after heart or lung transplantation. Am J Phys Med Rehabil 1999;78(2):108–110.

Doraisamy P. The management of spasticity—a review of options available in rehabilitation. Ann Acad Med Singapore. 1992;21(6):807–812.

Geis F, Viksne V. Touching: physical contact and level of arousal. Proceedings of the 80th Annual Convention of the American Psychological Association 1972;7:179–180.

Hayes JA. TAC-TIC therapy: a non-pharmacological stroking intervention for premature infants. Complement Ther Nurs Midwifery 1998;4(1):25–27.

Issurin VB, Tenenbaum G. Acute and residual effects of vibratory stimulation on explosive strength in elite and amateur athletes. J Sports Sci 1999;17(3):177–182.

Kuntz A. Anatomic and physiologic properties of cutaneo-visceral vasomotor reflex arc. J Neurophysiol 1945;8:421–430.

MacManaway B, Turcan J. Healing. Wellingborough, England: Thorsons, 1983.

Malaquin-Pavan E. [Therapeutic benefit of touch-massage in the overall management of demented elderly] (French). Rech Soins Infirm 1997;(49):11–66. Abstract.

Mansour AA, Beuche M, Laing G, Leis A, Nurse J. A study to test the effectiveness of placebo Reiki standardization procedures developed for a planned Reiki efficacy study. J Altern Complement Med 1999;5(2): 153–164.

Matthew PBC. The reflex excitation of the soleus muscle of a decerebrated cat caused by vibration applied to its tendon. J Physiol 1966;184:450–472.

Naliboff BD, Tachhiki KH. Autonomic and skeletal muscle responses to non-electrical cutaneous stimulation. Percept Motor Skills 1991;72(2):575–584.

Tyler DO, Winslow EH, Clark AP, White KM. Effects of a one minute back rub on mixed venous saturation and heart rate in critically ill patients. Heart Lung 1990;19(5): 562–565.

Ulm G. The current significance of physiotherapeutic measures in the treatment of Parkinson's disease. J Neural Transm Suppl 1995;46:455–460.

Vickers A, Ohlsson A, Lacy JB, Horsley A. Massage for promoting growth and development of preterm and/or low birth-weight infants. Cochrane Database Syst Rev 2000;(2): CD000390.

6

Superficial Fluid Techniques

Superficial fluid techniques are massage techniques that are applied to tissues superficial to muscle to increase the return flow of lymph. These techniques include superficial effleurage and superficial lymph drainage technique. This chapter describes each of these techniques, how to perform the technique, and how to apply it in a practice sequence. It also includes a discussion of the indications, contraindications, cautions, outcomes of care, and postintervention care associated with each technique.

Table 6-1
Summary of Impairment-Level Outcomes of Care for Superficial Fluid Techniques

Impairment-Level Outcome of Care	Technique	
	Superficial Effleurage	Superficial Lymph Drainage Technique
Systemic sedation	✓	✓
Decreased anxiety	✓	✓
Counterirritant analgesia	P	P
Increased venous return	?	✓
Decreased edema	P	✓
Increased lymphatic return	P	✓

✓, the outcome is supported by research summarized in this chapter; P, the outcome is probable; ?, the outcome is debatable (research results are not consistent).

Superficial Effleurage

OTHER NAMES USED FOR THIS TECHNIQUE

"Effleurage," "gliding," "stroking," "deep stroking."[1–8]

DEFINITION

Superficial effleurage: a gliding manipulation performed with light centripetal pressure that deforms subcutane-

ous tissue down to the investing layer of the deep fascia.[1–8]

NOTE

Some authors use the terms "effleurage" and "stroking" interchangeably.[1–5] This book follows the convention used in many texts, including *Beard's Massage*,[6] which distinguishes between effleurage and stroking on the basis of the pressure, direction, tissues engaged, and clinical effects of the strokes.[6–8] Although superficial effleurage may be used to produce similar reflex effects to those produced with superficial stroking (discussed in Chapter 5), it has additional effects on fluid dynamics.

The use of the word "effleurage" in current texts is (alas) highly variable with respect to the type and depth of tissues engaged by the stroke that is being described. Consequently, this book makes a further distinction between superficial effleurage and the similarly patterned deep effleurage, which uses sufficient pressure to engage and deform muscle (see Chapter 7, Neuromuscular Techniques). There is precedent and a clinical rationale for making this distinction; the clinician must learn to discriminate clearly among the various tissue layers—skin, subcutaneous fascia and fat, and muscle.[1,3,5,7] This ability will enable the clinician to selectively direct the force of a massage stroke toward each tissue layer, as required to achieve the desired treatment outcomes.

CLINICAL INDICATIONS AND IMPAIRMENT-LEVEL OUTCOMES OF CARE

This light, flowing technique can be used to facilitate the flow of interventions and to achieve circulatory effects, psychological effects, and a variety of physiological effects. Superficial effleurage is ideal for spreading lubricant and is commonly used as an introductory stroke in regional and general massage. It can also be used as a transitional stroke and between deeper techniques that engage the client's muscles (see Chapter 7, Neuromuscular Techniques).

Superficial effleurage is best known for its circulatory effects; numerous sources state that effleurage (in some form) increases lymphatic and venous return from the region to which it is applied.[1–8] One possible mechanism for this effect on lymphatic flow is that the gentle mechanical stresses of superficial effleurage produce a contraction of the lymphatic vessels, thereby increasing the formation and return of lymph.[9] Furthermore, superficial effleurage may produce direct movement of lymph when the pressure of the stroke is light and the rate of glide is slow. Notwithstanding its mechanical effect on lymphatic vessels, superficial effleurage does not appear to affect local arterial or venous flow, at least in healthy tissues.[10–12]

Effects on lymphatic flow make superficial effleurage an indicated treatment for conditions of lymphatic congestion, including dependent edema; edema or effusion associated with the acute and subacute phases of common musculoskeletal injuries such as bursitis,

sprains, strains, contusions, dislocations, separations, and fractures; reflex sympathetic dystrophy; and congestion of the breast associated with menses or lactation. It may also be of use when treating venous stasis[12] and related conditions, such as varicosities and venous ulcers. Finally, superficial effleurage is useful in the treatment of lymphedema following surgical excision of lymphatics.[13] In light of its range of effects on lymphatic flow, superficial effleurage is a component technique in some systems of manual lymph drainage.

Superficial effleurage also has a variety of other psychological and physiological effects. As with superficial stroking, superficial effleurage can be used to decrease anxiety, induce relaxation,[14,15] temporarily decrease lower motor neuron excitability,[16,17] and stimulate peristalsis.[18–19] Because of its mild mechanical effects, superficial effleurage can be used with superficial reflex techniques to induce sedation, increase general comfort, and reduce the perception of pain in postoperative situations. It is also indicated for infant colic.[19] The main impairment-level outcomes of care for superficial effleurage are summarized in Table 6-1.

CAUTIONS AND CONTRAINDICATIONS

Clinical training and supervised practice are critical for the proper application of superficial effleurage. Advanced training may be advisable in certain situations, particularly when dealing with pathological conditions. Although superficial effleurage only uses enough pressure to deform superficial fat and fascia, with their associated superficial vessels, the clinician should consider all contraindications and cautions to massage (see Chapter 2, The Clinical Decision-Making Process).[1] There are several contraindications for clients with cardiac, orthopedic, and metabolic conditions. Superficial effleurage is generally well tolerated by critically ill clients.[20,21] For acute cardiac conditions, however, although light massage is beneficial after myocardial infarction, there is a caution to allow a 48-hour wait after coronary artery bypass surgery before using massage.[15,20] Furthermore, the clinician must exercise caution when the client presents with cardiac insufficiency or congestive heart failure, since an increase in venous return can compromise cardiac or pulmonary function. Local application of superficial effleurage may be contraindicated or not well tolerated by clients with acute orthopedic injuries or reflex sympathetic dystrophy. In these situations, the clinician should apply the technique proximal to the site of the injury to enhance drainage. In general, the clinician should not apply superficial effleurage over newly forming scars,[22] areas of confirmed or suspected infection, cellulitis, and thrombus. The use of superficial effleurage may increase the rate of kidney filtration in clients with serious kidney pathology or nutritional deficiency and lead to complications. Finally, even the use of light massage may reduce the duration of effectiveness of epidural anesthesia.[23]

Prerequisite Skills for Superficial Effleurage

Before practicing superficial effleurage technique, students should know how to

Recognize major vascular disease

Recognize major lymphatic dysfunction

Use standing aligned, lunge, and lunge and reach postures

Palpate the thickness of superficial fascia and fat

Accurately locate the investing layer of deep fascia

Manual Technique begins on next page

MANUAL TECHNIQUE

Superficial Effleurage

In the following figures (Figs. 6-1 to 6-9), superficial effleurage is applied to the various regions of the body. Figures are ordered from head to foot in supine and then prone. Each figure illustrates most of the guidelines for manual technique outlined below.

1. Lubricant is preferred when performing superficial effleurage. However, unless the skin is moist or very hairy, the clinician can perform superficial effleurage effectively without lubricant.

2. Hand(s) are as softly relaxed as possible while gliding over the skin. The entire palmar surface molds continuously to the changing contours of the client's body, like water flowing over substrate. Fingers may be spread apart, but not so widely that the hand becomes tense. The thumb may be abducted to enable the clinician to use the web space to encircle a limb.

3. The hand points in the general direction of the pressure stroke. Small deviations of the wrist are used to enable the hand to conform to local body contours. The clinician must make every effort to minimize the amount of radial or ulnar wrist deviation, to prevent repetitive strain injury.

4. Pressure of the stroke is toward axillary or inguinal lymph nodes on the trunk (Fig. 6-3) and centripetal on the limbs (Figs. 6-4A and B, 6-5, and 6-7). When the clinician applies this technique to the client's back, the stroke most commonly begins at the sacrum and moves toward the axilla (Fig. 6-6), although it can also be applied from the head down.

5. With each repetition, the centripetal pressure stroke engages progressively deeper layers of tissue, advancing as deep as the investing layer of the deep fascia. The clinician repeats strokes 5 to 10 times or more, to overcome the inertial resistance of fluid. Using the same pattern of movement, the clinician can gradually increase the amount of pressure applied and engage underlying muscle if this is indicated (see Chapter 7, Neuromuscular Techniques).

6. Some authors suggest that the pressure of each stroke can be increased with increasing proximity of the hand(s) to the heart.[6,8] The clinician can also use a distinct pause with slight overpressure at the proximal end of the stroke, preferably over a set of lymph nodes.

7. The rate of the stroke can vary from 5 to 50 cm/sec. One author specifies a rate of 15 cm/sec or 6 to 7 inches/sec.[6]

8. There are varying opinions on the use of the return stroke. The return stroke may be omitted, since the production of even a slight centrifugal pressure conflicts with the aim of assisting fluid return (Figs. 6-1 and 6-2A). Alternatively, the clinician may allow the hand(s) to remain in contact with the client's body for the return stroke but use minimal pressure while performing dragless superficial stroking with either palmar or fingertip contact (Fig. 6-2 B and C). If the clinician chooses to use a return stroke, the transition from one direction to the other must not be abrupt.

9. Alternating, two-handed superficial effleurage, with the return strokes performed in the air, is a useful variation.

10. Thumb or finger contact is used on smaller parts or around the periphery of swelling, with the same general intention (Figs. 6-8 and 6-9). Forelimbs and digits may be encircled with a "bracelet" or "ring" contact.

Manual Technique continues on page 150

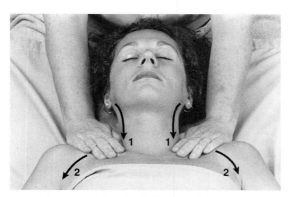

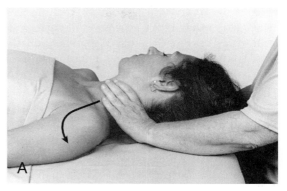

Figure 6-1. Bilateral superficial effleurage of the neck and shoulders. The stroke moves down the neck, over the clavicles toward the axillae, finishing at the deltoid, and settling the shoulders with a gentle downward pressure.

Figure 6-2. A. Unilateral superficial effleurage of the rotated neck. The stroke may end at the root of the neck or continue over the clavicle toward the axilla.

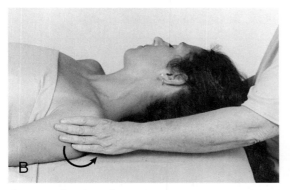

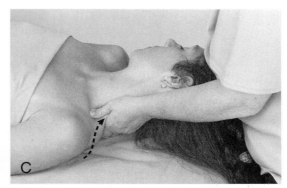

Figure 6-2 (continued). B. A light return stroke may be added at the end of the stroke. To perform this, the forearm supinates while the hand maintains contact with the client's skin. **C.** And the hand draws lightly back toward the occiput.

Manual Technique Figures continue on next page

11. When the clinician is using superficial effleurage to treat localized swelling, it is preferable to treat proximal regions first and to ensure that the individual strokes begin at the proximal margin or the periphery of the swelling so that no attempt is made to push fluid into or through an area of congestion. Later chapters discuss the design of comprehensive massage sequences to increase lymphatic and venous return.

Components of Superficial Effleurage

Contact: Whole relaxed palmar surface of hand

Pressure: Light

Engages: Skin, superficial fascia, and fat

Direction: On limbs, centripetal; on torso, toward axillary or inguinal lymph nodes

Amplitude: Length of the region

Rate: 5 to 50 cm/sec

Duration: 2 min or longer

Intergrades[a] with: Petrissage and superficial stroking

Context: Used for extended periods alone or alternating with superficial lymph drainage technique to facilitate return of lymph and possibly blood; commonly used as a prelude and postlude to extended application of neuromuscular techniques

---

[a]To merge gradually into one another.

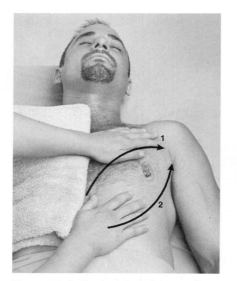

Figure 6-3. On the chest, for both men and women, strokes are directed toward the axilla while avoiding the region of the client's nipple. (For concepts related to the ethics of touching the breast, see Chapter 2, The Clinical Decision-Making Process and Chapter 4, Preparation and Positioning for Treatment.)

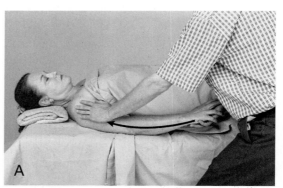

Figure 6-4. During superficial effleurage of the arm, the clinician alternates application of the stroke to the lateral and medial surfaces of the client's arm. **A.** The lateral surface.

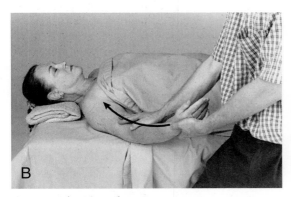

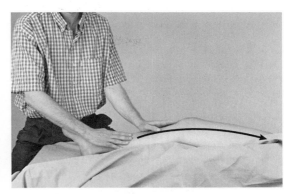

Figure 6-4, (continued). B. The medial surface. Note the change in the clinician's stance.

Figure 6-5. Medial and lateral surfaces of the client's leg can often be included in the same stroke. Note the clinician's upright posture.

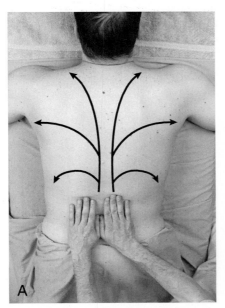

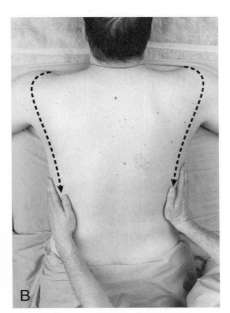

Figure 6-6. A, B. Bilateral superficial effleurage of the back begins at the sacrum and can follow different paths. The clinician may alternate these different paths on consecutive strokes.

Manual Technique Figures continue on next page

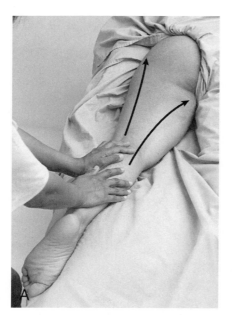
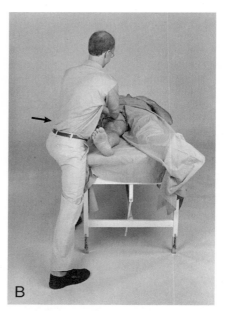

Figure 6-7. **A.** Superficial effleurage of the posterior leg, including the gluteals. **B.** For this technique, which requires light pressure, the clinician should achieve the stroke length primarily through leg movement while maintaining an upright torso. Here, on the other hand, the clinician is reaching and leaning; if repeated, this action will place unnecessary strain on the lower back.

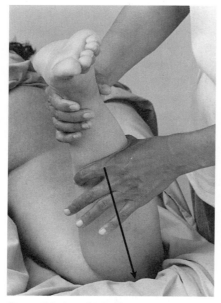

Figure 6-8. Superficial effleurage applied to the ankle with an encircling "bracelet" contact.

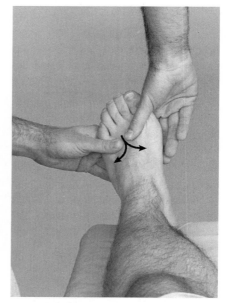

Figure 6-9. Superficial effleurage with short thumb strokes will increase lymphatic return from the foot. Similar short strokes can be used to drain posttraumatic edema in a centrifugal direction, away from the periphery of swelling.

CLINICIAN'S POSITION AND MOVEMENT

1. The basic positions used by the clinician are described in Chapter 4, Preparation and Positioning for Treatment, in the sections on standing aligned posture, lunge, and lunge and reach.
2. When applying superficial effleurage to a large region such as the back or the legs, the clinician achieves the full length of the strokes through appropriate movement of the legs, rather than through overreaching with the arms. Throughout the stroke, the clinician's torso remains upright to minimize repetitive flexion and extension of the lumbar spine (Figs. 6-5, 6-7B).

PALPATE

As he performs the technique, the clinician palpates the client for the following:

1. Skin texture
2. Skin temperature
3. Presence of perspiration and moisture
4. Horizontal stretch of the skin and subcutaneous fascia, which occurs in the direction of movement; however, because lubricant reduces drag, these superficial tissues are not stretched to their elastic limit
5. Subcutaneous fatty lipomas that are common on the back[24] and floating, hard fibrositic nodules that are common around the iliac crest and occiput; both of these can be tender on palpation
6. Surface contours
7. Increased pliability that reflects the reduction of viscosity of healthy superficial subcutaneous tissues, which normally occurs with continued application
8. Inertial resistance of the subcutaneous tissue, which reflects its fluid content (i.e., interstitial fluid pressure)
9. Resorption of fluid from edematous tissue, which is accompanied by changes in surface contours and the viscosity and inertial resistance of the subcutaneous tissues

OBSERVE

As he performs the technique, the clinician observes the client for signs of reduction of swelling or of relaxation. The signs listed below may signal this.

REDUCTION OF SWELLING

1. Normalization of skin color and texture
2. Change of surface contours
3. Visible reduction of swelling, which may often occur within 15 to 45 min; cumulative reduction of swelling will occur during the course of the treatment regimen, with resolution of an inflammatory process, or with resolution of circulatory and lymphatic dysfunction

RELAXATION

1. Decrease in rate and depth of breathing
2. Deeper voice tone
3. Changes in skin color, such as flushing; pallor may indicate an undesirable sympathetic response
4. Systemic reduction of muscle resting tension, as evidenced by softening of the tissue contours or broadening and flattening of body segments
5. Muscle twitches and jerks
6. Increases in peristaltic noises
7. Decreases in heart rate, as evidenced by change in pulses that are visible at the neck, wrist, and foot
8. Agitation or sweating, which may indicate an undesirable sympathetic response

COMMUNICATION WITH THE CLIENT

The clinician uses communication that seeks feedback on the client's level of comfort during the technique. Some examples of statements that the clinician can use are listed below.

1. "Let me know if this pressure becomes uncomfortable." When the clinician is treating close to areas of acute or subacute inflammation, he must ensure that the pressure of the technique does not increase the client's level of pain.
2. "What is happening with your pain." This statement can be used when the technique is being applied to reduce pain, to check periodically how the client perceives that the client's pain has been affected by the intervention.
3. The clinician should also encourage the client to perform deep diaphragmatic breathing during the intervention.

COMPLEMENTARY MODALITIES

There are several modalities that the clinician can use in a complementary manner with superficial effleurage.

1. For edema secondary to trauma that the clinician is treating in the acute stage, the appropriate regimen (RICE) includes rest, ice or the application of cold for 10 to 15 min, compression, and elevation of the

limbs to 30 or 45 degrees. Passive relaxed movements and gentle joint mobilization techniques (grade 1 sustained and grades 1 and 2 oscillating) can be used to reduce pain. The clinician should also encourage the client to perform deep diaphragmatic breathing.

2. The comprehensive treatment of lymphedema involves client education on appropriate hygiene, the regular use of compression bandages and garments, and specialized active exercises. Depending on the nature and extent of lymphedema, any of the following direct interventions may be indicated: gait, locomotion, balance, and posture awareness training; strengthening; and functional training in self-care and home management, including the use of assistive and adaptive devices.[2] Neuromuscular and connective tissue massage techniques may be useful for fibrosed edema.

SELF-CARE INSTRUCTIONS

1. For hydrostatic edema related to acute orthopedic injuries, the clinician instructs the client on the uses of elevation, compression, rest, and ice.
2. Clients with lymphedema require detailed, expert instruction on skin care, bandaging, and exercise.

A Practice Sequence for Superficial Effleurage

The following sequence of body regions is generally ordered from proximal to distal, and can be completed in 30 min. Apply superficial effleurage to each region in succession. Begin the strokes distally within each region and cover the entire region with centripetal strokes that run the full length of the region. Repeat strokes several times.

Supine: Neck, face, chest, arm, abdomen, anterior legs

Prone: Back, gluteals, posterior legs

Try variations that

Use only the centripetal pressure stroke

Use superficial stroking to return to the starting position

Use constant pressure

Increase pressure slightly as the strokes move proximally

Pause over lymph nodes at the proximal end of the stroke

Use different rates (5–50 cm/sec)

How you would apply the technique using only sidelying positions while working from proximal to distal regions?

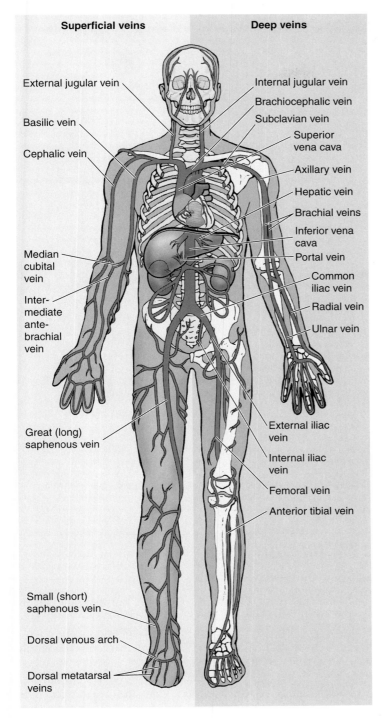

Superficial veins   **Deep veins**

External jugular vein

Basilic vein

Cephalic vein

Median cubital vein

Intermediate antebrachial vein

Great (long) saphenous vein

Small (short) saphenous vein

Dorsal venous arch

Dorsal metatarsal veins

Internal jugular vein

Brachiocephalic vein

Subclavian vein

Superior vena cava

Axillary vein

Hepatic vein

Brachial veins

Inferior vena cava

Portal vein

Common iliac vein

Radial vein

Ulnar vein

External iliac vein

Internal iliac vein

Femoral vein

Anterior tibial vein

Principal veins

Figure 6-10. Venous return to the heart. Reprinted from Moore, K. Clinically Oriented Anatomy, 4th Edition, (1999) p. 33 with the permission of Lippincott Williams & Wilkins.

Figure 6-11. Lymphatic watersheds with indication of the direction of flow of lymph. (Redrawn from Tappan FM, Benjamin PJ. Tappan's Handbook of Healing Massage Techniques, 3rd Edition, p 227. Copyright 1998. Adapted with permission from Prentice-Hall, Inc, Upper Saddle River, NJ).

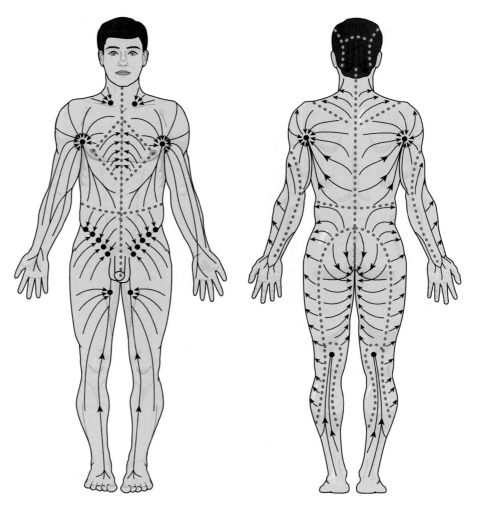

Superficial Lymph Drainage Technique

DEFINITION

Superficial lymph drainage technique: a nongliding technique performed in the direction of lymphatic flow, using short, rhythmical strokes with minimal to light pressure, which deforms subcutaneous tissue without engaging muscle.[25–33]

NOTE

Superficial lymph drainage technique is a variant of superficial effleurage that was developed in the 20th century by Emil Vodder and subsequently elaborated on by several schools of manual lymph drainage (MLD).[25–33] Superficial lymph drainage and superficial effleurage have in common the application of light pressure that is directed centripetally through the same tissue layer. During superficial effleurage, however, the clinician's hands glide over the skin—it is a faster and more general manipulation. Conversely, during superficial lymph drainage technique the clinician very gently stretches the client's skin, superficial fascia, and accompanying lymphatics to their elastic limit in the direction of lymphatic flow, without compressing deeper structures, and then carefully releases the stretched tissues.

Superficial lymph drainage technique is a principal technique of the various schools of MLD, which may also use superficial effleurage, compression, and other techniques, with variable emphasis in their treatment regimens.

CLINICAL INDICATIONS AND IMPAIRMENT-LEVEL OUTCOMES OF CARE

Local applications of superficial lymph drainage technique can increase lymphatic return from the region to which it is applied. When the clinician applies this technique to larger areas of the client's body, it can produce an increase in the volume of lymph that is returned to the venous system. The proposed mechanism for these effects is that the slow, delicate, rhythmical stretching of the tissues stimulates contraction of the lymphatic vessels,[9,25,29] propels lymph through the collapsible superficial lymphatics,[25,29,34] increases local blood flow,[35] and reduces the time required for alternative pathways (anastamoses) to form after lymphatic pathways have been interrupted by damage. When this technique is performed skillfully, it can result in sedation (parasympathetic activity), reduced pain (counterirritant analgesia), and improvement in general immune function.[25,36]

Superficial lymph drainage technique can be used as part of a comprehensive treatment regimen known as complex or complete decongestive therapy or physiotherapy, (CDT, CDP, or CDMT). This treatment regimen includes bandaging or compression garments, specific exercises, and education on hygiene.[31–33] It is a well-documented regimen that extensive research suggests is effective in the treatment of lymphedema,[37–51] particularly lymphedema that arises after surgical intervention in breast cancer.[32,52–64] Superficial lymph drainage is effective for traumatic edema,[65,66] venous insufficiency,[67,68] acne,[25,29] and a variety of other conditions.[69–76] The main impairment-level outcomes of care for superficial lymph drainage are summarized in Table 6-1.

CAUTIONS AND CONTRAINDICATIONS

Clinical training and supervised practice are critical for the proper application of superficial lymph drainage technique. Advanced training may be advisable in certain situations, particularly when dealing with pathological conditions. The contraindications to the use of techniques with mechanical effects apply to the use of superficial lymph drainage (see Chapter 2, The Clinical Decision-Making Process).

The contraindications to the use of superficial lymph drainage technique include acute systemic or local inflammation due to bacterial or viral infection, untreated metastatic disease, allergic reactions, recent thrombosis, and edema due to right-sided heart failure (the client may be massaged outside the area of the edema).[25,27,29,77–78]

There are several cautions to the use of superficial lymph drainage technique. The clinician must exercise caution when the client presents with cardiac insufficiency or congestive heart failure, since an increase in venous return can compromise cardiac or pulmonary function. When the client presents with thyroid hyperactivity, avoid local application in the area of the thyroid. If the client has asthma, then treat between attacks, use shorter interventions, and avoid applying around the area of the sternum. The clinician should avoid the client's abdomen during menstruation and reduce or omit treatment during pregnancy. If the client has low blood pressure, use caution and shorten interventions in early stages of treatment.[25,27,29] When treating traumatic edema—as with any condition—the application of superficial lymph drainage must be painless and pleasant. If the client is unable to tolerate a local application of this technique, only apply it proximally. Using superficial lymph drainage technique on chronic inflammation may stimulate a transient acute inflammation.[27] Finally, the client may experience slight nausea or fatigue following full-body sessions.[29]

Prerequisite Skills for Superficial Lymph Drainage Technique

Before practicing superficial lymph drainage technique, students should know how to

- Recognize major vascular disease
- Recognize major lymphatic dysfunction
- Use standing aligned, seated aligned, and lunge postures
- Palpate the thickness of subcutaneous fat
- Find the elastic barrier in the skin and in the superficial fat and fascia
- Accurately locate the investing layer of the deep fascia

Manual Technique begins on next page

MANUAL TECHNIQUE

Superficial Lymph Drainage

In the following figures (Figs. 6-12 to 6-20), superficial lymph drainage technique is applied to the various regions of the body. Figures are ordered from head to foot in supine and then prone. Each figure illustrates most of the guidelines for manual technique outlined below.

1. No oil is used. If the skin of either the clinician or the client is moist, the clinician may apply enough unscented fine talc, cornstarch, or chalk to his hands to prevent sticking.

2. This technique demands supreme relaxation of the hands, which only comes from extensive practice. Any part of the hand can be used, as long as the manual contact is soft and evenly distributed (e.g., Figs. 6-15, 6-16, and 6-19). The clinician may abduct his thumb so the web space forms part of the contact surface (Fig. 6-15). When he is treating smaller parts of the body, fingerpad or thumb contact is useful (Figs. 6-12, 6-13, and 6-20).

3. Two hands placed side by side can create a larger contact that is suitable for broad areas like the torso or thigh (Fig. 6-16).

4. The clinician uses minimal pressure to engage the skin and sink slightly into the subcutaneous fat; little or no indentation should be visible. He then gently stretches the skin and superficial fascia in the general direction of lymphatic flow, without engaging underlying muscle, by applying pressure that is directed parallel to the surface. He can obtain better results if the stroke shape is semi-elliptical or semicircular, so that stretch of the tissues occurs in two directions on the plane of the surface of the client's skin while he maintains a general centripetal orientation.[25,29]

5. The working surface of the clinician's hand does not glide over the skin.

6. At the end of each slow, short stroke, when the skin and superficial fascia have been stretched in a manner that takes the slack out of these tissues, the clinician pauses, then gradually releases the pressure he exerted and allows the skin to return to its original position.

7. Hands may remain in one place on the client's skin, so that the clinician can perform several strokes on the same location. In that situation, he must take care to ensure that no centrifugal pressure is exerted as his hand follows the skin back to its original position (Figs. 6-12, 6-14, 6-16, and 6-18). Alternatively, he may gently break contact with the client's body and move his hand(s) slightly proximally with each successive stroke, essentially "walking" his hands along the client's body part (Figs. 6-15 and 6-17). In either case, he should repeat strokes or series of strokes several times to overcome the inertial resistance of the fluid. Bear in mind that developing the requisite fine control of pressure while performing this technique takes considerable practice.

8. The order of the intervention is important when using superficial lymphatic drainage technique. The clinician should begin intervention at the proximal junction between the lymphatic and venous systems (Fig. 6-12), treat the client's neck, and drain the client's related trunk quadrant before proceeding to an affected limb. If time for the session is constrained, he reduces the amount of time he spends treating the affected area rather than that spent on the proximal areas.[31] He will begin work on the limb by opening axillary or inguinal areas, whether or not the associated lymph nodes are intact (Fig. 6-14). Furthermore, he should treat proximal portions of an affected region before distal portions. Finally, he should make frequent returns to the proximal areas that he cleared earlier in the intervention, thus achieving a frequent movement back and forth from proximal areas to distal areas.

Manual Technique continues on page 160

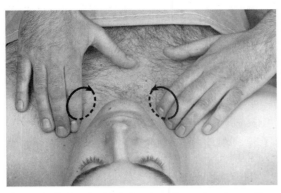

Figure 6-12. A series of strokes down the neck ends near the junction of the venous and lymphatic systems; pressure is directed inferiorly under the clavicle and medially toward the "terminus." This sequence clears the most proximal portion of the lymphatic system and begins any intervention. The clinician should repeat this stroke several times.

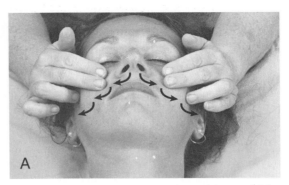

Figure 6-13. A. Fingerpad contact can be used for superficial lymph drainage of the face.

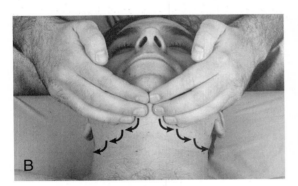

Figure 6-13 (continued). B. Fingerpad contact can also be used for the submandibular region.

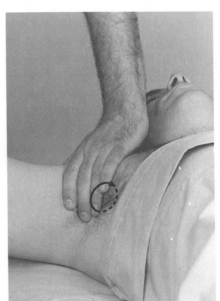

Figure 6-14. Axillary and inguinal areas are treated prior to work on the related limb, and the clinician returns frequently to these areas during work on the client's limb. The hand directs pressure toward the midline of the arm and superiorly.

Manual Technique Figures continue on next page

9. If the client's lymphatic passages have been obstructed or recently irradiated, the strokes performed by the clinician are directed across normal lymphatic watersheds to the nearest group of nodes that have intact drainage, often the contralateral axillary or inguinal nodes, or the ipsilateral abdomen, since these areas must be thoroughly drained first to prepare them to receive lymph.[31]

10. Once the clinician has become familiar with the delicate contact required for performing superficial lymphatic drainage, he can strive to attain regularity of stroke rhythm, to enhance the technique's sedative effect.

11. Superficial lymphatic drainage technique and its related complementary modalities are time consuming to deliver. During the initial stages of treatment, daily interventions of up to 45 to 90 min are often desirable, depending on the client's condition and the severity of her edema.[29,31]

Components of Superficial Lymph Drainage Technique

Contact: The entire relaxed palmar surface of the hand, heel of the hand, grouped fingers

Pressure: Minimal to light (5 mm Hg, "the weight of a nickel")

Engages: Skin, superficial fascia, and fat only

Direction: Centripetal, in the direction of lymphatic pathways

Amplitude/length: Short, less than 2.5 cm (1 inch)

Rate: Slow, about 2.5 cm/sec

Duration: 5 to 60 min or longer

Intergrades with: Superficial effleurage

Combines with: May be combined with varying amounts of compression (for fibrosed edema)

Context: Used alone for extended periods or alternated with superficial effleurage

---

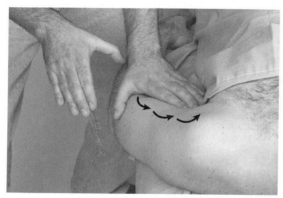

Figure 6-15. The index finger, abducted thumb, and adjacent palm form a surface that can fit the arm well. The hands alternate and move proximally with each stroke. The sequence from elbow to axilla may be repeated several times. (A similar sequence uses the ulnar border of the palm to make contact.)

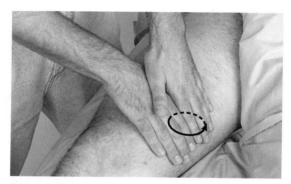

Figure 6-16. Stationary ellipses on the anterior thigh. The return stroke *(dotted line)* must be applied without centrifugal pressure. Instead, the clinician's hand should follow the elastic recoil of the skin.

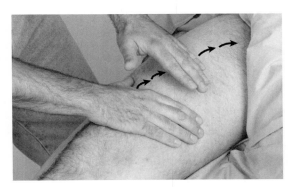

Figure 6-17. The two hands can work together: one moving the lymph forward and the second holding the lymph as the first hand moves more proximally in preparation for the next stroke.

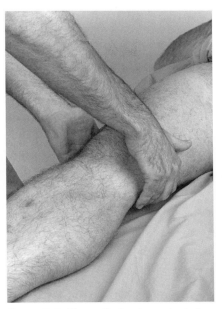

Figure 6-18. The popliteal nodes are treated with the client in supine.

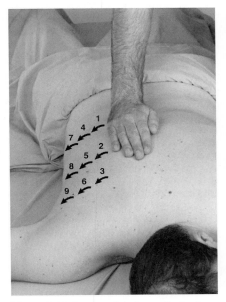

Figure 6-19. A series of strokes on the back directs pressure toward the axilla.

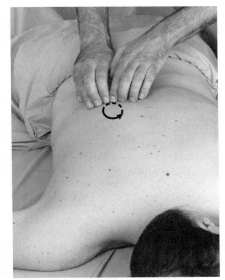

Figure 6-20. Fingerpad technique along the intercostal spaces; pressure is gently directed into the rib spaces and toward the spine to access deeper intrathoracic lymphatics.

CLINICIAN'S POSITION AND MOVEMENT

1. The basic positions used by the clinician are described in Chapter 4, Preparation and Positioning for Treatment, in the sections on standing aligned, seated aligned, and lunge postures. Since superficial lymph drainage technique strokes are short, relatively little reaching is required.

2. Adjusting the manual contact to the contours of the client and the region of application requires flexibility in the movement of the clinician's shoulders and elbows. Consequently, the clinician may use relatively large movements of the arm to achieve small manual movements.

PALPATE

As he performs the technique, the clinician palpates the client for the following:

1. Skin texture
2. Skin temperature
3. Presence of perspiration and moisture
4. Stretch in skin and subcutaneous fascia; because the rate of movement is slow, the end feel of this gentle stretch of the superficial tissues can be palpated; the clinician works up to, but not through, this barrier
5. Subcutaneous fatty lipomas, which are common on the back,[24] and floating, hard fibrositic nodules, which are common around the iliac crest and occiput; both of these can be tender on palpation
6. Surface contours
7. Increased pliability that reflects the reduction of viscosity of healthy superficial subcutaneous tissues, which normally occurs with continued application
8. Inertial resistance of the subcutaneous tissue that reflects its fluid content (i.e., interstitial fluid pressure)
9. Density of edematous tissue, related to its degree of fibrosis
10. Resorption of fluid from edematous tissue, which is accompanied by changes in surface contours, tissue stretch, tissue density, and the viscosity and inertial resistance of the subcutaneous tissues

OBSERVE

As he performs the technique, the clinician observes the client for signs of reduction of swelling. The signs listed below may signal this.

1. Normalization of skin color and texture
2. Reduction of trophic changes
3. Reduction of surface contours
4. Visible reduction of swelling, which may often occur within 15 to 45 min; cumulative reduction of swelling will occur during the course of the treatment regimen, with resolution of an inflammatory process, or with resolution of circulatory and lymphatic dysfunction

COMMUNICATION WITH THE CLIENT

The clinician uses communication that seeks feedback on the client's level of comfort during the technique. Some issues that the clinician needs to address and examples of statements that the clinician can use are listed below.

1. "Let me know if this pressure becomes uncomfortable." When the clinician is treating near areas of acute or subacute inflammation, he should ensure that the mechanical stimulus of the technique is tolerable. This technique should be painless at all times.

2. The clinician should advise the client to urinate before the intervention and inform her that she may still need to urinate during or soon after its conclusion.[50]

3. The clinician should explain to the client that it is not uncommon to experience fatigue after the initial intervention. In addition, he should request that the client report the occurrence of other sequelae, such as nausea if it is more than slight, shivering, or postintervention pain, which suggest overtreatment.

COMPLEMENTARY MODALITIES

There are several modalities that the clinician can use in a complementary manner with superficial lymph drainage technique.

1. For edema secondary to trauma that the clinician is treating in the acute stage, the appropriate regimen (RICE) includes rest, ice or the application of cold for 10 to 15 min, compression, and elevation of the limbs to 30 or 45 degrees. Passive relaxed movements and gentle joint mobilization techniques (grade 1 sustained and grades 1 and 2 oscillating) can be used to reduce pain. The clinician should also encourage the client to perform deep diaphragmatic breathing during the intervention.

2. For edema related to dependency or venous stasis, raised leg exercises may be helpful.[79]

3. The comprehensive treatment of lymphedema involves client education on appropriate hygiene, the regular use of compression bandages and garments,

and specialized active exercises.[28,32,33,53,62] Depending on the nature and extent of lymphedema, any of the following direct interventions may be indicated: gait, locomotion, balance, and posture awareness training; strengthening; and functional training in self-care and home management, including the use of assistive and adaptive devices.[2] Neuromuscular and connective tissue massage techniques may be useful for fibrosed edema.

SELF-CARE INSTRUCTIONS

1. For hydrostatic edema related to acute orthopedic injuries, the clinician instructs the client on the uses of elevation, compression, rest, and ice.
2. Clients with lymphedema require detailed expert instruction on skin care, bandaging, and exercise.
3. Clients with edema related to dependency or venous stasis can benefit from raised leg exercises.[79]

Practice for Superficial Lymph Drainage

As with superficial effleurage, the best sequence of regions to facilitate return of lymph begins with proximal regions and proceeds to distal ones. However, because superficial lymph drainage technique is slow, a complete full-body sequence like the one below will take anywhere from 1.5 to 3 hr, depending on the amount of repetition that is used.

Apply the technique to each region in succession. Begin the strokes distally within each region, and cover the entire region with short centripetal strokes that gradually move proximally. For shorter practice periods, any region, preceded by the neck, may be covered within half an hour.

Supine: Neck, face, chest, arm, abdomen, anterior legs

Prone: Back, gluteals, posterior legs

Finding soft, comfortable, relaxed hand contacts that best conform to regional contours can take some experimentation. Try variations that use

- The full palmar surface
- The ulnar border of the hand
- The thumb, index, and included web space
- Flat hands, including the fingers

How would you apply the technique using only sidelying positions while working from proximal to distal regions?

Clinical Example

Client profile	A 45-year-old female with breast cancer in remission presents 1 month postmastectomy with chronic lymphedema of the right arm and hand. She has had 50% of axillary lymph nodes and some breast tissue removed, and has had no radiation.
Summary of clinical findings	Subjective 1. Complains of right-handed pain and swelling that interferes with function 2. Complains of pain on activity 3. Reports feeling self-conscious about appearance of arm Objective Impairments 1. Gross edema, pitting from shoulder to fingers; girth recorded 2. Limb volume R > L; measured with volumetric analysis 3. Strength: Grade 3– for shoulder, elbow, and wrist movements on right 4. Range of motion R shoulder: flexion = 85 degrees, extension = 5 degrees, abduction = 70 degrees, adduction = 10 degrees, external rotation = 30 degrees, internal rotation = 5 degrees

continued

	R elbow: flexion = 95 degrees, extension = neutral, pronation = 45 degrees, supination = 30 degrees R wrist: flexion = 25 degrees, extension = 35 degrees, radial deviation = 5 degrees, ulnar deviation = 10 degrees R hand MCPs: flexion = 45 degrees, extension = neutral; IPs: flexion = 50 degrees, extension = neutral
	Functional limitations 1. Unable to comb hair with R arm 2. Difficulty dressing and performing self-care 3. Unable to reach object placed above shoulder level 4. Unable to carry objects in R hand
Treatment planning	Treatment rationale To reduce the client's edema and address the secondary weakness, pain, distorted body image, and functional limitations

Impairment	Role of massage
Edema (impaired lymph drainage)	Primary treatment, direct effect on lymphatic drainage
Range of motion	Primary treatment, direct effect since range is limited by edema
Strength	Possible secondary effect; weakness is primarily due to disuse; decreased edema may facilitate strengthening and will provide increased range for strengthening
Altered body image	Possible secondary effect, since gross edema contributes to altered body image

Massage techniques	Superficial effleurage, briefly, and then superficial lymph drainage technique. These are applied in sequence each session, thoroughly to the contralateral quadrant first (including intercostal and sternal areas), and then to proximal areas of the affected quadrant especially to axillar, intercostal and parasternal areas. The clinician gradually works more distally into the client's arm, then alternates back and forth between proximal and distal segments. In addition, at the outset of each intervention, repetitive broad-contact compression delivered over the junctions of the R lymphatic and thoracic ducts with the vena cava may also be useful (see Chapter 7, Neuromuscular Techniques).
Complementary techniques and other interventions	Medical management, bandaging or pressure garments, skin hygiene, range-of-motion exercises, functional activity, strengthening exercises, adaptive equipment for short-term use
Functional outcomes of care	1. Client will be able to carry a 10-lb object in her R hand while ambulating 100 ft, as required for carrying groceries 2. Client will be able to perform self-care activities (dressing, bathing, toileting) without adaptive equipment 3. Client will be able to reach object placed 3 ft above head with her R hand, as required for hanging laundry on the clothesline 4. Client will be able to lift 1-lb object from overhead shelf with her R hand, as required for placing and removing groceries on an overhead kitchen shelf 5. Client will demonstrate increased social interaction with fewer complaints of self-consciousness regarding the appearance of her arm

References

1. Fritz S. Fundamentals of therapeutic massage. St Louis: Mosby-Lifeline, 1995.
2. American Physical Therapy Association. The guide to physical therapist practice. Phys Ther 1997;77(11):1155–1674.
3. Tappan FM, Benjamin P. Tappan's handbook of healing massage techniques. 3rd ed. Stamford, CT: Appleton & Lange, 1998.
4. Loving J. Massage therapy. Stamford, CT: Appleton & Lange, 1999.
5. Salvo SG. Massage therapy. Philadelphia: WB Saunders, 1999.
6. de Domenico G, Wood EC. Beard's massage. 4th ed. Philadelphia: WB Saunders, 1997.
7. Holey E, Cook E. Therapeutic massage. London, England: WB Saunders, 1997.
8. Hollis M. Massage for therapists. 2nd ed. Oxford, England: Blackwell Science, 1998.
9. Schmid-Schonbein GW. Microlymphatics and lymph flow. Physiol Rev 1990;70(4):987–1028.
10. Tiidus PM, Shoemaker JK. Effleurage massage, muscle blood flow and long-term post-exercise strength recovery. Int J Sports Med 1995;16(7):478–483.
11. Shoemaker JK, Tiidus PM, Mader R. Failure of manual massage to alter limb blood flow: measures by Doppler ultrasound. Med Sci Sports Exerc 1997;29(5):610–614.
12. Yates J. A physician's guide to massage therapy; its physiological effects and their application to treatment. British Columbia, Canada: The Massage Therapists Association of British Columbia; 1990.
13. Mason MP. The treatment of lymphoedema by complex decongestive physiotherapy. Aust J Physiother 1993;39:41–45.
14. Groer M, Mozingo J, Droppleman P, et al. Measures of salivary secretory immunoglobulin A and state anxiety after a nursing back rub. Appl Nurs Res 1994;7(1):2–6.
15. Labyak SE, Metzger BL. The effects of effleurage backrub on the physiological components of relaxation: a meta-analysis. Nurs Res 1997;46(1):59–62.
16. Goldberg J, Sullivan SJ, Seaborne DE. The effect of two intensities of massage on H-reflex amplitude. Phys Ther 1992;72(6):449–457.
17. Sullivan SJ, Seguin S, Seaborne D, et al. Reduction of H-reflex amplitude during the application of effleurage to the triceps surae in neurologically healthy subjects. Physiother Theory Pract 1993;9:25–31.
18. Larsen JH. Infants' colic and belly massage. Practitioner 1990;234(1487):396–397.
19. Emly M. Abdominal massage. Nurs Times 1993:89(3):34–36.
20. Dunbar S, Redick E. Should patients with acute myocardial infarctions receive back massage? Focus Crit Care 1986;13(3):42–46.
21. Tyler DO, Winslow EH, Clark AP, White KM. Effects of a one minute back rub on mixed venous saturation and heart rate in critically ill patients. Heart Lung 19 1990(5):562–565.
22. Leduc A, Lievens P, Dewald J. The influence of multidirectional vibrations on wound healing and on regeneration of blood and lymph vessels. Lymphology 1981;14(4):179–185.
23. Ueda W, Katatoka Y, Sagara Y. Effect of gentle massage on regression of sensory analgesia during epidural block. Anesth Analg 1993;76(4):783–785.
24. Grieve GP. Episacroiliac lipoma. Physiotherapy 1990;76(6):308–310.
25. Wittlinger H, Wittlinger G. Textbook of Dr Vodder's manual lymphatic drainage, vol 1: basic course. 3rd ed. Heidelberg, Germany: Karl F Haug Verlag, 1982.
26. Kurz I. Textbook of Dr. Vodder's manual lymph drainage, vol 2: therapy. 4th ed. Heidelberg: Karl F Haug Verlag, 1997.
27. Kurz I. Textbook of Dr. Vodder's manual lymph drainage, vol. 3: treatment manual. 2nd ed. Heidelberg: Karl F Haug Verlag, 1990.
28. Kasseroller RG. The Vodder School: the Vodder method. Cancer 1998;83(12 suppl American):2840–2842.
29. Harris R. An introduction to manual lymph drainage: the Vodder method. Massage Ther J 1992;winter:55–66.
30. Fritsch C, Tomson D. [The usefulness of lymphatic drainage.] Schweiz Rundsch Med Prax. (French) 1991;80(15):383–386. (Abstract)
31. Casley-Smith JR, Boris M, Weindorf S, Lasinski B. Treatment for lymphedema of the arm—the – Casley-Smith method: a noninvasive method produces continued reduction. Cancer 1998;83(12 suppl American):2843–2860.
32. Leduc O, Leduc A, Bourgeois P, Belgrado JP. The physical treatment of upper limb edema. Cancer 1998;83(12 suppl American):2835–2839.
33. Lerner R. Complete decongestive physiotherapy and the Lerner Lymphedema Services Academy of Lymphatic Studies (the Lerner School). Cancer 1998;83(12 suppl American):2861–2863.
34. Francois A, Richaud C, Bouchet JY, et al. Does medical treatment of lymphedema act by increasing lymph flow? VASA 1989;18(4):281–286.
35. Hutzschenreuter P, Brummer H, Ebberfeld K. [Experimental and clinical studies of the mechanism of effect of manual lymph drainage therapy.] Z Lymphol (German) 1989;13(1):62–64. (Abstract)
36. Hutzschenreuter P, Ehlers R. [Effect of manual lymph drainage on the autonomic nervous system.] Z Lymphol (German) 1986;10(2):58–60. (Abstract)
37. Ko DS, Lerner R, Klose G, Cosimi AB. Effective treatment of lymphedema of the extremities. Arch Surg 1998;133(4):452–458.
38. Franzeck UK, Spiegel I, Fischer M, et al. Combined physical therapy for lymphedema evaluated by fluorescence microlymphography and lymph capillary pressure measurements. J Vasc Res 1997;34(4):306–311.
39. Herpertz U. [Outcome of various inpatient lymph drainage procedures.] Z Lymphol (German) 1996;20(1):27–30. (Abstract)
40. Boris M, Weindorf S, Lasinski B, Boris G. Lymphedema reduction by noninvasive complex lymphedema therapy. Oncology (Huntingt) 1994;8(9):95–106.

41. Foldi M. Treatment of lymphedema. Lymphology 1994; 27(1):1–5. (Editorial)

42. Gillham L. Lymphedema and physiotherapists: control not cure. Physiotherapy 1994;80(12):835–843.

43. Ruger K. [Lymphedema of the head in clinical practice.] Z Lymphol (German) 1993;17(1):6–11. (Abstract)

44. Barrellier MT. [Lymphedema: is there a treatment?] Rev Med Interne (French) 1992;13(1):49–57. (Abstract)

45. Lerner R. The ideal treatment of lymphedema. AMTA Massage Ther J 1992;winter:37–39.

46. Clodius L, Foldi E, Foldi M. On nonoperative management of chronic lymphedema. Lymphology 1990;23(1):2–3.

47. Cluzan R, Miserey G, Barrey P, Alliot F. [Principles and results of physiotherapeutic therapy in mechanical lymphatic insufficiency of secondary or primary nature.] Phlebologie (French) 1988;41(2):401–408. (Abstract)

48. Einfeld TH, Henkel M, Schmidt-Aufurth T, et al. [Therapeutic and palliative lymphdrainage in the treatment of face and neck edema.] HNO (German) 1986;34(9): 365–367.

49. Foldi E, Foldi M, Weissleder H. Conservative treatment of lymphoedema of the limbs. Angiology 1985;36: 171–180.

50. Kurz W, Kurz R, Litmanovitch YI, et al. Effect of manual lymph drainage massage on blood components and urinary neurohormones in chronic lymphedema. Angiology 1981;32(2):119–127.

51. Kurz W, Wittlinger G, Litmanovitch YI, et al. Effect of manual lymph drainage massage on urinary excretion of neurohormones and minerals in chronic lymphedema. Angiology 1978;29(10):764–772.

52. Enig B, Mogensen M, Jorgensen RJ. [Lymphedema in patients treated for breast cancer. A cross-sectional study in the county of Ribe. The need of manual lymph drainage; risk factors.] Ugeskr Laeger (Danish) 1999;161(22):3293–3298. (Abstract)

53. Johansson K, Albertsson M, Ingvar C, Ekdahl C. Effects of compression bandaging with or without manual lymph drainage treatment in patients with postoperative arm lymphedema. Lymphology 1999;32(3):103–110.

54. Fiaschi E, Francesconi G, Fiumicelli S, et al. Manual lymphatic drainage for chronic post-mastectomy lymphoedema treatment. Panminerva Med 1998;40(1): 48–50.

55. Foldi E. The treatment of lymphedema. Cancer 1998;83(12 suppl American):2833–2834.

56. Johansson K, Lie E, Ekdahl C, Lindfeldt J. A randomized study comparing manual lymph drainage with sequential pneumatic compression for treatment of postoperative arm lymphedema. Lymphology 1998;31(2):56–64.

57. Ferrandez JC, Laroche JP, Serin D, et al. [Lymphoscintigraphic aspects of the effects of manual lymphatic drainage.] J Mal Vasc (French) 1996;21(5):283–289. (Abstract)

58. Cluzan RV, Alliot F, Ghabboun S, Pascot M. Treatment of secondary lymphedema of the upper limb with CYCLO 3 FORT. Lymphology 1996;29(1):29–35.

59. Mirolo BR, Bunce IH, Chapman M, et al. Psychosocial benefits of postmastectomy lymphedema therapy. Cancer Nurs 1995;18(3):197–205.

60. Gruffaz J. [Management by the angiologist of sequellae of radiosurgical treatment of breast cancer.] J Mal Vasc (French) 1995;20(2):150–152. (Abstract)

61. Bunce IH, Mirolo BR, Hennessy JM, et al. Post-mastectomy lymphoedema treatment and measurement. Med J Aust 1994;161(2):125–128.

62. Bertelli G, Venturini M, Forno G, et al. An analysis of prognostic factors in response to conservative treatment of postmastectomy lymphedema. Surg Gynecol Obstet 1992; 175(5):455–460.

63. Casley-Smith JR, Casley-Smith JR. Modern treatment of lymphoedema. 1. Complex physical therapy: the first 200 Australian limbs. Aust J Dermatol 1992;33(2):61–68.

64. Zanolla R, Monzeglio C, Balzarini A, Martino G. Evaluation of the results of three different methods of postmastectomy lymphedema treatment. J Surg Oncol 1984;26: 210–213.

65. Weiss JM. Treatment of leg edema and wounds in a patient with severe musculoskeletal injuries. Phys Ther 1998; 78(10):1104–1113.

66. Trettin H. [Craniocerebral trauma caused by sports. Pathogenic mechanism, clinical aspects and physical therapy with special reference to manual lymph drainage.] Z Lymphol (German) 1993;17(2):36–40. (Abstract)

67. Valentin J, Leonhardt D, Perrin M. [Prevention of venous thromboses and cutaneous necroses using physical methods and pressure therapy in the surgery of chronic venous insufficiency of the lower limbs.] Phlebologie (French) 1988;41(3):690–696. (Abstract)

68. Asdonk J. [Physical lymph drainage and therapy of edema in chronic venous insufficiency.] Z Lymphol (German) 1981;5(2):107–111. (Abstract)

69. Chomard D, Habault P, Ledemeney M, Haon C. Prognostic aspects of TcPO2 in iloprost treatment as an alternative to amputation. Angiology 1999;50(4):283–288.

70. Husmann MJ, Roedel C, Leu AJ, et al. [Lymphoedema, lymphatic microangiopathy and increased lymphatic and interstitial pressure in a patient with Parkinson's disease.] Schweiz Med Wochenschr (German) 1999;129(10):410–412. (Abstract)

71. Klyscz T, Bogenschutz O, Junger M, Rassner G. [Microangiopathic changes and functional disorders of nail fold capillaries in dermatomyositis.] Hautarzt (German) 1996; 47(4):289–293. (Abstract)

72. Zahumensky E, Rybka J, Adamikova A. [New aspects of pharmacologic and general prophylactic care of the diabetic foot]. Vnitr Lek (Russian) 1995;41(8):531–534. (Abstract)

73. Bringezu G. [Combatting fatigue in sports physical therapy with reference to manual lymph drainage.] Z Lymphol (German) 1994;18(1):12–15. (Abstract)

74. Joos E, Bourgeois P, Famaey JP. Lymphatic disorders in rheumatoid arthritis. Semin Arthritis Rheum 1993;22(6): 392–398.

75. Trettin H. [Neurologic principles of edema in inactivity.] Z Lymphol (German) 1992;16(1):14–16. (Abstract)

76. Kaaja R, Tiula E. Manual lymph drainage in nephrotic syndrome during pregnancy. Lancet 1989;Oct 21:990.

77. Preisler VK, Hagen R, Hoppe F. [Indications and risks of manual lymph drainage in head-neck tumors.] Laryngorhinootologie (German) 1998;77(4):207–212. (Abstract)

78. Herpertz U. [Malignant lymphedema.] Z Lymphol (German) 1990;14(1):17–23. (Abstract)

79. Ciocon JO, Galindo-Ciocan D, Galindo DJ. Raised leg exercises for leg edema in the elderly. Angiology 1995;46(1):19–25.

Suggested Readings

Adcock J. Rehabilitation of the breast cancer patient. In: Physical therapy for the cancer patient. ed. Charles L. McGarvey III New York: Churchill Livingstone, 1990: 67–84.

Asdonk J. [Effectiveness, indications and contraindications of manual lymph drainage therapy in painful edema] (German). Z Lymphol. 1995;19(1):16–22. (Abstract)

Bauer WC, Dracup KA. Physiologic effects of back massage in patients with acute myocardial infarction. Focus Crit Care 1987;14(6):42–46.

Bertelli G, Venturini M, Forno G, et al. Conservative treatment of postmastectomy lymphedema: a controlled study. Ann Oncol 1991;2(8):575–578.

Browse NL. The diagnosis and management of primary lymphedema. J Vasc Surg. 1986;3(1):181–184.

Calnan JS, Pflug JJ, Reis ND, Taylor LM. Lymphatic pressures and the flow of lymph. Br J Plast Surg 1970;23(4):305–317.

Carriere B. Edema: its development and treatment using lymph drainage massage. Clin Manage 1988;8(5):119–121.

Casley-Smith JR. Estimation of optimal massage pressure: is this possible? Folia Angiol 1981;29:154–156.

Casley-Smith JR. Measuring and representing peripheral oedema and its alterations. Lymphology 1994;27(2):56–70.

Drinker CK, Yoffey JM. Lymphatics, lymph, and lymphoid tissue: their physiological and clinical significance. Cambridge, MA: Harvard University Press, 1941.

Dubois F. Use of a new specific massage technique to prevent the formation of hypertrophic scars. In: Cluzan RV, Pecking AP, Lokiec FM, eds. Progress in Lymphology XIII, Exerpta Medica. Int. Congress Series no. 994. Amsterdam: Elsevier Science Publishers BV, 1992:635.

Eliska O, Eliska M. Ultrastructure and function of the lymphatics in man and dog legs under different conditions—massage. In: Cluzan RV, Pecking AP, Lokiec FM, eds. Progress in Lymphology XIII, Exerpta Medica. Int. Congress Series no. 994. Amsterdam: Elsevier Science Publishers BV, 1992:97.

Flowers KR. String wrapping versus massage for reducing digital volume. Phys Ther 1998;68(1):57–59.

Foldi E, Sauerwald A, Hennig B. Effect of complex decongestive physiotherapy on gene expression for the inflammatory response in peripheral lymphedema. Lymphology. 2000;33(1):19–23.

Foldi E. Massage and damage to lymphatics. Lymphology 1995;28:1–3.

Foldi M. Anatomical and physiological basis for physical therapy of lymphedema. Experentia 1978;33(suppl):15–18.

Francois A. Use of isoptic lymphography in the evaluation of manual lymphatic drainage effects in chronic lower limb edema. In: Partsch H, ed. Progress in Lymphology XI, Exerpta Medica Int. Congress Series no. 779. Amsterdam: Elsevier Science Publishers BV, 1987:555.

Giardini D, Bohimann R. [Le drainage lymphatique manuel.] Lausanne: Ed. Payot; 1991. (French)

Gruffaz J. [Le drainage lymphatique manuel.] J Mal Vasc (French) 1985;10:187–191.

Herpertz U. [Significance of radiogenic damage for lymphology.] Z Lymphol (German) 1990;14(2):62–67.

Hurst PAE. Venous and lymphatic disease—assessment and treatment. In: Downie PA, ed. Cash's textbook of chest, heart and vascular disorders for physiotherapists. London: Faber and Faber, 1987:654–665.

Kirshbgaum M. Using massage in the relief of lymphoedema. Prof Nurse 1996;11(4):230–232.

Leduc A, Caplan I, Lievens P. [Traitment physique de l'oedeme du bras.] Paris, 1981. (French)

Lindemayr H, Santler R, Jurecka W. [Compression therapy of lymphedema.] MMW Munch Med Wochenschr (German) 1980;122(22):825–828. (Abstract)

Little L, Porche DJ. Manual lymph drainage (MLD). J Assoc Nurses AIDS Care 1998;9(1):78–81.

Morgan RG, Casley-Smith JR, Mason MR, Casley-Smith JR. Complex physical therapy for the lymphoedematous arm. J Hand Surg 1992;17(4):437–441.

Mortimer PS. Therapy approaches for lymphedema. Angiology 1997;48(1):87–91.

Mortimer PS, Simmonds R, Rezvani M, et al. The measurement of skin lymph flow by isotope clearance—reliability, reproducibility, injection dynamics, and the effect of massage. J Invest Dermatol 1990;95(6):677–682.

Rinehart-Ayres ME. Conservative approaches to lymphedema treatment. Cancer 1998;83(12 suppl American): 2828–2832.

Robert L. [Therapie manuelle des oedemes]. Paris: Ed Spek, 1992. (French)

Ruger K. [Diagnosis and therapy of malignant lymphedema.] Fortschr Med (German) 1998;116(12):28–30, 32, 34.

Stahel HU. Manual lymph drainage. Curr Probl Dermatol. 1999;27:148–152.

Swedborg I. Effectiveness of combined methods of physiotherapy for post-mastectomy lymphoedema. Scand J Rehabil Med 1980;12(2):77–85.

Thiadens SR. Current status of education and treatment resources for lymphedema. Cancer 1998;83(12 suppl American):2864–2868.

Uher EM, Vacariu G, Schneider B, Fialka V. [Comparison of manual lymph drainage with physical therapy in complex regional pain syndrome, type I. A comparative randomized controlled therapy study] (German). Wien Klin Wochenschr. 2000;112(3):133–137. (Abstract)

Vasudevan SV, Melvin JL. Upper extremity edema control: rationale of the techniques. Am J Occup Ther 1979;33(8):520–523.

Vodder E. Lymphdrainage. Aesthet Med 1965;14:6.

Williams C. Compression therapy for lymphoedema from Vernon-Carus. Br J Nurs 1998;7(6):339–343.

Worthington EL Jr, Martin GA, Shumate M. Which prepared-childbirth coping strategies are effective? JOGN Nurs 1982;11(1):45–51.

Xujian S. Effect of massage and temperature on the permeability of initials. Lymphology 1990;23:48–50.

7

Neuromuscular Techniques

Neuromuscular techniques are those massage techniques that palpate muscle, affect the level of resting tension of muscles, and have additional psychoneuroimmunological effects. These techniques include broad-contact compression, petrissage, stripping, and specific compression. This chapter describes each of these techniques, how to perform the technique, and how to apply it in a practice sequence. It also includes a discussion of the indications, contraindications, cautions, outcomes of care, and postintervention care associated with each technique.

Table 7-1
Summary of Impairment-Level Outcomes of Care for Neuromuscular Techniques

Impairment-Level Outcome of Care	*Technique*			
	Broad-Contact Compression	*Petrissage*	*Stripping*	*Specific Compression*
Increased perceived relaxation and decreased levels of stress hormones	P	✓	P	P
Decreased perceived anxiety and levels of stress hormones	P	✓	P	P
Stimulated immune function	P	✓	P	P
Systemic sedation	P	✓	P	P
Sensory arousal	P	✓	–	–
Counterirritant analgesia	P	✓	✓	✓
Increased venous return (direct effect)	P	P	–	–
Increased lymphatic return (direct effect)	P	P	–	–
Decreased edema (direct effect)	P	P	–	–
Normalized muscle resting tension and neuromuscular tone	–	P	P	P
Decreased muscle spasm	–	P	P	P
Increased muscle extensibility	–	✓	✓	✓
Enhanced muscle performance (secondary effect)	–	✓	✓	✓
Balance of agonist/antagonist function	–	P	P	P

continued

Table 7-1 *(continued)*

Impairment-Level Outcome of Care	Technique			
	Broad-Contact Compression	Petrissage	Stripping	Specific Compression
Improved movement responses	–	P	P	P
Decreased trigger point activity	–	✓	✓	✓
Increased tissue mobility	–	P	P	P
Increased joint mobility	–	✓	P	P
Separation and lengthening of fascia	–	P	P	–
Normalized postural alignment	–	P	P	P
Decreased dyspnea	P	P	P	P
Increased rib cage mobility	P	P	P	P
Increased airway clearance/mobilization of secretions	✓	–	–	–
Stimulated peristalsis	P	P	P	P

✓, the outcome is supported by research summarized in this or other chapters; P, the outcome is probable; –, nonexistent, negligible, or improbable effects.

Broad-Contact Compression

OTHER NAMES USED FOR THIS TECHNIQUE

"Compression," "pressure," "pressing."[1–8]

DEFINITION

Broad-contact compression: A nongliding technique that is delivered with a broad-contact surface. This technique engages the client's muscle, and the pressure and release of the stroke is perpendicular to the surface of the client's body.[1–3]

NOTES

Broad-contact compression owes its current classification as an independent technique largely to its applications in athletics.[1–3,5,9] The technique is not usually discussed in older texts[10–12] and is still omitted from some modern ones.[6–8] Nevertheless, this stroke is the technical foundation and prerequisite for many classical gliding techniques that engage muscle (see "Petrissage," below in this chapter). Although broad-contact compression lacks the component of "drag" (horizontal tension) that characterizes petrissage, it is an extremely versatile technique in its own right.

CLINICAL INDICATIONS AND IMPAIRMENT-LEVEL OUTCOMES OF CARE

Broad-contact compression is a useful introductory stroke that can be used to assess the general quality and the level of resting tension of larger skeletal muscles. This technique can also be used to achieve effects on circulation, muscle resting tension, and rib cage mobility.

Although various texts state that the repetitive, rhythmic nature of broad-contact compression results in "increased circulation,"[1–3] this postulated direct mechanical effect may be an increase in lymphatic and possibly venous return. For example, when broad-contact compression is applied to the rib cage—especially in the region of the upper anterior and posterior ribs, over the junctions of the right lymphatic and thoracic ducts with the venous circulation—it may assist systemic lymphatic return.[13,14] In addition, when it is performed on the soles or palms, it may assist lymphatic return from the limb.[13,14] The circulatory effects of broad-contact compression have not, however, been evaluated systematically in the research on massage. Furthermore, research on the effect of the similar compressive petrissage technique on fluid flow is inconclusive (see later in this chapter).[15]

Nevertheless, there are two extensive areas of related research that support circulatory effects of broad-contact compression that should be considered: closed chest cardiac massage and pneumatic devices that apply compression. Vigorous compression of the rib cage in the context of closed chest cardiac massage (CPR) produces forward blood flow.[16–18] Pneumatic devices that apply compression ("intermittent pneumatic compression," or "impulse compression") to clients' limbs increase venous return and are useful in the treatment of a variety of circulatory conditions.[19–22] Moderate circumferential pressure on the limbs applied with a pneumatic cuff has also been shown to increase lymphatic return.[24–26] In one study the rate of lymphatic return increased with the pressure applied (up to 320 mm Hg), and a wait of at least 8 seconds was required after each local compression to permit refilling of terminal lymphatics.[26]

Compression of the rib cage is used in a variety of ways in cardiopulmonary rehabilitation. Rib cage compression is incorporated into breathing retraining techniques that improve breathing patterns and promote increased respiratory volume during inspiration and expiration.[27] When broad-contact compression is performed vigorously and repetitively on the rib cage ("shaking" or "rib springing"), it facilitates the movement of secretions through the bronchial tree.[6,28,29] This technique can be used alone or combined with postural drainage (see Chapter 10, Percussive Techniques).

Texts are inconsistent on whether broad-contact compression increases or decreases muscle resting tension.[1–3,5] It is possible that broad-contact compression may result in a transient and marginal increase or decrease in muscle resting tension, depending on the rate and vigor of the application of the technique. Broad-contact compression is commonly used in precompetition sports massage for several reasons: it has a possible effect on tone, it does not require a lubricant or the removal of clothing, and it can be adapted to be either sedative or stimulating.[1–3,9] It is possible to perform effective full-body massage sequences that have specific effects on several of the clients' systems with the skillful use of only broad-contact compression. The main impairment-level outcomes of care for broad-contact compression are summarized in Table 7-1.

CAUTIONS AND CONTRAINDICATIONS

Clinical training and supervised practice are critical for the proper application of broad-contact compression. Advanced training may be advisable in certain situations, particularly when dealing with pathological conditions. All of the general and local contraindications noted for massage techniques apply to the use of broad-contact compression (see Chapter 2, The Clinical Decision-Making Process).[30] There are also specific contraindications to the use of this technique that include clients with hemophilia; local sites of acute inflammation and infection; and clients with confirmed or suspected thrombus, thrombophlebitis, or malignancy. If the clinician is applying broad-contact compression to the client's rib cage to mobilize bronchial secretions and enhance airway clearance, some contraindications include a flail chest, an immobile rib cage, fractured or brittle ribs, and recent chest or spinal surgery.[6] The clinician should perform a careful examination and moderate her use of pressure with clients who have confirmed or suspected osteoporosis, clients with wounds that are in the early stages of healing, and clients who are taking anticoagulants. Caution is also required when treating areas of spasm, hypotonia, or active trigger points and when treating the rib cage, if there is potential for bronchospasm.

Prerequisite Skills for Broad-Contact Compression

Before practicing broad-contact compression, students should know how to

  Describe the spatial relationship between bones and major groups of skeletal muscle throughout the body

  Identify major groups of skeletal muscle and major bony prominences using contour alone

  Describe the movement of the rib cage during relaxed and forced breathing

  Assess muscle resting tension

  Use a postural scan to assess muscular bulk, tone, and balance

  Use wide-stance knee bend, lunge, lunge and lean, and standing controlled lean postures

See Chapter 4, Preparation and Positioning for Treatment, and Appendix B, Selected Soft-Tissue Examination Techniques.

Manual Technique begins on next page

Broad-Contact Compression

In the following figures (Figs. 7-1 to 7-8), broad-contact compression is applied to the various regions of the body. Figures are ordered from head to foot in supine and then prone. Each figure illustrates several of the guidelines for manual technique outlined below.

1. Broad-contact compression is best done with no or little lubricant.

2. The technique is usually applied to areas where there is muscle tissue (Figs. 7-4 to 7-7), but it can also be applied over bone to achieve specialized effects (Figs. 7-1 and 7-3).

3. The hand is relaxed to facilitate palpation, and pressure is evenly distributed over the entire contact surface. When the palmar surface is used, fingers may be spread apart slightly to increase the size of the contact surface (Fig. 7-4). When the stroke is being applied with significant force, however, it is not advisable to use the palmar surface, since the wrist will be placed in considerable extension. In this case, use a fist or the proximal forearm to apply the technique (Figs. 7-5A and B, 7-6, and 7-7).

4. The compression and release portions of the stroke are performed gradually and smoothly when the rate of application is slow. When the clinician performs the technique quickly, it should still be performed smoothly.

5. The initial direction of application of pressure is perpendicular to the surface of the client's body, with no effort to direct the stroke in a horizontal direction or parallel to the surface. Pressure applied in this manner will cause the individual muscle fibers to be spread apart. As the pressure of application increases, the tissues in large muscle groups, such as the gluteals, may tend to roll and produce some horizontal movement (Fig. 7-5A and B).

6. Stroke rate will vary with the clinical use of the technique. The rate can be fast and rhythmical (1 to 2 strokes per sec) as is often the case in precompetition sports massage. Alternatively, a single compression can be sustained for 10 to 20 sec, allowing time to gradually apply and release the pressure (Fig. 7-7). This will often achieve a more sedative effect and may more readily affect connective tissue elements of the muscle if the compression is taken to the end of range of the tissues.

7. The clinician can lift the client's tissues between each stroke when applying faster rhythmical compression to large muscle groups, such as the hamstrings or quadriceps.

8. Rhythmical compression can produce a rocking motion that has its own clinical effects, particularly when it is applied around the pelvis (see Chapter 9, Passive Movement Techniques).

9. To enhance venous and lymphatic return from a limb, the clinician begins compression proximally at the junction between the limb and the limb girdle and then applies a series of compression strokes that move from distal to proximal; each successive series of compressions begins distal to the previous series (Fig. 7-8). When performing the technique to increase lymphatic return, it may be advisable to wait at least 8 sec before compressing the same local area again.[26]

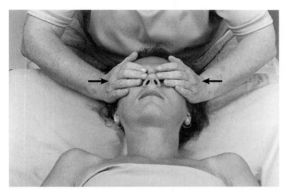

Figure 7-1. Gentle bilateral palmar compression of the head can assist sinus drainage.

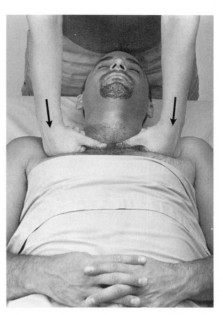

Figure 7-2. Compression of the upper thorax to assist expiration.

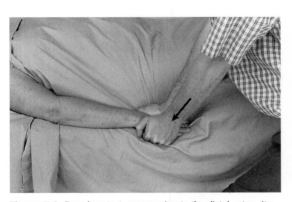

Figure 7-3. Broad-contact compression to the distal extremity promotes general mobility of the small joints.

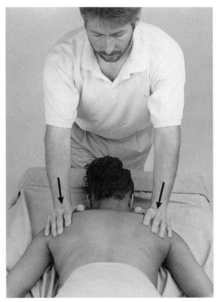

Figure 7-4. Bilateral palmar compression of the shoulders using a standing controlled lean. The heels of the hands are in contact with the acromial portion of the upper trapezius muscle.

Manual Technique Figures continue on next page

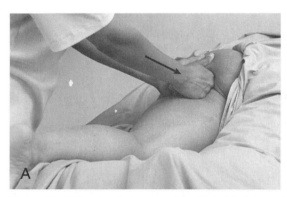

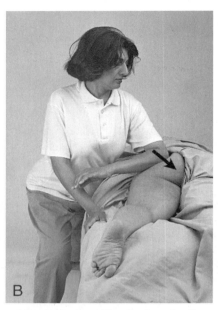

Figure 7-5. A. Broad-contact compression of the gluteals to produce sedation can be done either directly on the client's skin or through fabric. The clinician has a choice of contact surfaces: reinforced or doubled fists or palms. **B.** Gluteal compression using the forearm in a lunge and lean posture. The clinician uses her free hand to further stabilize the posture.

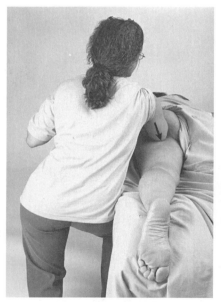

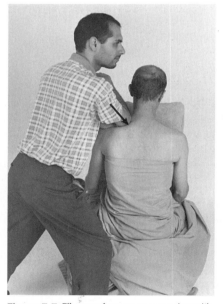

Figure 7-6. Compression with the forearm or elbow is one of the few techniques that gives the clinician enough leverage to produce a mechanical effect on the superior attachment of the hamstring muscle. The technique must be executed carefully and should be done bilaterally to avoid producing a pelvic rotation in the client.

Figure 7-7. Elbow or forearm compression with the client seated is an effective approach to soften a chronically indurated upper trapezius muscle. The clinician bends his knees, inclines his trunk slightly, and maintains relaxed shoulders to transfer his body weight to the client's body in a controlled manner.

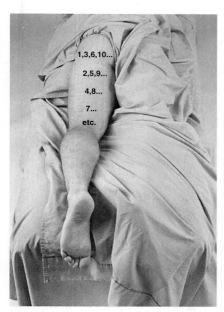

Figure 7-8. The numbers indicate the sequence in which compressions are performed to enhance fluid return from the limb. (See Manual Technique, item #9, page 172, for description.)

Components of Broad-Contact Compression

Contact: Whole palmar surface of the hand, heel of the hand, dorsal surface of proximal phalanges together (fist), or forearm

Pressure: Light to heavy

Tissues engaged: Muscle, associated tissues, and the underlying structures, such as the rib cage, that are reached through muscle; if compression is sustained, connective tissue elements are engaged

Direction: Perpendicular to surface of the client's body

Amplitude/length: NA

Rate: 1 to 10 or more seconds per cycle of compression/release

Duration: 20 to 60 sec or longer

Intergrades[a] with: Petrissage, specific compression

Combined with: May be combined with rocking, although neither technique is improved by this combination

Context: May be used alone extensively; it is commonly used after effleurage and/or as a prelude to more-specific neuromuscular techniques

---

[a]To merge gradually one into another.

CLINICIAN'S POSITION AND MOVEMENT

1. The basic positions used by the clinician are described in Chapter 4, Preparation and Positioning for Treatment, in the sections on standing aligned posture, standing controlled lean, lunge and lean, and wide-stance knee bend postures. The clinician can increase the pressure applied by shifting or rocking a stable center of gravity forward over the compressed segment of the client's body. Alternately, the clinician can bend both knees to lower upper body weight down onto the client (Figs. 7-4, 7-5B, 7-6, and 7-7).
2. Regardless of the working posture that the clinician selects, the clinician adopts the following positions: both feet remain flat on the floor, hands and forearms remain as relaxed as possible, elbows are flexed, and shoulders are as relaxed as possible.
3. The clinician uses contact surfaces other than the hands to apply the large amounts of pressure to the client that are required for this technique. Consequently, as the clinician performs palpation during the application of deeper compression, the clinician must gauge how the client's compressed tissues are deforming under body weight (Figs. 7-4 to 7-7). This type of palpation might be termed "proprioceptive palpation"—as opposed to strict manual palpation per se, since the clinician is using proprioceptive sense to judge the movement of the client's tissues. The development of this "proprioceptive palpation" skill is essential to learning how to apply higher-force neuromuscular and connective tissue techniques.

PALPATE

When performing the technique, the clinician palpates the client's tissues for the following:

1. General resistance or resilience of soft tissues
2. Localized areas of hardness or tautness that may require the use of a more specific technique
3. Increased pliability that reflects the reduction in viscosity of healthy superficial subcutaneous tissues, which normally occurs with continued application of the technique
4. Resorption of fluid from edematous tissue, which is accompanied by changes in surface contours, and the viscosity and inertial resistance of the subcutaneous tissues
5. Change in resting muscle tension with continued application of the technique
6. Change in the mobility of the rib cage when the technique is applied locally

OBSERVE

When performing the technique, the clinician observes the client for changes in muscular tension, circulation, or breathing pattern. The signs listed below may signal this.

1. Reduction of muscle tension, as evidenced by softening of the tissue contours or broadening and flattening of body segments
2. If the technique is used to treat respiratory conditions, note abnormalities in the client's usual breathing pattern and changes in these patterns with continued application of the technique.
3. If the technique is used to treat edema proximal to the site of edema, visible reduction of swelling may often occur within 15 to 45 min. Cumulative reduction of swelling will occur during the course of the treatment regimen, with resolution of an inflammatory process, or with resolution of circulatory and lymphatic dysfunction.
4. Normalizing of skin color and texture that reflects circulatory changes

COMMUNICATION WITH THE CLIENT

The clinician uses communication that may elicit the client's feedback on his level of comfort during the application of techniques. Some examples of statements that the clinician can use are listed below.

1. "Let me know if you begin to feel uncomfortable." Ensure that the client finds the depth of the compression comfortable.
2. "Notice where I am applying pressure on your rib cage. Now breathe into my hand(s)." If the clinician is applying the technique to the client's rib cage (Figs. 7-2, 7-4), she ensures that the client's breathing is not impeded by the resistance that is provided by the compression stroke.

COMPLEMENTARY MODALITIES

1. Physical agents. With chronic orthopedic conditions, the clinician can appropriately apply deep moist heat, such as a hot pack, for 5 to 20 min (until a mild hyperemia appears on the client's skin) prior to the application of compression.
2. In situations in which the client presents with a generalized elevation of resting muscle tension because of stress, the clinician may use diaphragmatic breathing or progressive relaxation as an adjunct to the intervention.

A Practice Sequence for Broad-Contact Compression

Allow 30 minutes per person

Allow 4 to 5 sec per stroke, including the phases of gradual compression, hold, and gradual release; synchronize the strokes with your breathing to achieve an even, relaxing tempo; bend your knees and slowly rock your body weight over the contact surface to produce a deep, even compressive force; use relaxed, broad contact

Supine

Partially rotate the client's head and gently apply techniques in the following manner:

1. Down the sides of his neck from the mastoid process to the clavicle (this is a sensitive area on many people)
2. Across the upper chest from sternum to the axilla inferior to the clavicle
3. From the anterior deltoid down each arm; compress the hand as a unit
4. Down the sternum (use a narrower contact surface, such as the ulnar border of the hand, to avoid the client's breast tissue)
5. Across the lower ribs from midline toward the axilla (avoid direct pressure on the xiphoid process)
6. Gently, with soft hands, around the abdomen in clockwise circles
7. From the inguinal line to just above the client's knee; repeat to cover the anteromedial and anterolateral surfaces of the thigh

Prone

Gently apply techniques in the following manner:

1. Bilaterally along upper trapezius to the acromion process while you are standing at the head of the table (considerable pressure can be used here)
2. From the posterior deltoid move down each arm
3. Down either side of the spine from occiput to sacrum; repeat, moving slightly more laterally on the back with each new series of compressive strokes
4. Unilaterally and bilaterally on the lumbar musculature with broad palmar contact
5. From the iliac crest on one side, down the gluteals, and distally to the knee, repeat to cover the posteromedial and posterolateral surfaces of the thigh; if pressure on the posterior surface causes the client to report patellar pain, place additional pillows under his ankles or lower leg from the popliteal space to the feet

SELF-CARE INSTRUCTIONS

1. There is no specific self-care that the client is required to perform after the application of broad-contact compression. Depending on the clinical situation, stretching, range of motion, isometrics, diaphragmatic breathing, or progressive relaxation exercises may be indicated.

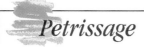

Petrissage

OTHER NAMES USED FOR THIS TECHNIQUE

"Kneading."[1-8]

DEFINITION

Petrissage: A group of related techniques that repetitively compress, shear, and release muscle tissue with varying amounts of drag, lift, and glide[1-8]

NOTES

1. Petrissage (from the French *petrir*, to knead)[3,6] is one of two techniques that are almost invariably used in classical massage interventions (the other is effleurage). It is an indispensable technique when the clinician is treating muscle.
2. The term *petrissage* was formerly used to refer to techniques that repetitively grasp, lift, shear, and release muscle tissue between the hands (see

"wringing," "squeezing," and "picking up" below in this chapter). Related techniques that repetitively compress, shear, and release muscle against underlying muscle and bone were defined separately as "kneading," although sometimes these definitions were reversed! It is common now for both lifting and compressive forms of these techniques to be grouped under the single name petrissage,[1,2,6–8] although slightly differing usages persist (one recent text drops the French term entirely[5]).

3. Contemporary author's opinions differ as to how much skin glide should occur when applying compressive or kneading forms of this technique.[2,6–8]

4. Observation shows that the different types of petrissage intergrade. The mechanical forces applied to the muscle are basically similar for all forms of petrissage described in this chapter. Slowing the rate of application and using less lubricant will, however, increase the amount of drag, or sustained horizontal force, that results and may produce greater effects on connective tissue.

5. There is agreement among authors that petrissage, in either lifting or kneading forms, repetitively compresses and releases muscle. However, some authors[3] follow Kellogg's usage[12] and classify other techniques that compress and release muscle as forms of "friction." We prefer to reserve the term friction for a precise, specific technique directed toward connective tissue (see Chapter 8, Connective Tissue Techniques).

6. A regrettable drawback of the massage literature is that researchers do not always provide detailed descriptions of the interventions that were performed. Consequently, the word petrissage rarely shows up in methodological descriptions, although it is commonly the predominant technique of classical massage. In summarizing the literature for this text, the authors have assumed the predominant use of petrissage (which, in our view, includes "deep effleurage") that is directed toward skeletal muscle in situations in which the techniques performed in the intervention were not specifically mentioned or were characterized broadly as "massage," "standard massage," "Swedish massage," or "classical massage." As a result, the discussion of the research base for petrissage and the list of related impairment-level outcomes of care is larger for this technique than for other massage techniques. The reader is advised that some of the following discussion may be applicable to other techniques, especially the other neuromuscular techniques in this chapter.

CLINICAL INDICATIONS AND IMPAIRMENT-LEVEL OUTCOMES OF CARE

Much of the recent research on massage focuses on the psychoneuroimmunological effects of classical massage. Nevertheless, petrissage may also have physical effects on muscle resting tension and connective tissue extensibility, in addition to effects on pain, cardiopulmonary function, and immune function. Finally, its effects on circulation and reflex effects on visceral function are less certain.

Classical massage may reduce anxiety (measured by state-trait questionnaires and salivary cortisol levels), reduce stress, and improve relaxation.[31–41] This anxiolytic effect has been observed in a wide variety of clinical settings and clinical conditions. In addition, petrissage may be useful in alleviating the behavioral symptoms of depression,[15,33,37,39,41–43] hyperactivity,[44] and other conditions with affective components.[36,40,44,45] Several studies have shown improved immune function and positively altered allergic responses.[46–48]

The effect of petrissage on the level of resting muscle tension can probably not be considered apart from its psychological effects.[49] Anxiety has a well-documented generalized effect of increasing the level of resting tension of skeletal muscle;[50,51] as a result, interventions that reduce anxiety may have indirect effects on resting level of tension. Beyond this generalized effect, there is little recent research. Although some authors state that petrissage can reduce the level of muscle resting tension in the area to which it is applied, because of mechanical stress on proprioceptors,[1,3,5,6] others are equivocal or do not mention this effect.[2,7,8] Related research suggests that petrissage decreases motoneuron excitability, but only during the application of the technique.[52–58] This may be of limited clinical usefulness,[59,60] except when treating patterns of abnormal movement and abnormal neuromuscular tone (spasticity) that are associated with lesions of the brain or spinal cord.[8,54]

Other related research notes that increases in joint range of motion may occur after the application of petrissage,[61,62] although it is unclear whether the effect is due to increased mobility of connective tissue or decreased muscle resting tension. Increased extensibility and mobility of connective tissue is noted as an effect of petrissage in several texts[1,3,6,7] and research studies.[63–65] However, it is unlikely that petrissage will lengthen connective tissue to the same degree as connective tissue techniques, which apply more-sustained tensional load or drag (see Chapter 8, Connective Tissue Techniques). The observed positive effects of petrissage on pulmonary conditions such as asthma, chronic obstructive pulmonary disease (COPD), and cystic fibrosis may be a result of the combined effects of decreased anxiety and increased chest wall mobility.[66–68]

Clients who received petrissage reported a significant reduction in their perception of pain during labor,[69,70] after surgery,[71] with cancer,[72,73] and with chronic orthopedic conditions.[74,75] Petrissage may also be of value in the reduction of low back pain.[76] To date, the mechanisms of the analgesia resulting from the application of petrissage are not thoroughly understood. Current theories include the gating of pain impulses, increased serotonin levels, and improved restorative sleep.[15,77,78]

While most texts state that petrissage increases venous return,[2–4,6,7] research suggests otherwise. This technique may have marginal effects on blood chemistry and local blood flow,[79–80] but its effects on regional and systemic flow are likely to be both small and transient, if they occur at all.[81–85] A more likely effect is an increase in lymphatic return, although the studies documenting this effect used repetitive compressive techniques produced by machines.[86–88] Reduction of edema is a possible effect when the technique is applied proximal to the edema and around the periphery of swelling (if tolerable). Consistent with the finding of a marginal effect of petrissage on blood flow is the observation that "sports massage" (including petrissage) does not often increase the rate of removal of lactate from muscle after exercise above that for passive rest.[89–92] In fact, although massage has experienced much recent popularity among athletes, recent reviews are generally skeptical about its ability to enhance many types of function in a sports context.[93–95] For example, research has not shown that petrissage before athletic activity can greatly enhance performance;[96–98] its effects on delayed-onset muscle soreness are equivocal;[99–101] and postperformance reports on repair of damage, recovery of function, and mood are mixed.[102–107] By contrast, the effects of petrissage on rehabilitation and mood have been consistently demonstrated in other contexts.[31–43,61,63,65,74–76,108–114]

Petrissage has been used in conjunction with a variety of other techniques in multimodal treatment programs for clinical conditions such as headaches, trigger point syndromes, low back pain, fibromyalgia, and emphysema.[108–114] In these situations, the positive effects of petrissage appear to be enhanced in programs that include the use of modalities and client participation.[109,114] Finally, foreign studies (lamentably available in English only in abstract) intriguingly suggest that classical massage (including petrissage) can be used to achieve reflex effects on circulation and visceral function that are not mentioned in the English literature.[115–122]

The main impairment-level outcomes of care for petrissage are summarized in Table 7-1.

CAUTIONS AND CONTRAINDICATIONS

Clinical training and supervised practice are critical for the proper application of petrissage. Advanced training may be advisable, particularly when dealing with pathological conditions. All of the general and local contraindications noted for massage techniques apply to the use of petrissage (see Chapter 2, The Clinical Decision-Making Process).[30] In addition, there are several specific contraindications to the application of petrissage: clients with hemophilia, local sites of acute inflammation and infection, confirmed or suspected thrombus,[123] thrombophlebitis, and potentially metastatic malignancy. Clients who have confirmed or suspected osteoporosis or wounds in early stages of healing or who are taking anticoagulants require careful examination and moderation of the pressure with which the petrissage is applied. The clinician must exercise care when treating areas of spasm, hypotonia, and active trigger points. The use of excessive pressure may damage delicate terminal lymphatics, although this damage itself may facilitate the drainage of edema.[124] Lastly, difficulties may arise with the application of any massage techniques to clients who have profound learning disabilities or dementia.[125,126]

Prerequisite Skills for Petrissage

Before practicing petrissage, students should be able to

- Describe the spatial relationship between bones and major groups of skeletal muscle throughout the body
- Specify the proximal and distal attachments, action, fiber direction, and spatial relationships of major skeletal muscles
- Palpate the fiber directions, borders, and tendons of superficial muscles
- Assess muscular tone
- Use a postural analysis to assess muscular bulk, tone, and balance
- Use wide-stance knee bend, lunge, and lunge and lean postures

See Chapter 4, Preparation and Positioning for Treatment, and Appendix B, Selected Soft-Tissue Examination Techniques.

Manual Technique begins on next page

MANUAL TECHNIQUE

Petrissage 1: Muscle Squeezing

In the following figures (Figs. 7-9 to 7-15) muscle squeezing is applied to the various regions of the body. Figures are ordered from head to foot in supine and then prone. Each figure illustrates most of the guidelines for manual technique outlined below.

PETRISSAGE 1: MUSCLE SQUEEZING

Other Names Used for This Technique

"Squeezing," "squeeze-kneading."[1–8]

1. This nongliding technique is best performed without lubricant and can be applied effectively through fabric (Fig. 7-12).

2. One or both hands are used to grasp, lift, and squeeze a muscle, muscle group, or body segment, with minimal glide. It is easiest to perform on mid-sized body segments such as the calf (Fig. 7-15), upper arm, upper trapezius (Fig. 7-13), hand, and foot (Fig. 7-12).

3. Smaller muscles such as the sternocleidomastoid may be squeezed between the thumb and index finger (Figs. 7-9 and 7-10).

4. If two hands are used, a bowing action may be added to further shear the muscle.

5. Because this technique uses mostly hand and forearm strength, extended application is not recommended, especially if it is being applied to large muscle groups like the quadriceps (Fig. 7-11).

Components of Muscle Squeezing

Contact: The entire palmar surface; the thumb and index finger and included web space

Pressure: Light to moderate

Engages: Muscle and associated fascia

Direction: Applied around the (partial) circumference of the muscle belly or limbs

Amplitude/length: NA

Rate: 1 to 3 sec or more per cycle of compression/release

Duration: 10 to 20 sec or more

Intergrades with: Other forms of petrissage

Context: Usually used as an introductory muscular technique that is preceded by superficial effleurage and followed by more-specific forms of petrissage; may be used as a finishing stroke or by itself to address a region in a short time

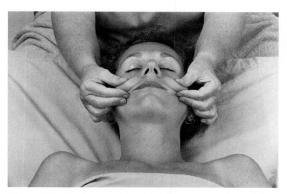

Figure 7-9. Gentle squeezing of facial muscles and superficial tissues between index and thumb.

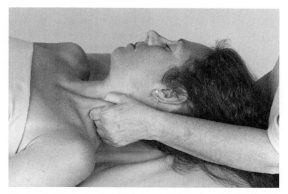

Figure 7-10. Squeezing either head of the sternocleidomastoid between thumb and index may elicit pain from latent myofascial trigger points (see later in this chapter). The clinician must be able to distinguish between the two divisions of the muscle.

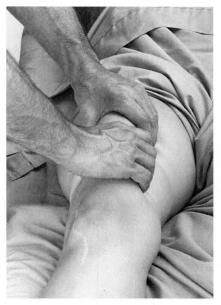

Figure 7-11. Two-handed squeezing of bulky muscle groups, such as the quadriceps, taxes the hands, and should not be done for long periods.

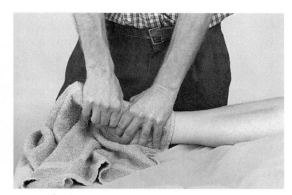

Figure 7-12. Squeezing the whole foot through the sheet or a towel often gives the clinician a better grip and thus yields a deeper application of technique than working directly on the skin.

Manual Technique Figures continue on next page

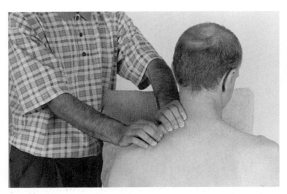

Figure 7-13. Squeezing of the upper trapezius muscle can be done with the client prone, supine, sidelying, or seated. An additional bowing force may be added.

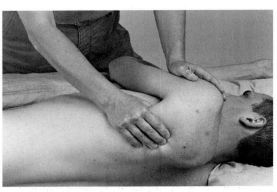

Figure 7-14. The muscles of the posterior axillary wall (teres major and latissimus dorsi) are easily accessible for squeezing when the client is in sidelying. One hand squeezes while the other hand positions the scapula, as desired, to increase accessibility of the muscles.

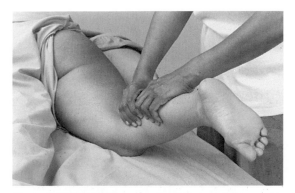

Figure 7-15. Two-handed squeezing of the posterior compartments of the leg may be combined with passive flexion/extension of the knee or with shaking of the ankle and foot.

Clinician's Position and Movement for Muscle Squeezing

1. The basic positions used by the clinician are described in Chapter 4, Preparation and Positioning for Treatment, in the sections on standing aligned posture and seated aligned posture. The clinician's position is quite variable. When treating larger body segments, the clinician usually faces the long axis of the muscle(s) to be squeezed (Figs. 7-12 to 7-15).

Manual Technique begins on next page

MANUAL TECHNIQUE

Petrissage 2: Wringing

In the following figures (Figs. 7-16 to 7-22), wringing is applied to the various regions of the body. Figures are ordered from head to foot on the anterior surface and then the posterior surface. Each figure illustrates most of the guidelines for manual technique outlined below.

PETRISSAGE 2: WRINGING

1. For large body segments, the hands rest on opposite sides of the circumference of the body segment to be wrung and compress toward each other (Fig. 7-18A).

2. Maintaining compression, the hands slide toward each other, lifting and shearing the muscle between them as they pass each other (Figs. 7-17, 7-18B, 7-20, and 7-22).

3. The hands continue to slide without exerting pressure until they rest on opposite sides of the body segment on which they began, and a new stroke is initiated (Fig. 7-18C). After two complete cycles, the hands will be in the position in which they started.

4. The clinician must be careful to apply pressure gradually at the beginning of the strokes, to avoid jerking.

5. To wring large body segments, such as the torso or quadriceps muscles, the thumbs should be adducted to avoid strain on the carpometacarpal joints (Figs. 7-17, 7-18A to C, and 7-20). For smaller body segments, such as arms, hands, or feet, the thumbs may be abducted so that the entire web space between the thumb and index remains in contact during the technique (Figs. 7-16 and 7-19). Wringing with abducted thumbs places undue strain on the joints of the thumb and should be avoided except for short treatment periods.

6. As with other forms of petrissage that use the whole hand, begin wringing proximally on the limb and proceed in a distal direction. Return proximally with wringing or with superficial effleurage and repeat. This is thought to maximize lymphatic return by clearing proximal areas first.[60]

7. Areas of elevated resting tension can benefit from extended (5 or more min) periods of wringing, although this involves a lot of work on the part of the clinician.

8. *Note:* Considerable pressure is needed to lift and shear the bulk of large muscle groups between the hands as the hands pass each other. The clinician must avoid the tendency to produce a superficial effleurage which is oriented across the body segment and has no mechanical effect on the muscle itself.

Components of Wringing

Contact: Palmar surface of both hands

Pressure: Light to heavy

Engages: Muscle, associated fascia, and contained tissues

Direction: Across the long axis of the body segment

Amplitude/length: Half circumference of the body segment to which wringing is being applied

Speed: 1 to 3 sec per cycle of compress/release

Rate: 20 to 60 sec or more

Intergrades with: Other forms of general petrissage

Context: Usually used as an introductory muscular technique that is preceded by superficial effleurage and followed by more-specific forms of petrissage

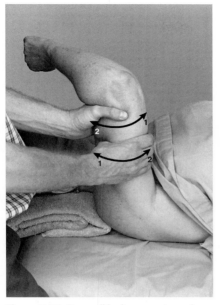

Figure 7-16. On small body segments, such as the upper arm, wringing may be done with thumbs abducted. In this position, the client's arm must be completely relaxed.

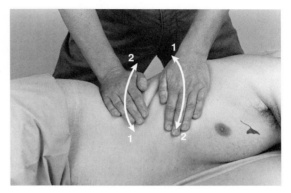

Figure 7-17. Wringing the lower rib cage in prone, supine, or sidelying is an indirect way of loosening the respiratory diaphragm.

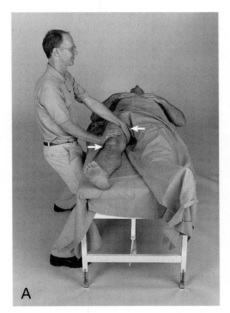

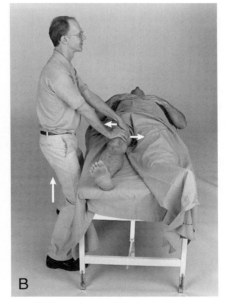

Figure 7-18. A. For bulky regions, such as the quadriceps, the hamstrings, and the back, effective wringing requires that the clinician use correct body mechanics. At the start of the stroke, the hands are diametrically opposed. They then begin to compress together. The clinician's posture is wide-stance ("horse stance") with bent knees. **B.** The clinician's legs straighten, adding force to the lift and shear produced by the passing hands.

Manual Technique Figures continue on next page

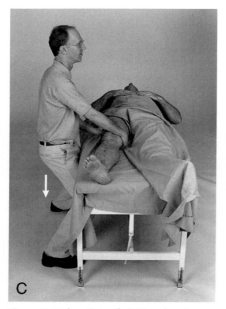

Figure 7-18 (continued). C. The relaxation phase: the hands pass each other, release tissue, and move to a position opposite the starting position. Simultaneously, the knees bend again in preparation for the next stroke.

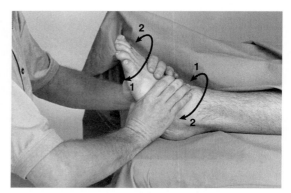

Figure 7-19. Wringing an entire foot or hand engages many structures with each stroke and is a good choice of technique when time is limited.

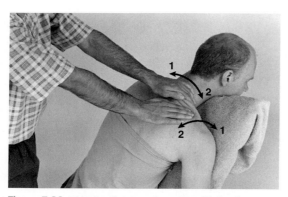

Figure 7-20. Wringing the upper trapezius with the client seated.

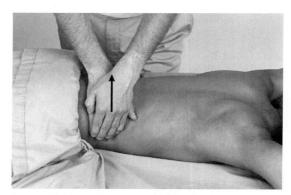

Figure 7-21. A variation of wringing involves one- or two-handed lifting of the torso in prone or supine. Gravity provides the opposing force.

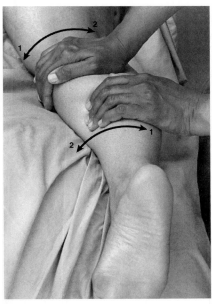

Figure 7-22. Wringing the calf.

Clinician's Position and Movement for Wringing

For large body segments such as the torso or thighs, wringing must be performed with correct leg movement, to generate sufficient force to compress, lift, and shear large masses between the hands. The clinician achieves this leg movement with the following steps:

1. Stand facing the long axis of the body segment to be wrung (Fig. 7-18A).
2. Begin in the wide-stance knee-bend posture with the knees flexed between 30 and 45 degrees. The lowered position allows some palmar contact of the near hand while reducing extension of the wrist (Fig. 7-18A).
3. During the pressure phase of the stroke, as the hands compress and slide toward each other, straighten the legs without hyperextending the knees (Fig. 7-18B). During the relaxation phase of the stroke, as the hands slide apart, flex the knees again (Fig. 7-18C). Thus for each stroke, the knees flex and extend; much of the power for the application of the technique is generated by the extension of knees.
4. Coordination of the leg and arm movements takes practice. The reward is a secure, smooth, very deep, and effective technique.
5. Initially, the clinician's legs may fatigue or become sore; this passes as the clinician's leg strength increases.

When wringing smaller body segments, the clinician can use a variety of aligned postures that are described in Chapter 4, Preparation and Positioning for Treatment.

Manual Technique begins on next page

MANUAL TECHNIQUE

Petrissage 3: Picking Up ("C-Kneading")

In the following figures (Figs. 7-23 to 7-28,) picking up is applied to the various regions of the body. Figures are ordered from head to foot in supine and then prone. Each figure illustrates most of the guidelines for manual technique outlined below.

A. One-handed technique for smaller body segments such as the arms, forearms, and calves (Figs. 7-23 to 7-24C)

 1. The thumb is abducted so the hand forms a C-shape, with the four fingers grouped together in adduction.

 2. Grasp and squeeze while gliding in a centripetal direction. Most of the hand remains in contact with the client's body, with the focus on the thumb, index finger, and web space. The client's tissues are squeezed through the closing web space for the power stroke, and the thumb is progressively adducted toward the end of the stroke ("squeezing off the stroke").

 3. During the power stroke, the clinician can make an effort to lift the tissues off the underlying bone (Fig. 7-24A, B, and C).

 4. The hand reopens to a C-shape while gliding back to its original position with minimal pressure (return stroke).

 5. One author suggests using a four count as follows: compress on one, grasp and lift on two, release on three, and move/glide on four.[8]

B. Alternate two-handed technique for larger or flatter body segments such as the thighs and back (Figs. 7-25, 7-27, and 7-28)

 1. The two hands face each other in an open C position as described above (Fig. 7-28).

 2. The individual motion of each hand is similar to the one-handed technique described above. However, the two hands work in contrary motion: one hand performs a short power stroke while the other is performing a short return stroke. Power strokes are delivered toward the opposing hand; return strokes move away from the opposing hand.

 3. For optimal effectiveness, the clinician should sustain some compression between the hands throughout the application of this technique. This results in a continuous lifting of the tissue between the hands.

 4. On limbs, begin the sequence of strokes proximally and gradually move the focus of the strokes distally.[60]

 5. Coordination between the hands takes practice; once mastered, it yields a technique that clients perceive as very pleasant.

 6. The prolonged application of picking up (one- or two-handed) is not advisable because of wear on the clinician's hands and forearms.

Components of Picking Up

Contact: Palmar surface, especially the web space between the thumb and index finger

Pressure: Light to moderate

Engages: Muscle and associated fascia

Direction: Parallel to the long axis of the body segment

Amplitude/length: 5 to 20 cm or more

Rate: 1 to 3 sec per cycle of compression/release

Duration: 20 to 60 sec or more

Intergrades with: Other forms of general petrissage

Context: Usually preceded by superficial effleurage and more-general forms of petrissage and followed by more-specific forms of petrissage

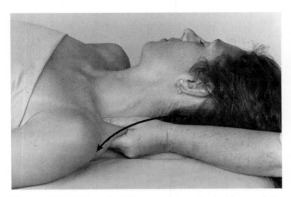

Figure 7-23. Unilateral picking up of upper trapezius muscle in supine.

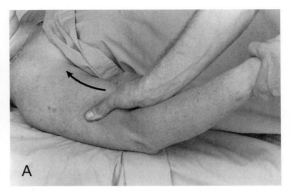

Figure 7-24. Upper arms are an ideal size for one-handed picking up. **A.** The biceps brachii.

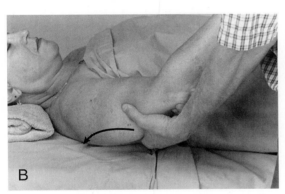

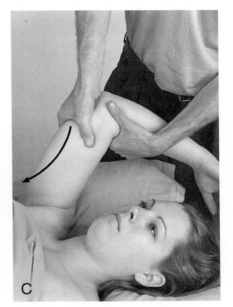

Figure 7-24 (continued). B. The triceps brachii (with the glenohumeral joint in the loose-packed position). **C.** The triceps with the shoulder and elbow flexed. Apply pressure in a centripetal direction and lift the tissues away from the underlying bone.

Manual Technique Figures continue on next page

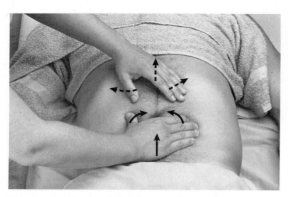

Figure 7-25. Two-handed picking up of rectus abdominus. Return stroke is shown in a *dotted line.* Practice is required to attain good contact during two-handed picking up on flat surfaces like the abdomen or the back.

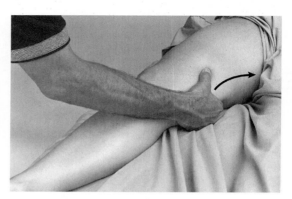

Figure 7-26. One-handed picking up of the adductors of the hip.

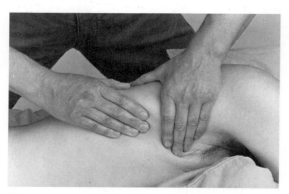

Figure 7-27. Two-handed picking up is a good technique for the lateral edge of the latissimus dorsi. The clinician can work her way down to the iliac crest. Placing the client's arm overhead also improves access to the abdominal oblique and quadratus lumborum muscles.

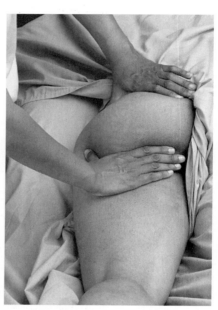

Figure 7-28. Hand position to begin two-handed picking up of the gluteals.

Clinician's Position and Movement for Pickiing Up

1. The basic positions used by the clinician are described in Chapter 4, Preparation and Positioning for Treatment, under standing aligned posture, wide-stance knee bend, and wide-stance knee bend with trunk rotation.

2. To generate more force during the application of one-handed forms, shift or lean forward into the client's body during the compression and lift portion of the stroke; then shift or lean back during the release and move portion.

3. For the application of two-handed forms, the clinician stands facing the long axis of the body segment in the wide-stance knee bend, as for wringing. Knee flexion in this position may reduce hyperextension of the wrists by bringing the clinician closer to the level of the client (Fig. 7-27).

4. To generate more power for two-handed forms, rotate the ipsilateral shoulder, to lean slightly into each power stroke (wide-stance knee bend with trunk rotation). This increases the force and effectiveness of the technique, minimizes hand and forearm fatigue, and results in a smooth upper body rhythm.

5. Do not let the shoulders elevate during the application of the technique.

Manual Technique begins on next page

Petrissage 4: Broad-Contact Kneading and "Deep Effleurage"

In the following figures (Figs. 7-29 to 7-36), broad-contact kneading is applied to the various regions of the body. Figures are ordered from head to foot in supine and then prone. Each figure illustrates most of the guidelines for manual technique outlined below.

1. As with wringing and picking up, there is a pressure stroke and a return stroke. The pressure stroke and return stroke combine to form circles or ellipses that are oriented along or across the fibers in the different muscle layers (Figs. 7-30A and B and 7-33). Most often, the long axis of the stroke runs parallel to the long axis of the body segment or muscle to which the technique is being applied, especially when significant pressure is required (Figs. 7-30A and 7-33). Elongating the ellipse results in "deep effleurage," provided the pressure is centripetal (Figs. 7-33 and 7-34).

2. Maintain the wrist in neutral (no radial or ulnar deviation). This is critical to reduce joint stress with high-pressure applications of broad-contact kneading (Figs. 7-29, 7-30A and B, 7-33, 7-35, and 7-36).

3. Other options are to reinforce the dorsal surface of the hand or wrist with the other hand (Figs. 7-30A, and 7-33) or to bring the hands together so that they reinforce each other (Fig. 7-35).

4. More-specific contact can be obtained by bridging or arching the hand slightly (flexing the metacarpophalangeal and interphalangeal joints), which produces two contact surfaces—broader at the heel and more specific at the fingertips. (Fig. 7-33).

5. As with the application of all types of petrissage, begin proximally and proceed in a distal direction while maintaining centripetal pressure to maximize lymphatic return.

6. Variations: Some authors describe a form of circular kneading in which no glide occurs over the skin.[7] This technique engages muscle and is, in other respects, the same as kneading that glides over the skin.

7. Other variations: Some authors describe a two-handed form of kneading, termed fulling or broadening, in which the hands compress in a direction that is down and away from each other to spread or broaden the muscle belly, and then lift the muscle up on the return stroke.[3,5]

8. Other variations: Some authors describe a two-handed form of kneading, termed box kneading, in which the hands are positioned so that they are diametrically opposed on a limb, then compress toward each other, and then move proximally. This stroke is recommended to increase fluid return (Fig. 7-30B).[7]

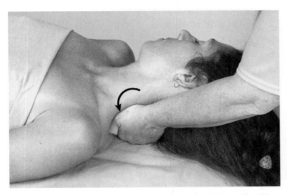

Figure 7-29. Kneading the posterior triangle of the neck with the heel of the hand.

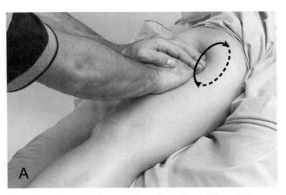

Figure 7-30. **A.** Reinforced palmar kneading of the anterior thigh. Return stroke is shown in a *dotted line*.

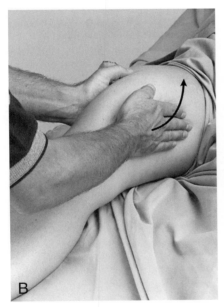

Figure 7-30 (continued). **B.** One version of "box-kneading." The hands can work in opposition, lifting tissue and/or pushing it proximally.

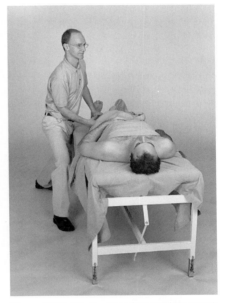

Figure 7-31. Effective kneading requires correct application of the clinician's body weight. This is especially true when kneading the iliotibial band, which is composed of dense connective tissue. The clinician stabilizes his elbow against his iliac crest and carefully shifts his body weight toward the client.

Manual Technique Figures continue on next page

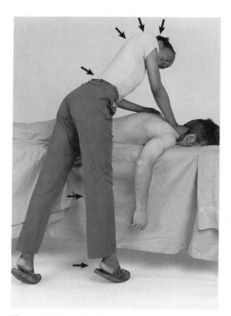

Figure 7-32. This clinician is committing at least five common errors of body mechanics while attempting a forceful kneading of trapezius. Common errors of body mechanics are detailed in Chapter 4, Preparation and Positioning for Treatment.

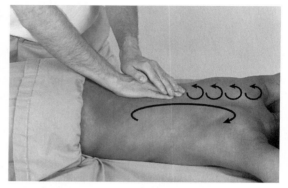

Figure 7-33. Reinforced palmar kneading to the erector spinae muscles performed with a slightly arched hand. The strokes may take the form of smaller circles or of one long ellipse that covers the erector spinae muscles in a single stroke ("deep stroking" or "deep effleurage").

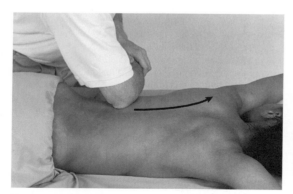

Figure 7-34. Using the forearm along the erector spinae muscles. The clinician must be careful to avoid compressing the spinous processes. The return stroke is often omitted.

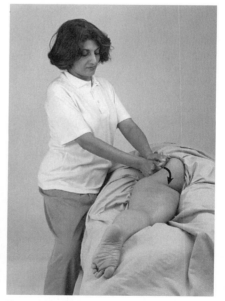

Figure 7-35. Reinforced fist kneading of the superior gluteal attachments is most effective when tissue is moved away from the sacrum or iliac crest.

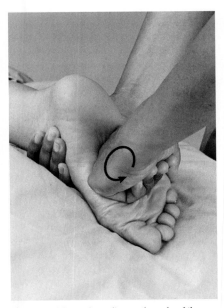

Figure 7-36. Fist kneading to the sole of the foot is easier to control if the fist is rotated during the stroke. A deeper but less comfortable technique is obtained if the foot is passively dorsiflexed.

Components of Broad-Contact Kneading

Contact: Full palmar surface of the hand, often reinforced on the wrist and/or metacarpals, fist/knuckles, or proximal forearm

Pressure: Light to heavy

Engages: Muscle and associated tissues; slower strokes and greater drag (horizontal tension) will lengthen connective tissue elements of the muscle more

Direction: Circular or elliptical; the long axis of ellipses is often oriented parallel to the long axis of muscles or muscle groups

Amplitude/length: 10 cm or more

Rate: 10 to 25 cm/sec

Duration: 20 to 60 sec or more

Intergrades with: Superficial effleurage and other forms of petrissage; a notable, commonly used variation sometimes called "deep effleurage" or "deep stroking" has the same long, gliding template of superficial effleurage, but engages muscle with a considerable amount of pressure; this is not a superficial maneuver and has much in common with the broad-contact kneading described here; nongliding forms using fingertip contact intergrade with friction (see Chapter 8, Connective Tissue Techniques).

Context: Usually preceded by superficial effleurage, alternated with other general forms of petrissage, and followed by more-specific forms of petrissage

Clinician's Position and Movement

1. The basic positions used by the clinician are described in Chapter 4, Preparation and Positioning for Treatment, in the sections on lunge, lunge and reach, lunge and lean, and standing controlled lean. In these positions, the clinician's torso is pointed toward the point of contact (Figs. 7-31 and 7-35).

2. The power portion of the stroke occurs through partial extension of the elbows, which may be coupled with a forward movement during the lunge or the inclining of the body toward the contact point during the lunge and lean (Figs. 7-31 and 7-35).

3. Shoulders and arms transmit the force from the correct lower body movement; they do not generate it. Consequently, greater force of application of this technique can be generated through the correct use of the legs and body weight.

4. Common errors that occur, especially when the clinician is trying to generate more pressure, are:

   Hyperextension of the elbows ("straight-arming")
   Excessive elevation and/or protraction of the shoulders
   Tilting of the head
   Excessive leaning forward at the waist (Fig. 7-32)

   All of these errors are more likely to occur if the table is too high.

Petrissage 5: Specific Kneading

In the following figures (Figs. 7-37 to 7-44B), specific kneading is applied to the various regions of the body. Figures are ordered from head to foot in supine and then prone. Each figure illustrates most of the guidelines for manual technique outlined below.

PETRISSAGE: SPECIFIC KNEADING (THUMBS, FINGERPADS, FINGERTIPS)

A. Fingertip and Fingerpad Technique (Figs. 7-37, 7-39, 7-42, 7-43)

1. Unless the surface to be kneaded is relatively small (Fig. 7-37), the fingers of the hand are usually held together (Fig. 7-42 and 7-43). The heel or the entire rest of the hand may remain in contact with the client's body to provide stability (Fig. 7-42). When light pressure is required, as when kneading the face, this stabilization may be omitted.

2. Repetitive circles are commonly performed, with the pressure being applied during the portion of the stroke that pushes away from the clinician; this potentially allows the use of body weight to augment the force of application.

3. The other hand may reinforce across the carpals and metacarpals of the working hand to stabilize the wrist and enhance the force of the technique (Fig. 7-43).

B. Thumb Technique (Figs. 7-38, 7-40, 7-41, 7-44A and B)

1. The hand lies close to or flat on the surface of the client's body, with the fingers parallel (Fig. 7-38). Fingertips remain loosely in contact, and depending on the shape of the region to be kneaded, the heel of the hand may also remain in partial contact (Fig. 7-40).

2. The ventral surface of the distal first phalanx delivers pressure in small ellipses, the long axis of which is parallel to the long axis of the thumb. The thumbs are not widely abducted during this motion (Figs. 7-41 and 7-44A).

3. The clinician must be careful to ensure that the pressure is exerted along, rather than across, the long axis of the thumb.

4. Usually both thumbs are used in a technique known as alternate thumb kneading. One thumb performs a pressure stroke while the other performs a return stroke (Figs. 7-38, 7-41, and 7-44A & B).

5. The technique described above may seem awkward at first, but it places a minimum amount of stress on the mobile, vulnerable joints of the thumb.

6. Specific kneading should be performed sparingly for short periods and be frequently alternated with other techniques that place different stresses on the joints of the hand.

Components of Specific Kneading

Contact: Fingertips, fingerpads, or thumbs form the working surface; in either case the heel of the hand remains in contact to stabilize the hand

Pressure: Light to moderate

Engages: Muscle and associated tissues; slower strokes and greater drag (horizontal tension) will likely lengthen connective tissue elements of the muscle more than faster strokes

Direction: Circular or elliptical; the long axis of ellipses is often oriented parallel to the long axis of muscles or muscle groups

Amplitude/length: Up to 10 cm (determined by size of clinician's hand)

Rate: 0.5 to 2 sec per cycle of compression/release

Duration: Up to 20 sec at one time, provided clinician does not experience hand fatigue

Intergrades with: Stripping

Context: Usually preceded by, alternated with, and followed by superficial effleurage and more-general forms of petrissage such as wringing or palmar kneading

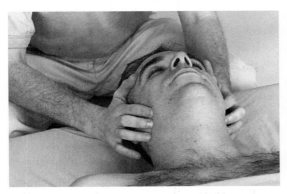

Figure 7-37. Fingertips and finger pads are ideal for petrissage of the face, which is usually done without applying lubricant. Finger pad kneading of the masseter muscle.

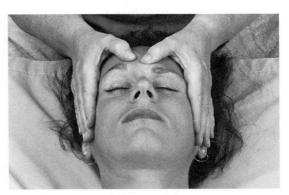

Figure 7-38. Alternate thumb-kneading to the belly of the frontalis muscle.

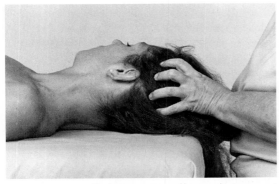

Figure 7-39. Fingertip kneading of the scalp may be performed lightly with glide over the skin and through the hair or with more pressure and no glide.

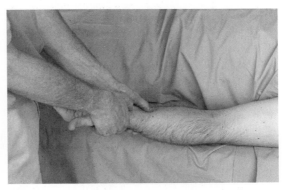

Figure 7-40. Alternate thumb-kneading is a technique that fits onto forelimbs beautifully. Begin proximally, proceed distally, and return with a long centripetal stroke to the starting position. On the calf, the return stroke will "split" the heads of the gastrocnemius muscle.

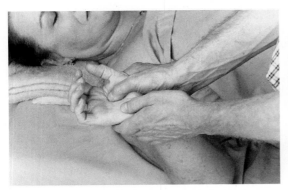

Figure 7-41. Slow, rhythmical thumb-kneading of the thenar and hypothenar eminences is deeply relaxing. Because of the large number of structures in the hand (or the foot), thorough petrissage can take 30 min or longer.

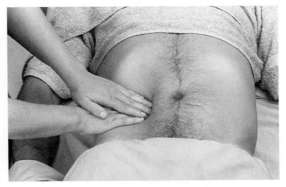

Figure 7-42. Finger pad kneading to the lateral border of rectus abdominus muscle.

Manual Technique Figures continue on next page

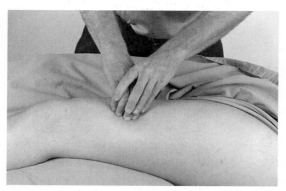

Figure 7-43. Reinforced fingertip kneading of the quadriceps muscle.

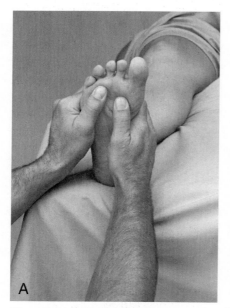

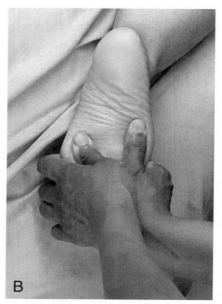

Figure 7-44. A. The clinician kneels at the foot of the table to perform alternate thumb-kneading to the sole of the foot in supine. **B.** The same technique in prone.

Clinician's Position and Movement for Specific Kneading

1. The basic positions used by the clinician are described in Chapter 4, Preparation and Positioning for Treatment, in the sections on standing, seated, or kneeling aligned posture. The clinician is positioned facing the body segment.
2. During thumb kneading, the movement of the thumbs is quite constrained as described above. The force of the technique is derived from small movements at the carpometacarpal, carpal, and elbow joints, which bring the weight of the forearm and upper arm into play.
3. During fingertip kneading, the clinician can increase the force of application by leaning slightly into the stroke while pushing the fingers away.

PALPATE (FOR ALL FORMS OF PETRISSAGE)

As she performs the technique, the clinician palpates the client's skin and tissues for the following:

1. General resistance and resilience of soft tissues
2. Mobility of the interfaces between the muscles and muscle layers
3. Resistance to further stretch toward the end of the excursion of each stroke
4. Localized areas of hardness that may require use of more-specific techniques
5. Taut bands in muscle, which may reflect trigger point activity (see later in this chapter)
6. Fibrosis, adhesions, and induration within and between muscle layers, which can indicate chronic inflammation
7. Decrease in local fluid viscosity with continued application of the technique
8. The palpable softening of muscle tissue, which often results when petrissage is applied for several minutes; this may reflect a decrease in the viscosity of superficial tissues, caused by increased temperature; an increase in the hydration of the connective tissue matrix; a softening of taut bands, which is consistent with reduced activity of trigger points; and a marginal systemic decrease in the level of resting tension of skeletal muscle, if the massage is relaxing
9. The clinician slows the rate of petrissage when working in deep layers, to facilitate palpation and to allow superficial tissue to move aside with each stroke

OBSERVE (FOR ALL FORMS OF PETRISSAGE)

As she performs the technique, the clinician observes the client for changes in the level of resting muscle tension and edema. Some of these signs are listed in the following:

1. Systemic reduction of muscle tension, as evidenced by softening of the tissue contours or broadening and flattening of body segments
2. General consistency and resting level of tone; How fluid does the tissue appear as it is being moved?
3. Taut, visible bands in resting muscle; a muscle with a visibly well-defined anatomical form when not in use is probably hypertonic
4. Hyperemia; a reactive hyperemia may accompany the application of this technique
5. If petrissage is used to treat edema (proximal to the edema) or fibrosed edema (on-site), note signs of resorption of fluid from edematous tissue: changes in surface contours, reduction in size or hardness of edema, and changes in the viscosity and inertial resistance of the subcutaneous tissues
6. The depth of the penetration of the effect of the stroke; as the client's muscles relax and the fluid viscosity of the tissues decreases, the same force will produce effects deeper into and further along the client's tissues; consequently, it does not require greater force to achieve a greater penetration of effects, simply the appropriate application of the technique for longer periods

COMMUNICATION WITH THE CLIENT

The clinician uses communication to ensure the client's comfort during the application of the technique. Some examples of statements that the clinician can use are listed below.

1. "Is this pressure OK?" "Would you like it deeper?" "Would you like less pressure?" "Which feels better . . . this . . . (adjust depth) or this?" Ensure that the depth of technique is comfortable for the client.
2. "Is it tender here?" "When I work here, do you feel it anywhere else?" In cases in which the client examination suggests that there is elevated muscle resting tension, slowly increase the depth of application of the technique while inquiring about tenderness and possible referral of pain.

COMPLEMENTARY MODALITIES

There are several modalities that the clinician can use in a complementary manner to enhance the effects of petrissage.

1. Physical agents. With chronic orthopedic conditions, the clinician can appropriately apply deep moist heat, such as a hot pack, for 5 to 20 min (until a mild hyperemia appears on the client's skin) prior to the application of compression.

2. In situations in which there is a generalized elevation of the level of resting tension in skeletal muscle because of stress, the clinician may use diaphragmatic breathing, progressive relaxation, or other appropriate relaxation techniques.
3. Petrissage is an excellent elude to passive stretching, proprioceptive neuromuscular facilitation techniques, and joint mobilization.

POSTINTERVENTION SELF-CARE INSTRUCTIONS

1. Extensive deep petrissage may occasionally produce mild local soreness during a 24- to 48-h period following intervention. The clinician can advise the client that a warm bath, a warm Epsom salts bath, or the application of moist heat may reduce this soreness.
2. More-severe or persistent postintervention pain or pain that arises in adjacent areas may indicate activation of a latent or satellite trigger point (see later in this chapter) or the generalized reactive tightening of antagonist muscle groups. The clinician should always instruct clients to contact the clinician when more than mild, transient pain results from the application of any massage technique.
3. Depending on the clinical situation, the use of therapeutic exercise, automobilization techniques, diaphragmatic breathing, or progressive relaxation exercises may be indicated.
4. Clients can be taught self-massage of accessible areas.
5. Family members can be taught to perform basic petrissage and the cautions involved in applying this within a home program.[68]

A Practice Sequence for Petrissage

First, attempt each technique individually until you are confident of the basics of the manual technique and body movement. You can then apply the following basic sequence, initially allowing 15 to 20 min for any region. The same sequence can be adapted with minor variations for all regions.

1. Apply a small amount of lubricant to the client's body using superficial effleurage.
2. Begin by applying wringing proximally on the region, then move distally.
3. Once you reach the most distal part of the region, either apply wringing on the way back up, or return with superficial effleurage.
4. Using a similar pattern, which begins proximally and proceeds distally, introduce in turn

Muscle squeezing

Picking up

Broad-contact kneading

Specific kneading

Whenever possible maximize centripetal pressure. At the end, finish with wringing and then superficial effleurage.

Regional modifications:
Back: Proximal and distal can be designated as being at either end of the back.

Abdomen: Where possible (i.e., with effleurage and kneading), apply the techniques in a generally clockwise direction and sequence.

Face: Use light pressure and no lubricant. Most of the techniques can be applied as described with slight adaptations. Use only two fingers or finger and thumb for "smaller" versions of wringing and picking up squeezing where tissue can be lifted. Fingertip kneading is the most useful technique.

Hands and feet: Many small muscles, ends of tendons, and fascial sheaths can be addressed individually to great effect. As with the face, the amplitude of the techniques is smaller; however, considerable pressure can be used because of the density of connective tissue in these regions.

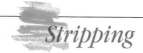

Stripping

OTHER NAMES USED FOR THIS TECHNIQUE

"Stripping massage," "deep stroking," "deep stroking massage."[127–129]

DEFINITION

Stripping: A very slow and specific gliding technique that is applied from one attachment of a muscle to the other for the purpose of reducing the activity of myofascial trigger points.[1-8]

NOTES

1. Travell and Simons first coined the term stripping massage.[127] Technically, it is related to specific petrissage (see above in this chapter), because it involves the compression and release of muscle fibers, and to direct fascial technique (see Chapter 8, Connective Tissue Techniques) because of the slow rate of glide. In this text, it is considered separately because of its well-defined method and excellent effect on trigger point activity.

2. As defined by Chaitow[130] and others, "neuromuscular technique" is a complex system of techniques that includes, among other techniques, finger and thumb strokes that resemble stripping, as it is defined above.

3. "Strumming" is a form of direct fascial technique that is directed along[131] or more commonly across[129,131] muscle fibers, which may sometimes resemble stripping and which may have effects on trigger point activity.

CLINICAL INDICATIONS AND IMPAIRMENT-LEVEL OUTCOMES OF CARE

A myofascial trigger point is a hyperirritable area in skeletal muscle that is associated with a hypersensitive and palpable nodule located in a taut band. The area is painful on compression and can give rise to a variety of symptoms, such as referred pain, referred tenderness, motor dysfunction, and autonomic phenomena.[129] Trigger points are categorized as active or latent, of primary location or a satellite. A trigger point has a characteristic response to palpation: a local twitch response of the taut muscle fibers, and referred pain in a specific pattern for that muscle, which occurs or increases on direct compression of the trigger point.[127-129,131] An active trigger point in a muscle refers pain whether the muscle is working or at rest, can weaken a muscle, and can prevent it from lengthening fully. By contrast, a latent trigger point is painful only when it is palpated. The application of specific compression to a latent trigger point will evoke the characteristic pain referral pattern for that trigger point. A muscle containing a latent trigger point can also be shortened and weakened.

Primary trigger points arise in response to trauma, acute and chronic overload (tendinopathies and repetitive strain disorders), postural imbalance, fatigue, and emotional stress and are exacerbated by a variety of factors.[129-131] Satellite trigger points may develop in response to altered biomechanics, in the pain referral area

of a primary trigger point, or in the synergist and antagonist muscle groups of the muscle that contains the primary trigger point.[131] Key trigger points are responsible for activating satellites; consequently, inactivation of a key trigger point will inactivate its associated satellites.[131] Trigger points may also occur in connective tissue, such as fascia, ligaments, and periosteum, and produce a variety of symptoms.[129,131]

Trigger points located in muscle are frequently the cause or the consequence of common musculoskeletal complaints, such as tension headache, temporomandibular joint problems, spinal pain, chronic low back pain, disk herniation, chronic pelvic pain, painful rib syndrome, nonarticular pain, and other myofascial pain syndromes.[130-142] Trigger points in muscle can cause nerve entrapments[128,129] and may also mimic nerve entrapments, radiculopathies, and visceral pathology.[128-129,142]

Stripping is indicated to reduce the activity, pain, and other symptoms of trigger points and to help restore the length and strength of the affected muscle.[129] It can be the preferred manual technique when trigger points are located near the center of a muscle. Inasmuch as stripping applies somewhat similar forces to the same tissue layer as petrissage, stripping may have many of the effects of petrissage when it is applied systematically to a region (see above in this chapter). Stripping may also share some effects with direct fascial technique (see Chapter 8, Connective Tissue Techniques). The main impairment-level outcomes of care for stripping are summarized in Table 7-1.

CAUTIONS AND CONTRAINDICATIONS

Clinical training and supervised practice are critical for the proper application of stripping. Advanced training may be advisable, particularly when dealing with pathological conditions. All of the general and local contraindications noted for massage techniques apply to the use of stripping (see Chapter 2, The Clinical Decision-Making Process).[1,30] Specific contraindications to the use of stripping include clients with hemophilia, local sites of acute inflammation and infection, confirmed or suspected thrombus,[123] thrombophlebitis, and potentially metastatic malignancies. Clinicians who are treating clients who have confirmed or suspected osteoporosis or wounds in early stages of healing or who use anticoagulants may choose to use a noncompressive manual method of inactivating trigger points, such as the combination of ice and stretching.[129] The clinician must also be careful when treating muscles that are adjacent to areas of spasm or acute inflammation.

Although Simons, Travell, and Simons[129] state that trigger points must be located by palpation, research suggests that latent trigger points cannot be reliably located using palpation.[143] Consequently, the clinician must make every effort to locate the points with precision. In addition, since trigger points can cause entrapments[128,129] and may mimic entrapments, radiculopathies, and visceral pathology,[128,129,140] the clinician must take particular care with her differential examination and promptly refer the client to his physician if a more serious clinical condition is suspected.

Active trigger points can cause excruciating, debilitating pain and be exquisitely sensitive to touch. In these cases, it is particularly important for the clinician to apply stripping with absolute respect for the client's pain tolerance. With long-standing or recurrent trigger points, the clinician must be careful to treat agonist, antagonist, and synergist muscle groups and to address the factors that may perpetuate the trigger points, such as structural asymmetry and repetitive ergonomic loading.[128–130] If an active trigger point remains after the correct application of treatment techniques, this may indicate that the trigger point is actually a satellite whose key trigger point must be addressed first. Extensive application of massage techniques to one muscle or muscle group around a joint may cause reactive tightening (reactive cramping) in the antagonist or synergist muscle groups or on the opposite side during or soon after the intervention.[129] Postintervention pain, which differs markedly from the client's presenting symptoms, is commonly a result of the activation of a latent or satellite trigger point and may indicate a need to treat the client's synergist and antagonist muscle groups more comprehensively.

Prerequisite Skills for Stripping

Before applying stripping students should be able to

Define the terms *latent, active, primary, key and satellite trigger points*

Describe the phenomenon of pain referral as it relates to trigger points (ideally students will recognize locations and referral patterns of common trigger points)

Describe fiber directions of all major skeletal muscles

Recognize a twitch response and jump sign

Identify a taut band

Solicit accurate feedback from client about pain referral

Use lunge and lean, and standing and seated controlled lean postures

See Chapter 4, Preparation and Positioning for Treatment, and Appendix B, Selected Soft-Tissue Examination Techniques.

MANUAL TECHNIQUE

Stripping

In the following figures (see Figs. 7-45 to 7-52), stripping is applied to the various regions of the body. Figures are ordered from head to foot in supine and then prone. Each figure illustrates most of the guidelines for manual technique outlined below. The manual technique presented largely follows Simons, Travell, and Simons.[129]

1. Place the client in a position that will comfortably allow full stretch of the target muscle. The target muscle should be neither slack nor tautly stretched.

2. If lubricant is not already present, apply a small amount either to the clinician's hands or to the client's skin.

Manual Technique continues on page 204

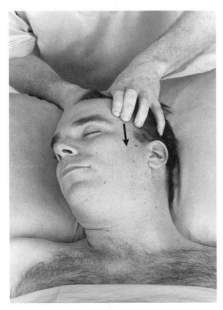

Figure 7-45. Fingertip stripping of the temporalis muscle, a common contributor to temporal headaches.

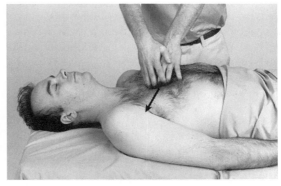

Figure 7-46. Reinforced fingertip stripping of the sternal head of pectoralis major muscle in a cross body position. If the client finds the pulling of hair uncomfortable, the clinician can add more lubricant or break the longer stroke into a series of shorter strokes, which follow the same line, at a comparable rate.

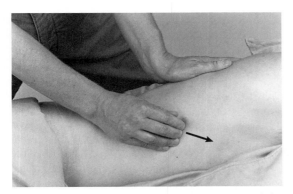

Figure 7-47. This stroke—very much like stripping except in its orientation to the intercostal muscle fibers—follows the intercostal spaces and will improve chest wall mobility.

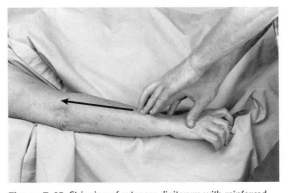

Figure 7-48. Stripping of extensor digitorum with reinforced fingertips.

Manual Technique Figures continue on page 205

3. Reinforce the fingers or thumbs whenever possible by placing the hands together (Figs. 7-46, 7-48, and 7-50) or use fingers as a group rather than individually (Figs. 7-47 and 7-52). Whenever possible, use pushing strokes, since they place less stress on the muscles of the hands and are easier to control than pulling strokes (all figures). When stripping larger or deeper muscles, using the elbow as the contact surface facilitates the use of body weight to increase the pressure of application of the technique (Figs. 7-49 and 7-51). Selected hand and body positions must be stable.

4. Beginning superficially and on one side of the trigger point, the clinician exerts sufficient pressure to engage the taut band then, in one continuous motion, glides slowly and with equal pressure along this layer across the trigger point all the way to the attachment of the muscle.[127,129] The next stroke starts on the other side of the trigger point and glides in the opposite direction toward the other attachment. If the taut band softens and the tenderness and pain referral diminish, the clinician can repeat this procedure again with the same pressure. Alternatively, the clinician can increase the pressure incrementally with each application.

5. The suggested rate of glide in the literature is 8 mm/sec,[127] or slowly enough to allow the nodule in the taut band to palpably release or soften beneath the advancing finger(s).[129] In either case the rate of glide is much slower than that of conventional petrissage.

6. The clinician must maintain exquisite control over the depth and pressure of application of this technique. During the initial pass along the taut band, the clinician may find it necessary to reduce pressure quickly and smoothly to a level that is tolerable for the client as the contact surface passes over the trigger point.

7. The clinician is advised not to persist with the application of this technique if the taut band and referral are unchanged after two or three passes. Lack of response to treatment may indicate that the trigger point may respond better to another technique or that the trigger point is a satellite and treatment of the key trigger point is required first.

8. Successful deactivation of a trigger point, as evidenced by elimination of pain referral on compression, must be followed with immediate, careful passive stretch (30 sec or more) and then careful active movement through the full range as soon as is practically possible.[129] If it is not possible to have the client perform active movement while he is on the treatment table, then it should be performed at the end of the intervention.

9. When treating several trigger points in an area, the clinician may find it advantageous to precede and follow stripping with petrissage and superficial effleurage. A regional intervention is indicated for a myotactic unit with multiple trigger points, especially if they are chronic or highly symptomatic.

Components of Stripping

Contact: Reinforced finger(s) and/or thumb(s), proximal interphalangeal joints (knuckles), olecranon process

Pressure: Light to heavy; pressure varies with the muscle layer engaged and the sensitivity of that layer; the range can be from scarcely more than the weight of the hand (when stripping a taut band harboring an active trigger point in a superficial muscle) to controlled upper-body weight reinforced with pressure from the legs (when stripping deep hamstring fibers)

Tissues Engaged: Muscle and related fascia

Direction: Along or parallel to fibers

Amplitude: Length of muscle

Rate: Very slow; Travell and Simons[127] give the rate as 0.8 cm/sec, or slow enough to obtain a palpable release[129]

Duration: 10 sec to several minutes

Intergrades with: Specific petrissage and direct fascial technique

Context: Follow inactivation of a trigger point with passive stretch for 30 sec and then with active range of motion to produce an isotonic contraction of the involved muscle; with severe or long-standing trigger points or those in deeper muscles, it is advantageous to apply regional petrissage before and after stripping

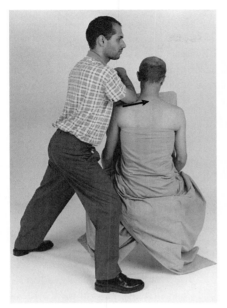

Figure 7-49. Upper trapezius muscle, the most common cause of myofascial pain felt in the temple, is best addressed with the client seated. The client maintains an upright seated posture and pushes with his feet against the floor for support.

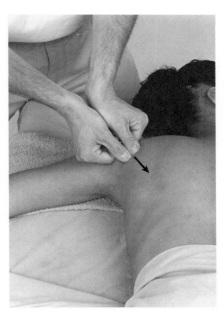

Figure 7-50. Stripping the infraspinatus muscle. With this contact, the thumbs are doubly reinforced against each other and against the flexed index fingers.

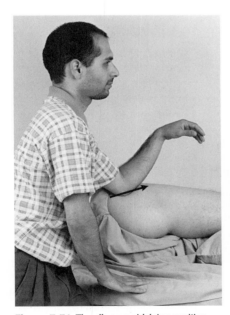

Figure 7-51. The elbow, a sidelying position, and considerable pressure may be needed when stripping the gluteus medius or minimus muscles. When trigger points are located near the iliac attachment (as with most gluteus medius trigger points), a superior-to-inferior path of application avoids pinching superficial tissue against the iliac crest.

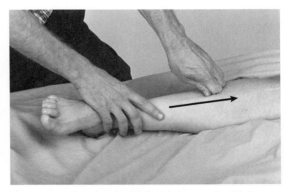

Figure 7-52. Stripping the tibialis anterior muscle with the knuckles. In addition to its effects on trigger point activity, stripping will likely lengthen the anterior fascial wall of the anterior compartment.

CLINICIAN'S POSITION AND MOVEMENT

1. The clinician's posture must be very stable, especially when stripping an active trigger point, since inadvertent small deviations in pressure may produce large increases in pain referral from the trigger point. Figures 7-49 and 7-51 show two variations of a standing controlled lean that allow the clinician the potential to transfer his body weight to the client in a controlled manner. Whatever position is chosen—and especially at higher pressures—the force of application of the technique must remain under the clinician's control at all times.[144]
2. Slight shifts in the angle of application of this technique can make a critical difference in whether the clinician can access a trigger point. For example, stripping of iliocostalis lumborum trigger points may yield no reproduction or increase in referral or pain (or therapeutic effect) when the clinician applies the pressure in a strictly anterior direction. On the other hand, a substantial increase in reproduction or referral of pain may occur when an equivalent amount of pressure is directed along the same taut band in an anteromedial direction (see Fig. 7-59).

PALPATE

As she performs the technique, the clinician palpates the client's tissues for the following:

1. Taut bands. The direction of muscle fibers (as well as the referral pattern) will permit the identification of the involved muscle. The taut band will often show approximately even levels of tension along its length; therefore, the clinician must develop an ability to identify layers of equal tension during palpation.
2. Local hardness. The trigger point itself may present as a very small area of local hardness (palpable nodule) in the taut band.
3. Twitch responses. Twitch responses may be palpated in superficial muscles.
4. Jump sign. A client may produce a large involuntary contraction and other gross affective signs of pain when the trigger point is palpated.
5. Generalized hardness. If there are adjacent trigger points in overlapping layers as, for example, commonly occur between the scapulae, the clinician may find it difficult to palpate anything other than a generalized hardness.
6. Softening of tissues. Softening of taut bands and regional hardness should occur with continued application of the technique.

As with petrissage, the clinician also palpates for:

7. Tissue resistance. General resistance or resilience of soft tissues.
8. Tissue mobility. Mobility of the interfaces between muscles and muscle layers.
9. Signs of inflammation. Fibrosis, adhesions, and induration within and between muscle layers, which is associated with chronic inflammation.

OBSERVE

As she performs the technique, the clinician observes the client for signs of trigger point activity. The signs listed below may indicate trigger point activity or a positive response to treatment.

1. Taut bands in superficial muscles are often easily visible.
2. Twitch responses are transient events (1/4 sec) that are often more easily seen than felt. They may occasionally appear as a "flutter" that cascades into adjacent muscles.
3. Softening of the contour of the taut band with continued application of the technique. Sometimes the contour of an entire muscle will soften, and more rarely, relaxation of the muscles throughout an entire region can occur as the activity of one trigger point diminishes.

As with petrissage, the clinician also observes:

4. Systemic reduction of muscle tension, as evidenced by softening of the tissue contours or broadening and flattening of body segments.
5. General consistency and resting level of tone.
6. Local hyperemia. A reactive hyperemia may accompany the application of this technique.

COMMUNICATION WITH THE CLIENT

The clinician uses communication to ensure the client's comfort during the application of the technique. Some examples of statements that the clinician can use are listed below.

1. "As I pass over the trigger point, you may notice that it intensifies the pain you've been feeling in your . . ." The clinician explains to the client what a trigger point is, what pain referral means, and that his symptoms may be temporarily reproduced or intensified as she passes over the trigger point. It is very important that the client understands that the discomfort of the technique is not gratuitous and that it has a therapeutic purpose.

2. "The pressure may feel somewhat uncomfortable, but it shouldn't be really painful . . . it should be tolerable. Tell me if at any time the discomfort is too great." The clinician ensures that the pressure of application of the technique is tolerable to the client; discomfort is acceptable, but outright pain is counterproductive, and the client (not the clinician) should establish the depth of the application of techniques. Recheck the client's tolerance with every increase in pressure. Obvious pain behavior indicates that pressure must be reduced. In addition, the clinician can explain the use of a 10-point pain scale and ask that the client not let the pain of stripping exceed level 3. If the resting pain of an active trigger point already exceeds level 3, then the application of the technique should not increase the client's pain more than a point and can only do so if the client shows no obvious pain behavior and clearly agrees to the procedure.

3. "Does this bring back the exact pattern of pain referral in your . . . ?" When the clinician locates a trigger point she may pause over it briefly and allow the client to compare the pattern of pain referral of the trigger point with the presenting symptoms.

COMPLEMENTARY MODALITIES

There are several modalities that the clinician can use in a complementary manner to decrease trigger point activity. When treating acute trauma, cold packs should be applied to assist resolution of the acute inflammation, regardless of the effect that this has on trigger points.[129]

Once the clinically acute stage has passed, the following massage techniques may also be useful.

1. Petrissage
2. Specific compression (trigger point pressure release)[129,131]
3. Connective tissue techniques such as skin rolling,[129] myofascial release,[129,131] and direct fascial technique

The following related techniques can also be used to treat trigger points effectively.[129,131]

1. Sustained gentle passive stretch (required after trigger point inactivation)
2. Active range of motion to produce an isotonic contraction of the affected muscle (required after trigger point inactivation)
3. Postisometric relaxation
4. Contract relax, hold relax, and related muscle energy techniques
5. Moist heat application
6. Ice (or vapocoolant spray) and simultaneous passive stretch; readers are referred to "Myofascial Pain and Dysfunction" for the necessary comprehensive instructions
7. Therapeutic ultrasound
8. High-voltage galvanic stimulation
9. Transcutaneous electrical nerve stimulation; while this is not a specific intervention for trigger points, it may provide temporary relief of pain

A multidisciplinary approach to treatment that includes appropriate medical management is most effective for the treatment of myofascial pain syndromes and trigger points.[127–131,145]

SELF-CARE INSTRUCTIONS

The clinician can instruct the client in many of the aforementioned complementary modalities for home use. Of particular importance are:

1. Correct self-stretch techniques and postisometric relaxation
2. Gentle active range of motion through the full range of motion; isotonic contraction of the affected muscle
3. Moist heat application to the trigger point (not the area of referral)
4. Clients may also selectively be taught how to apply stripping in accessible areas
5. Ergonomic education related to posture or repetitive activity

---

A Practice Sequence for Stripping

Allow at least 30 min per person.

Many people have latent trigger points in the fibers of the upper and middle trapezius and the rhomboids. If your client does not happen to have these, you can still practice stripping in this regional exercise.

Before you start, assess the range and ease of motion of glenohumeral and scapular movements.

Prone
1. Apply a small amount of oil to the client's back, using superficial effleurage.
2. Perform regional petrissage to all the muscles of the upper back and posterior shoulder girdle using a sequence similar to that described in the box titled "A Practice Sequence for Petrissage." Begin with broad-contact techniques that cover a wide area and gradually proceed to more-localized techniques, such as fingertip kneading. Gradually progress deeper.
3. During this part of the massage, observe closely for muscles that appear to contain hard, taut bands, twitch responses, and spots that are tender or produce pain referrals.
4. If you think you have found a trigger point, confirm this using palpation.
5. Progressively strip all the fibers of the trapezius muscle, being attentive to the fiber directions. The muscle should be slightly stretched but not taut during this procedure. To effectively strip the upper trapezius in prone, you will have to sit at the head of the table and use substantial, reinforced pressure, which you apply in a caudal direction. Periodically intersperse stripping with broader strokes like palmar kneading or picking up.
6. On any active or latent trigger points, strip the taut band in alternating directions until the client's level of sensitivity decreases.
7. Repeat steps 5 and 6, focusing on the rhomboids. You will have to use marginally more pressure for this. The fiber direction as well as the pain referral patterns will help you identify which layer you are on.
8. Conclude with regional petrissage and then superficial effleurage.
9. Get feedback on how your client feels. If your client has begun to experience a temporal headache, you have likely activated a latent trigger point in the upper trapezius muscle.
10. Reassess range and ease of movement of the scapular movements.

Many people also have latent trigger points in the pectoral muscles on the anterior surface. How would you adapt this sequence to address those?

Specific Compression

OTHER NAMES USED FOR THIS TECHNIQUE

"Focal compression," "ischemic compression," "digital compression," "digital pressure," "sustained digital pressure," "direct pressure," "direct inhibitory pressure," "direct static pressure," "static friction," "deep touch."[1–9,127–131]

DEFINITION

Specific compression: A nongliding technique that is applied with a specific contact surface to muscle, tendon, or connective tissue; the compression and release is applied in a direction that is perpendicular to the target tissue, and the compression is often sustained

NOTES

Along with static contact, specific compression is probably the most widespread of all massage techniques. It is either used alone or as a component of more elaborate methods and systems, including positional release,[146] myotherapy,[147,148] trigger point pressure release,[129] neuromuscular technique,[130] shiatsu,[149,150] acupressure,[151,152] and reflexology.[1–3,5–7] Specific compression has been applied with a bewildering variety of rationales and names.

CLINICAL INDICATIONS AND IMPAIRMENT-LEVEL OUTCOMES OF CARE

Specific compression can be an effective manual technique for reducing the activity and symptoms of myofascial trigger points, especially for thin muscles that overlie bone.[127–129] For detailed definitions and descriptions relating to trigger points, see the preceding section on stripping or Table 7-2. During a "manual trigger point pressure release,"[129] specific compression is applied to the trigger point itself (not to the area of referral) and followed with passive stretch and active free movement. Since it can be used to reduce the activity of trigger points, specific compression has wide applicability when treating the effects of trauma; acute and chronic overload (e.g., tendinopathies and repetitive strain disorder); postural imbalance; fatigue; emotional stress; common musculoskeletal complaints such as tension headache, temporomandibular joint problems, spinal pain, chronic low back pain, disk herniation, chronic pelvic pain, painful rib syndrome, and nonarticular pain; and other myofascial pain syndromes.[127–142]

Specific compression can also be used as a proprioceptive stimulation technique.[153–157] Firm and moderate specific compression (inhibitory pressure) can be applied to tendons as a means of inhibiting the tone of the related muscle for a short time.[153] Intermittent or sustained application of specific compression to tendons (but not muscle) will also cause a reduction of motoneuron excitability (H-reflex), but only during the application of the stimulus.[154–157] The application of specific compression for the purpose of inhibiting muscle contraction has been integrated into many therapeutic techniques that seek to facilitate movement in conditions associated with abnormal neuromuscular tone, such as spasticity.

The authors' clinical observations suggest that specific compression may also be effective in softening adhesions and fibrosis in muscle, tendon, and fascia when it is applied in a slow and sustained manner.

Finally, foot reflexology[1–3,5–7,158,159] and Eastern-influenced massage systems[149–152] employ specific compression extensively to influence pain and physiological function at sites that are remote from application of the technique. These systems suggest that the effects of treatment occur through postulated complex somatovisceral reflexes. The main impairment-level outcomes

of care for specific compression are summarized in Table 7-1.

CAUTIONS AND CONTRAINDICATIONS

Clinical training and supervised practice are critical for the proper application of specific compression. Advanced training may be advisable, particularly when dealing with pathological conditions. As with other compressive neuromuscular techniques, all contraindications for massage techniques apply.[1,30] (See Chapter 2, The Clinical Decision-Making Process, for a detailed discussion of contraindications.) Specific contraindications to the use of specific compression include clients with hemophilia; local sites of acute inflammation and infection; and confirmed or suspected thrombus, thrombophlebitis, and malignancy. Specific compression can be very useful when applied on-site in the subacute stage of trauma, provided that edema has resolved. In this situation, the force of application must be reduced, and the technique must not cause the client pain. The clinician is advised not to perform sustained specific compression directly over superficial nerves, such as the radial or common peroneal nerves, since a compression neurapraxia can result.[160] Further cautions to the application of specific compression are osteoporosis, early-stage wounds, anticoagulant therapy, and areas of spasm and hypotonia.[1,2,6,7]

Common errors when treating trigger points with specific compression are listed in Table 7-3. When the clinician is using specific compression to treat trigger points, she must apply this technique with absolute regard for the client's pain tolerance and accompany the application of the technique with careful communication. In the case of long-standing or recurrent trigger

---

Table 7-2
Types of Trigger Points[129]

Trigger Point Type	Description
Active	Produces pain in a characteristic pattern at rest
Latent	Produces pain in a characteristic pattern only when palpated
Primary	Arises in response to trauma or acute or chronic overload
Key	Is responsible for activating (and inactivating) satellites
Satellite	Is activated by a key trigger point, by being in its area of referral, or by being its antagonist or synergist
Central	Is located near the center of muscle fibers
Attachment	Is located in a muscle's tendon or aponeurosis

points, the clinician can minimize the likelihood of recurrence of the trigger points by treating agonist, antagonist, and synergist muscle groups and addressing perpetuating factors, such as structural asymmetry and repetitive ergonomic loading.[128–130] Postintervention pain that differs markedly from the client's presenting symptoms is most often due to the activation of a latent or satellite trigger point and indicates a need to further address synergists and antagonists.[129] The clinician should be aware that specific compression may produce remote reflex effects that are out of proportion to the size of the area treated and the force applied.[7,130]

Table 7-3
Common Errors When Treating Trigger Points with Specific Compression

Error	*Result*
Pressure is applied too quickly	Client terminates technique
	Autonomic nervous system/sympathetic response
Pressure exceeds client's pain tolerance	Client terminates technique
	Autonomic nervous system/sympathetic response
Pressure is not maintained on the trigger point (sliding off)	No change in symptoms
Insufficient depth achieved	No change in symptoms
Too few repetitions of compression	No change in symptoms
Sustained accurate pressure does not diminish referral	Try a different trigger point
Passive stretch omitted	Recurrence of same trigger point symptoms
Perpetuating factors not addressed	Recurrence of same trigger point symptoms
Satellite and secondary trigger points not addressed	New symptoms appear

---

Prerequisite Skills for Specific Compression

Before applying specific compression to trigger points, students should be able to

Define the terms *latent, active, primary, key and satellite trigger points*

Describe the phenomenon of pain referral as it relates to trigger points (ideally will recognize locations and referral patterns of common trigger points)

Describe fiber directions of all major skeletal muscles

Recognize a twitch response and jump sign

Identify a taut band

Solicit accurate feedback from client about pain referral

Use lunge and lean, and standing and seated controlled lean postures

See Chapter 4, Preparation and Positioning for Treatment, and Appendix B, Selected Soft-Tissue Examination Techniques.

Manual Technique begins on page 212

MANUAL TECHNIQUE

Specific Compression

In the following figures (Figs. 7-53A to 7-61) specific compression is applied to the various regions of the body. Figures are ordered from head to foot in supine and then prone. Each figure illustrates most of the guidelines for manual technique outlined below.

For all applications of specific compression:

1. The contact chosen depends on the relative size of the clinician's and client's bodies, the area to be treated, and the hardness of the tissue. It is important that the contact fit the local "topography" of the client's body easily. The thumb and fingers are better suited to working smaller muscles, such as those in the rotator cuff, neck, and calves, and should be reinforced as necessary (Figs. 7-53A and B, 7-54, 7-55, and 7-58). The clinician's elbow is recommended as a contact when the client's tissues are very hard and also on larger muscles of the back, legs, and pelvis. This contact allows a greater use of upper body weight to sustain pressure and thus minimizes clinician fatigue (Figs. 7-56 and 7-57). The clinician may also use wooden or plastic tools (T-bars) that are gripped in the hand. Two such tools are shown in Figure 7-61.

2. The chosen contact must be stable, and the clinician must exercise exquisite control of both the direction and depth of pressure of application. For this reason the client's skin must be free of lubricant, to minimize slipping of the clinician's hands.

3. Pressure is slowly applied, increased gradually to the desired depth, sustained evenly, and then released gradually. The duration of compression will vary with the application; it can range from a few seconds to more than a minute.

When using specific compression to perform a trigger point pressure release:[129]

4. The pressure applied must be enough to reproduce or marginally increase the referred pain from the trigger point, but the level must be absolutely tolerable for the client. This amount of pressure will vary from being light, in the case of a highly active trigger point in a superficial muscle, to being heavy, in a less active trigger point in a deep muscle, such as the piriformis.

5. Once the clinician has established a tolerable initial depth/pressure in consultation with the client, there are basically two approaches to progressing the specific compression of a trigger point.

Progression using verbal client feedback: This approach relies on frequent client feedback and is recommended for novice clinicians. Maintain the compression at the initial depth of application until the referred pain subsides (i.e., "until you no longer feel pain, just the pressure of my thumb"), then increase the depth of application of the compression to a new level that re-creates a tolerable level of pain referral. Maintain the pressure of compression at that depth until the referral subsides, then repeat the application of the technique as needed. Depth of application is gradually increased in a series of stepwise increments until the client reports that tenderness and pain referral have disappeared.

Progression using feedback from palpation: Alternatively, the clinician can maintain the pressure of application at a constant level and exclusively use the barrier-release phenomenon to achieve the continuous progression of depth. As the trigger point releases and the tissues soften, the depth of penetration will gradually increase until the client reports that the referred pain has disappeared. This approach requires that the clinician accurately feel the presence of the tissue barrier to compression, and then sense and follow the release of the barrier into the client's tissue. This

Manual Technique continues on page 214

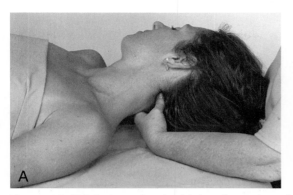

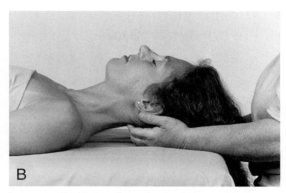

Figure 7-53. Digital compression of occipital attachments is an effective nonspecific technique for tension headaches and neck tension. This can be done (**A**) using the thumb, with the neck rotated or (**B**) on lined-up fingertips with the neck in neutral.

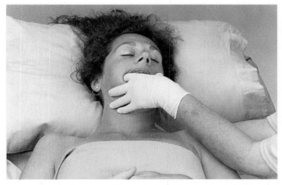

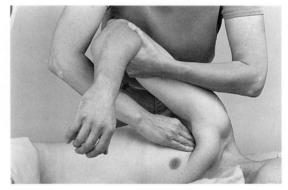

Figure 7-54. The lateral pterygoid muscle may be implicated in temporomandibular joint dysfunction. Intraoral specific compression of this muscle demands excellent communication skills and great sensitivity of execution.

Figure 7-55. Effective direct access to trigger points in the pectoralis minor muscle: slide under pectoralis major muscle, across the ribs, toward either the coracoid process or rib attachment. The approach must often be very slow because of tenderness. The other hand stabilizes the arm (and scapula) laterally. The technique can also be performed with the client in supine.

Manual Technique Figures continue on page 215

approach requires more-refined palpation skills than the first method.[129]

In the verbal feedback or palpatory feedback methods of progression, it may be more practical for the clinician to wait until the client reports that the pain referral is substantially diminished, rather than waiting for it to completely disappear. When applied correctly, both methods can provide clients with a demonstration of a correct and comfortable pressure of application that they can use at home.

6. There are differing opinions about how long to sustain specific compression of a trigger point, from 10 sec to more than 1 min.[127,129,146–148] For less-experienced clinicians, and especially when treating chronic or highly irritable trigger points, the authors recommend shorter, more frequent compressions that are sustained from 15 to 30 seconds and are interspersed with the application of petrissage, stripping, passive stretch, and other manual methods. This minimizes the possibility of overtreating the target muscle, activating latent satellites in synergist and antagonist muscle groups, or producing a biomechanical imbalance. Clinicians with higher levels of manual skill can use their judgment on the degree to which they extend the period in which they apply compression.

7. It is not always easy to maintain specific compression on the precise spot that reproduces the client's pain referral, even when lubricant has not been applied. The clinician must, therefore, determine whether a client's report of diminished pain referral reflects reduced trigger point activity or the movement of the clinician's contact off the trigger point. Stripping or stretching techniques may be better manual approaches for the treatment of "slippery" trigger points.

8. Following deactivation of the trigger point, perform a passive stretch of the treated muscle for 30 sec. As soon as possible after passive stretching, ask the client to carefully perform active range of motion through the available range to produce an isotonic contraction of the affected muscle.

9. When treating several trigger points within an area, the clinician may find it advantageous to precede and follow specific compression with petrissage and superficial effleurage. A regional approach to the intervention is indicated for a myotactic unit that has multiple trigger points, particularly if these trigger points are chronic or highly symptomatic.

Components of Specific Compression

Contact: Reinforced fingers or thumbs, reinforced proximal interphalangeal joints, olecranon process

Pressure: Light to heavy

Engages: Muscle and/or connective tissue

Direction: Perpendicular to the target tissue layer; this is often, but not always, perpendicular to the surface of the body; slight shifts in direction may facilitate access of individual trigger points

Amplitude/length: NA

Rate: 5 to 30 sec or more per compression

Duration: 5 min or more for a series of compressions applied to a muscle belly or region

Intergrades with: Broad-contact compression, specific petrissage, stripping

Context: Follow inactivation of a trigger point with passive stretch for 30 sec and then an active range of motion to produce an isotonic contraction of the involved muscle; if this technique is applied repetitively in a small area or to a deep muscle, it is advantageous to apply regional petrissage before and after application; follow specific compression that is being applied for the purpose of inhibition of abnormal neuromuscular tone with the desired movement or functional activity. Contexts for reflexology and acupressure are described in boxes near the end of this chapter.

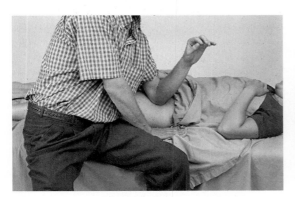

Figure 7-56. Specific compression of tensor fascia lata using the elbow, in a seated controlled lean.

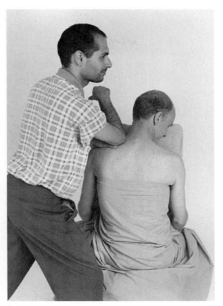

Figure 7-57. While applying specific compression with the elbow to the upper trapezius muscle, ask the client to adjust the head position to obtain the strongest pain referral. The clinician is using his left hand to stabilize the point of contact and to palpate for softening of the taut band.

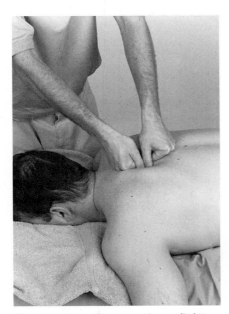

Figure 7-58. Specific compression applied to the rhomboids/midtrapezius muscle area with reinforced double-thumb contact.

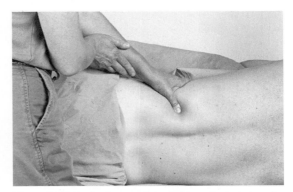

Figure 7-59. Angle of approach is often important when applying specific compression to trigger points. Here the clinician directs pressure anteromedially onto the iliocostalis lumborum muscle. A single thumb and light pressure may be adequate to accentuate pain referral from an active trigger point; reinforced thumbs or an elbow and some body weight might be required to elicit pain referral from latent trigger points.

Manual Technique Figures continue on next page

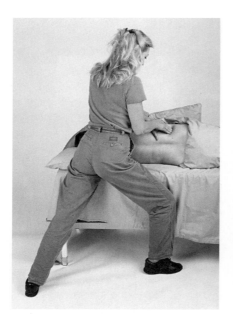

Figure 7-60. The lateral edge of the quadratus lumborum is accessible to specific compression in sidelying only with correct positioning. The client's ipsilateral arm is fully abducted, and the ipsilateral leg has been passively stretched downward, to open space at the waist. Doubled thumbs, reinforced fingers, or even the tip of the elbow may be used. Take care to avoid the poorly supported 11th and 12th (floating) ribs.

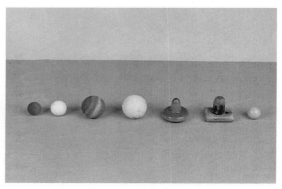

Figure 7-61. Devices that can assist with self-administration of specific compression of trigger points include balls of various sizes and densities and wooden or plastic massage tools.

CLINICIAN'S POSITION AND MOVEMENT

1. The clinician's selected posture must be stable, comfortable, and sustainable.
2. The basic positions used by the clinician are described in Chapter 4, Preparation and Positioning for Treatment, in the sections on lunge and lean (Fig. 7-60), standing controlled lean (Fig. 7-57), and seated controlled lean (Fig. 7-56). These positions allow controlled, sustained use of the clinician's upper-body weight to augment the force of application of the technique. The clinician should note that the client's body should not be used as a support when using these controlled-leaning positions. Instead, the clinician inclines the body toward the client in a controlled manner and applies precisely the desired amount of upper body weight to the contact surface, without becoming destabilized or unbalanced.
3. When the clinician uses the elbow as a contact (Figs. 7-56 and 7-57), the clinician assesses the degree of release that has occurred by gauging how the client's compressed tissue deforms under the clinician's body weight.

PALPATE

As she performs the technique, the clinician palpates the client's tissues for the following.

1. Taut bands. The fiber direction (as well as the pain referral pattern) will permit identification of the involved muscle.
2. Local hardness. The trigger point itself may present as a very small area of local hardness (palpable nodule) in the taut band. Compression is slowly applied to this nodule until the barrier to further compression is reached.
3. Twitch responses. Twitch responses may be palpated in superficial muscles.
4. Jump sign. A client may produce a large involuntary contraction and other gross affective signs of pain if the trigger point is palpated too forcefully.
5. Generalized hardness. If there are adjacent trigger points in overlapping layers as, for example, commonly occurs between the scapulae, the clinician may find it difficult to palpate anything other than a generalized hardness.
6. As the pressure of application is sustained at the tissue barrier, the palpable nodule or contraction knot associated with the trigger point will soften or release. The clinician may follow this release into the tissue without increasing the pressure of application.
7. Signs of inflammation. Fibrosis, adhesions, and induration within and between muscle layers, which are associated with chronic inflammation.

OBSERVE

As she performs the technique, the clinician observes the client for signs of trigger point activity. The signs listed below may indicate trigger point activity or a positive response to treatment.

1. Taut bands in superficial muscles are often easily visible.
2. Twitch responses are transient events (1/4 sec) that are often more easily seen than felt. They may occasionally appear as a "flutter" that cascades into adjacent muscles.
3. Softening of the contour of the taut band with continued application of the technique. Sometimes the contour of an entire muscle will soften, and more rarely, relaxation of the muscles throughout an entire region can occur as the activity of one trigger point diminishes.

As with petrissage, the clinician also observes:

4. Systemic reduction of muscle tension, as evidenced by softening of the tissue contours or broadening and flattening of body segments
5. General consistency and resting tension of muscle
6. Local hyperemia; a reactive hyperemia may accompany the application of this technique

COMMUNICATION WITH THE CLIENT

The clinician uses communication to ensure the client's comfort during the application of the technique. Some examples of statements that the clinician can use are listed below. When the clinician increases the pressure of application in an incremental manner, these communications are used with each change in pressure.

1. "As I put pressure on the trigger point, you may notice that it intensifies the pain you've been feeling in your . . ." The clinician explains to the client what a trigger point is, what pain referral means, and that his symptoms may be temporarily reproduced or intensified as she compresses the trigger point. It is very important that the client understands that the discomfort of the technique is not gratuitous and that it has a therapeutic purpose.
2. "Does this bring back the exact pattern of pain in your . . .?" When the clinician initially locates a trigger point, she may allow the client to compare the pattern of pain referral of the trigger point with his presenting symptoms. A client with a "single-point" syndrome will report that pressure on the trigger point reproduces the presenting symptoms exactly.
3. "The pressure may feel somewhat uncomfortable, but it shouldn't be really painful . . . it should be tolerable. Tell me if at any time the discomfort is too

great." The clinician ensures that the pressure of application of the technique is tolerable to the client; discomfort is acceptable, but outright pain is counterproductive, and the client (not the clinician) should establish the depth of the application of techniques. Recheck the client's tolerance with every increase in pressure. Obvious pain behavior indicates that pressure must be reduced. In addition, the clinician can explain the use of a 10-point pain scale and ask that the client not let the pain of specific compression exceed level 3. If the resting pain of an active trigger point already exceeds level 3, then the application of the technique should not increase the client's pain more than a point and can only do so if the client shows no obvious pain behavior and clearly agrees to the procedure. With practice, the clinician will develop an accurate sense of how much pressure to apply, which minimizes the necessity for verbal feedback.

4. "Let me know when the pain is gone and you can only feel the pressure of my thumb." Instruct the client to report when the pain referral disappears and only the sensation of pressure is felt.

OTHER APPROPRIATE TECHNIQUES

TRIGGER POINTS

There are several modalities that the clinician can use in a complementary manner to decrease trigger point activity. When treating acute trauma, cold packs should be applied to assist resolution of the acute inflammation, regardless of the effect that this has on the trigger points.[129] Once the clinically acute stage has passed, the following massage techniques may also be useful.

1. Petrissage
2. Stripping[129,131]
3. Connective tissue techniques such as skin rolling,[129] myofascial release,[129,131] and direct fascial technique

The following related techniques can also be used to treat trigger points effectively.[129,131]

1. Sustained gentle passive stretch (required after trigger point inactivation)
2. Active range of motion to produce an isotonic contraction of the affected muscle (required after trigger point inactivation)
3. Postisometric relaxation
4. Contract relax, hold relax, and related muscle energy techniques
5. Moist heat application

6. Ice (or vapocoolant spray) and simultaneous passive stretch; readers are referred to Myofascial Pain and Dysfunction for the necessary comprehensive instructions
7. Therapeutic ultrasound
8. High-voltage galvanic stimulation
9. Transcutaneous electrical nerve stimulation; while this is not a specific intervention for trigger points, it may provide temporary relief of pain

A multidisciplinary approach to treatment that includes appropriate medical management is most effective for the treatment of myofascial pain syndromes and trigger points.[127–131,145]

MOTOR CONTROL

When the clinician is using specific compression as a proprioceptive stimulation technique, several complementary techniques can be used to inhibit or stimulate neuromuscular tone and facilitate movement responses.

1. Prolonged cold, neutral warmth, and slow superficial stroking applied locally or over the posterior primary rami can be used to inhibit neuromuscular tone and facilitate movement responses (see Chapter 5, Superficial Reflex Techniques).[153]
2. Fine vibration, joint approximation and traction, light brushing, and static contact ("maintained touch") with both light and firm contacts can be used to increase neuromuscular tone and facilitate movement responses (see Chapter 5, Superficial Reflex Techniques).[153]

SELF-CARE INSTRUCTIONS

The clinician can instruct the client in many of the aforementioned complementary modalities for home use. Of particular importance in the management of trigger points are:

1. Correct self-stretch techniques and postisometric relaxation
2. Gentle active range of motion through the full range of motion; isotonic contraction of the affected muscle
3. Moist heat application to the trigger point (not the area of referral)
4. Self-administration of specific compression. Balls of varying sizes and hardness or handheld massage devices can be used to demonstrate this (Fig. 7-61). Clients must understand basic trigger point concepts prior to performing self-management programs. Clients should be advised not to repeat compression more than two to three times; to precede the

application of compression with some preparation of the muscle, such as superficial stroking; and to follow the application of pressure with an isotonic contraction of the muscle and the appropriate stretching exercise. Above all, clients must be advised not to compress the same trigger point for minutes at a time (which may feel good and afford temporary symptomatic relief).

5. Following is an example of a conservative and effective self-management program for a single trigger point that produced significant decreases in trigger point sensitivity, perceived pain levels, and frequency of self-care in adults with chronic myofascial neck pain follows.[161] Gentle superficial stroking of the muscle in which the trigger point occurs (2 to 3 min); application of specific compression to the location of the trigger point with a hand-held massage device for 15 to 60 sec; gentle isotonic contraction of the affected muscle (five repetitions); stretching of the affected muscle (two repetitions for 30 sec); and gentle superficial stroking and kneading of the affected muscle (2 to 3 min).[161] This intervention is performed once daily, and the client may use the application of moist heat to the site of the trigger point as an adjunct to this self-management program.

6. Ergonomic education related to posture or repetitive activity

---

A Practice Sequence for Specific Compression of Trigger Points (Trigger Point Pressure Release[129])

Allow 30 to 40 min.

The following practice sequence begins like the sequence for stripping, but substitutes specific compression for stripping at the point in the sequence when the trigger points are treated.

This sequence is directed to the hamstrings (another fairly common place to find latent trigger points) with the aim of performing the sequence with only one change of the client's position. Before you start, assess the length and strength of the hamstrings and consider how to perform the sequence with the minimum number of changes of position for the client.

1. Effleurage, begin superficial and progress to "deep"
2. Regional petrissage to posterior thigh with increasing depth and specificity
3. Using palpation, search for and confirm the presence of trigger points
4. Place the target muscle on a slight stretch and apply specific compression for 10 to 30 sec
5. Stretch the muscle passively for 30 sec
6. Repeat steps 4 and 5 until the referral declines or disappears and the full length of the muscle is restored
7. Regional petrissage including the antagonist and synergist muscle groups
8. Repeat steps 3 to 7 on other trigger points; do not do more than 3 or 4 repetitions unless you also do a few minutes of broad-contact petrissage on the lower back, gluteals, and calves; Why?
9. Finish with petrissage and superficial effleurage
10. You must treat the other leg for an equal time; Why?

Retest. Get feedback on how your client feels.

Reflex Effects of Specific Compression: Foot Reflexology

Foot reflexology is based on the premise that specific points on the feet (and hands) are reflexly related to other body segments or organs of the body (Fig. 7-62).[2,3,6,7,158,159] In reflexology, pain, tenderness, or soft-tissue hardening in particular areas of the foot is thought to reflect acute or chronic dysfunction of the related body segment or organ. On this basis, specific compression is applied to the reflex points on the foot to normalize function in the corresponding body segments or organs by "restoring lost balance" or "activating the movement of energy."[2]

The mechanisms by which the effects of reflexology occur are not known. Research and review on the subject are scant and mostly in untranslated European journals.[162-171] Results and opinions on the effects of reflexology are mixed, but some research does support the possibility of specific effects on organ function.[164,166,170] More-general outcomes that may result from the application of foot reflexology are reduced anxiety, increased relaxation, and improved mood and energy.[2,3,6,162]

Foot reflexology is logistically simple to perform and requires no oil, towels, or significant disrobing of the client. Contraindications and cautions to the application of reflexology are relatively few. They are mostly local contraindications, such as gout, peripheral vascular disease, and contagious or infectious foot conditions.[3] In addition, interventions may have to be shortened for weak, convalescent, or elderly clients. A full intervention consisting only of the application of foot reflexology may take from 30 to 60 min. Alternatively, the clinician may use foot reflexology for 5 or 10 min to precede or follow a massage sequence that addresses another area of the body.

Following the client examination, a typical intervention might proceed in the following manner. After a brief foot bath, the client is placed comfortably in sitting or lying. The clinician applies general, broad neuromuscular techniques such as wringing, compression, and passive joint movements of the ankles, metatarsals, and toes for several minutes.[2,6] Beginning with the toes and proceeding proximally,[6] the clinician applies specific compression systematically and thoroughly to all surfaces of the foot, using a slow, stable rhythm. The thumbs or knuckles are generally used for the plantar surface of the foot, while the fingers are used for the dorsal surface.[2,3] Pressure is sustained for several seconds on each point and may be prolonged for an additional 15 to 30 sec if a point is tender or hard.[3] The pressure is usually deep, but as with any massage technique, the clinician should moderate the pressure of application so that it feels pleasant or causes mild discomfort as opposed to pain.[3] The clinician can also use a short gliding stroke, similar to stripping or direct fascial technique.[2,3,6] More-detailed descriptions of the technique of foot reflexology are offered in books that address this subject exclusively.[158,159]

Clinical Significance

At the very least, reflexology provides a method for performing a thorough foot massage with associated general benefits.[31,162] The clinician who performs extended specific compression on the feet or hands should be mindful of its possible effects. Applying this type of massage technique on the client's feet or hands can produce systemic effects that are far greater than the area of the feet or hands that are treated might suggest, since altering patterns of tension and tenderness in the feet and hands may affect physiological processes elsewhere in the body.

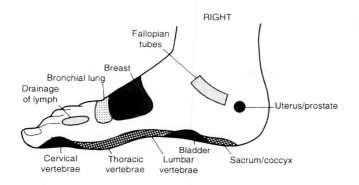

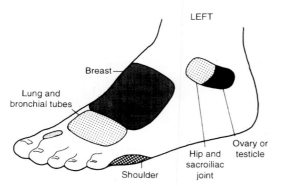

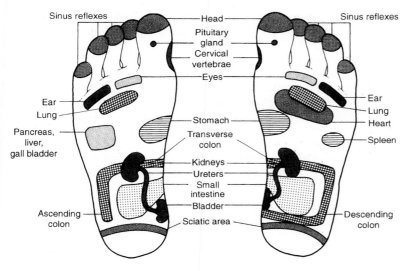

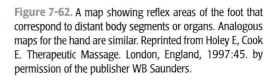

Figure 7-62. A map showing reflex areas of the foot that correspond to distant body segments or organs. Analogous maps for the hand are similar. Reprinted from Holey E, Cook E. *Therapeutic Massage.* London, England, 1997:45. by permission of the publisher WB Saunders.

Reflex Effects of Specific Compression: Meridian Theory and Acupoints

Traditional Chinese medicine is an ancient, vast, and sophisticated system of philosophy, clinical theory, and practice that has come to the attention of the West in recent decades primarily because of the evidence for the analgesic effects of acupuncture.[2,3,6,7,172,173] Fundamental to the system of Chinese medicine are several interrelated concepts that have no parallel concepts in Western medicine.

In Chinese medicine, energy *(qi, chi, ch'i)* circulates through the body in well-defined cycles through conduits or channels called meridians.[2,174] There are 12 bilateral paired meridians and 2 median sagittal meridians.[1,151,173] Each meridian is associated with an "organ," for which it is named, and has associated physiological functions, which do not correspond exactly to organ functions as defined in Western medicine. Each meridian also has a basic quality of energy that is characterized as being yin or yang.[1,151,174] Yin energy is metaphorically described as "female" and "negative," is ascending, and is associated with hollow organs such as the stomach. Yang energy is metaphorically characterized as "male" and "positive," is descending, and is associated with solid organs such as the liver.[1,151,174] Health is conceptualized as a dynamic balance between yin and yang energy flowing in precise diurnal patterns through the various meridians.[151,174] Pathways of the meridians do not consistently correspond to any material anatomical structure, though they sometimes follow intermuscular depressions and paths of major nerves.[2,7]

Strung along each meridian, at depths ranging from immediately below the surface up to 1 inch (2.5 cm) deep, are dozens of small points, or acupoints, that have lower electrical resistance and higher overlying skin temperature and that show altered sensitivity during states of imbalance or disease (Fig 7-63).[151,174] While the position of most acupoints coincides with locations of nerves, trigger points, or motor points,[2,7] there is debate as to how these various entities might correspond to each other.[130,175,176] Acupoints can be activated by a variety of precise approaches to achieve remote effects on the meridian, its associated organ, and related physiological processes.[151,174] Each meridian has several points of unusual clinical importance including activating points, soothing points, and stabilizing points.[130,151,174] Activating and soothing points, respectively, stimulate or sedate the meridian and its related organ and functions. Stabilizing points link the functions of one meridian with that of others. Finally, a variety of other points show sensitivity or tenderness when there is a dysfunction in the related meridian. Methods of stimulating acupoints include needling (acupuncture), massage, electrical current, laser, and moxibustion.[7] Manual systems that stimulate acupoints, such as acupressure and shiatsu, rely extensively on deep, sustained specific compression on the points themselves and may include small nongliding circular movements, tapping, and stretching.[1,2,149–152]

Recent research suggests a variety of clinical effects of stimulation of acupoints. Sustained (nonmanual) specific compression on individual acupoints (the pericardium-6 point, located in the middle of the ventral wrist crease) may be effective as an intervention for intraoperative and postoperative nausea and vomiting.[177–181] Acupressure may also be a useful intervention for sleep disorders, COPD, and women's reproductive disorders.[182–184] However, interventions aimed at restoring the harmonious flow of energy in states of imbalance or disease most commonly involve the stimulation of multiple acupoints in combination with other interventions following the use of complex diagnostic procedures. It must be emphasized that acupuncture, acupressure, and related modalities rely on elaborate, sophisticated, and radically different conceptual models of body processes than those used in Western medicine. Understanding the rationale of how to stimulate acupoints requires extensive study of these conceptual models and is beyond the scope of this book. The interested reader is referred to comprehensive texts.[172,173]

Clinical Significance

The clinician who uses specific compression extensively to treat trigger points should be aware of the following issues. Remote analgesic effects from specific compression may arise in patterns that do not always correspond to those suggested by the trigger points. This may occur because the clinician is treating an acupoint rather than a trigger point. In addition, patterns of pain and tension in the musculature, especially if they are recurrent, may reflect remote physiological and pathological processes. Specific compression should always be applied within the client's pain tolerance, and a palpable tissue response to the application of the technique should occur quickly. The clinician should avoid applying the technique if the client's tissues are extremely sensitive and should not persist with application if it fails to produce a quickly palpable tissue change. If the application of specific compression causes symptoms to abate for a short period followed by a recurrence of the symptoms, the clinician should identify the underlying causes of the symptoms before reapplying the technique.

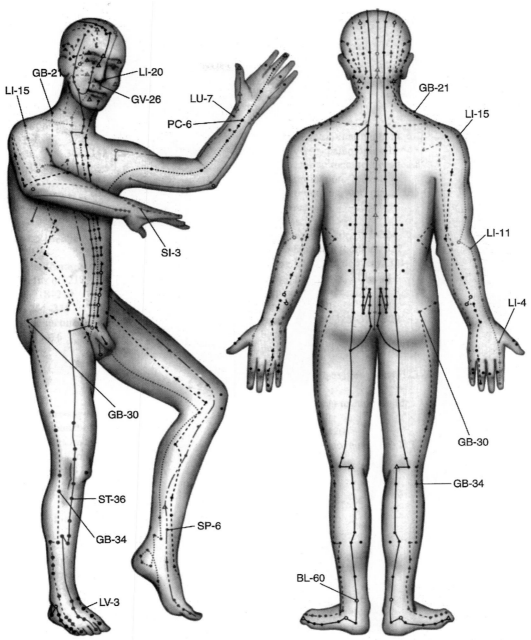

Figure 7-63. A map showing meridians with acupoints strung along it. Tappan FM, Benjamin PJ. Tappan's Handbook of Healing Massage Techniques, 3rd Edition. Copyright 1998. Reprinted by permission of Prentice-Hall, Inc., Upper Saddle River, NJ.

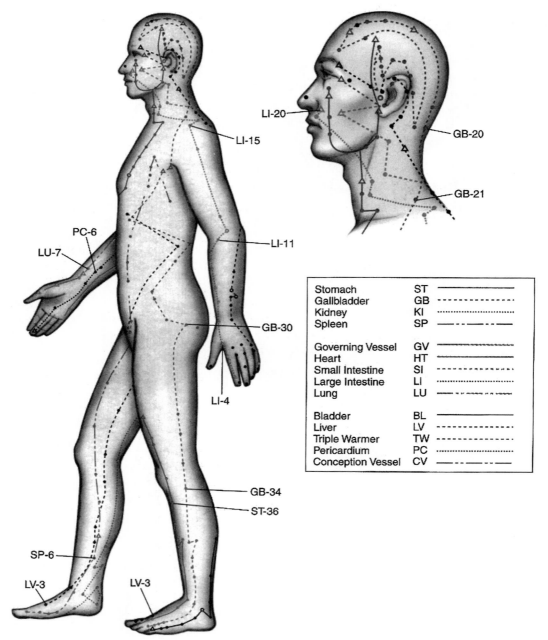

Stomach	ST	
Gallbladder	GB	
Kidney	KI	
Spleen	SP	
Governing Vessel	GV	
Heart	HT	
Small Intestine	SI	
Large Intestine	LI	
Lung	LU	
Bladder	BL	
Liver	LV	
Triple Warmer	TW	
Pericardium	PC	
Conception Vessel	CV	

Figure 7-63 *(continued).*

Clinical Example

Client profile	A 40-year-old woman with a high-risk pregnancy who has been hospitalized at 28 weeks' gestation for evaluation and modification of pharmacological management of premature onset of labor; prior to hospitalization she was bed bound for 6 weeks; medication: terbutaline (β-adrenergic stimulant).
Summary of clinical findings	*Subjective*

Subjective
1. Complaints of muscle and joint achiness
2. Complaints of generalized weakness
3. Complaints of stress related to the high-risk pregnancy
4. Rating of perceived stress using visual analog scale: 84
5. Reported stress-related symptoms
   · Physical: altered sleep patterns, fatigue, restlessness, headaches, achiness and tension in shoulder, neck, and back muscles
   · Emotional: Anxiety about the pregnancy, depression, and frustration; experiencing sudden shifts in mood
   · Mental: Forgetfulness, inability to concentrate
   · Behavioral: Frequent episodes of crying, disorganization, short temper, inability to sleep
6. Results of stress audit:[185] Scales include situational (family, individual roles, social being, environment, financial, work–school), symptoms (muscular system, parasympathetic nervous system, sympathetic nervous system, emotional, cognitive system, endocrine, immune system), vulnerability, total situational stress, total symptoms; measure not scored but used, as suggested, as a guide to the clinical interview; responses indicated a variety of stress-related symptoms and the need for stress management training

Objective
· Fetal monitor in situ.
· Client evaluated in lying; sitting and standing evaluated at return visit during permitted ambulation to the bathroom.

Impairments
1. Range of motion: Within normal limits for neck, upper and lower extremity range of motion; complaints of achiness during range of motion; lumbar spine range of motion not assessed
2. Strength: Unable to assess formally; resisted movement is contraindicated; risk of ongoing decrease in strength because of restricted activity level
3. Muscle resting tension: Increased level of muscle resting tension in neck, shoulder, and erector spinae muscles noted on palpation

Functional limitations
1. Bed mobility: Performed rolling side-to-side and scooting independently with use of monkey bar; complaints of achiness and weakness
2. Transfers: Performed lying-to-sit, sit-to-stand, stand-to-toilet, toilet-to-stand with contact guard assistance secondary to complaints of weakness and achiness
3. Ambulation: 10 feet with minimal assistance of one person secondary to poor balance and complaints of weakness

continued

(continued)

Treatment planning

Treatment rationale

Treatment is aimed at *(a)* preventing further deterioration of health status and functional level because of inactivity and *(b)* reducing stress-related symptoms as a means of increasing the client's comfort level and facilitating maternal and fetal well-being

Precautions

Monitor for maternal and fetal tachycardia and hypotension
Adhere to restrictions in physical activity: no sitting, standing or ambulation (other than to the bathroom with assistance)
Valsalva maneuver, resisted movements, abdominal exercises are contraindicated
Ensure adequate hydration during treatment and encourage frequent emptying of the bladder
Side effects of β-adrenergic medication: Maternal and fetal tachycardia and hypotension

Impairment	*Role of massage*
Anxiety	Primary treatment; direct effect of massage on reduction of perceived anxiety
Perceived stress	Primary treatment; direct effect of massage on increased perceived relaxation
Increased muscle resting tension	Primary treatment; localized primary effect of massage on reduction of level of muscle resting tension
	Secondary effect of general increase in relaxation and reduction of anxiety
Muscle and joint pain ("achiness")	Primary treatment; direct effect of massage on pain reduction through counterirritant analgesia and sedation
Fatigue	Secondary treatment; possible indirect effect of massage through increased sensory arousal
Other stress-related symptoms	Secondary treatment; possible indirect effect of massage through increase in perceived relaxation and reduction of perceived anxiety
Weakness	No effect

Massage techniques

General issues

The clinician works in close consultation with the attending physician throughout treatment. At least initially during treatment, the application of techniques to the abdomen is contraindicated. Depth of application of techniques is limited to the most superficial muscle layer. Passive movement techniques such as rocking are not included in the regimen. Intervention is initially as brief as 15 min. If this is well tolerated by the client, with no signs of fetal or maternal distress, the intervention time is increased in increments of 5 min up to 40 min. More areas of the client's body are included as the regimen is progressed.

(continued)

	Techniques
	· Apply gentle superficial effleurage and broad-contact petrissage in a rhythmical and soothing manner throughout the limbs, back, and shoulders for the specific aim of producing and sustaining sedation during the course of the massage. Rhythmical and gentle specific petrissage may also be applied to the hands, feet, and face. In areas of increased muscle tension, such as the shoulders, apply more-specific neuromuscular techniques, such as stripping and specific compression, in a manner that will elicit a pleasurable response from the client. Precede or follow the application of massage techniques with diaphragmatic breathing. Follow the application of massage techniques with gentle passive stretches of the muscles that were treated. Relaxing music of the client's choice may be used during the intervention.
	· As the client's impairments and mood improve, the clinician may instruct her on how to apply (nonmechanical) superficial reflex techniques, such as static contact and superficial stroking, to her own abdomen. This may be done in the context of applying lotion for skin care and may further improve the expectant mother's mood and her bonding with her child.
Other appropriate techniques and interventions[186]	· Medical management
	· Relaxation training (progressive muscle relaxation, guided imagery, meditation)
	· Stress management instruction (coping skills)
	· Therapeutic exercise in lying (stretching exercises and slow, smooth active range-of-motion exercise for neck, upper and lower extremity muscles in lying), especially ankle pumping to promote lower extremity circulation
	· Breathing training
	· Positioning instruction
	· Psychosocial counseling
	· Self-monitoring for signs of medication side effects and labor
	· Prenatal and postpartum education as required
Functional outcomes of care	Client will maintain ability to perform rolling side-to-side and scooting independently with use of monkey bar
	Client will maintain ability to perform transfers lying-to-sit, sit-to-stand, stand-to-toilet, toilet-to-stand with contact guard assistance
	Client will maintain ability to ambulate 10 feet to bathroom with minimal assistance of one person
	Client will demonstrate fewer complaints of achiness and weakness during functional activity
	Client will report increased sense of well-being and decreased stress-related symptoms

References

1. Fritz S. Fundamentals of therapeutic massage. St Louis: Mosby-Lifeline, 1995.
2. Tappan FM, Benjamin P. Tappan's handbook of healing massage techniques. 3rd ed. Stamford, CT: Appleton & Lange, 1998.
3. Salvo SG. Massage therapy. Philadelphia: WB Saunders, 1999.
4. American Physical Therapy Association. Guide to physical therapist practice. Phys Ther 1997;77(11).
5. Loving J. Massage therapy. Stamford, CT: Appleton & Lange, 1999.
6. de Domenico G, Wood EC. Beard's massage. 4th ed. Philadelphia: WB Saunders, 1997.

7. Holey E, Cook E. Therapeutic massage. London, England: WB Saunders, 1997.

8. Hollis M. Massage for therapists. 2nd ed. Oxford, England: Blackwell Science, 1998.

9. Benjamin PJ, Lamp SP. Understanding sports massage. Champaign, IL: Human Kinetics, 1996.

10. Murrell W. Massotherapeutics or massage as a mode of treatment. Philadelphia: Blakiston, 1890.

11. Palmer MD. Lessons on massage. 4th ed. London: Balliere Tindall and Cox, 1912.

12. Kellogg JH. The art of massage: a practical manual for the nurse, the student and the practitioner. Battle Creek, MI: Modern Medicine Publishing, 1929.

13. DiGiovanna EL, Schiowitz S. An osteopathic approach to diagnosis and treatment. Philadelphia: Lippincott-Raven, 1997.

14. Greenman PE. Principles of manual medicine. 2nd ed. Baltimore: Williams & Wilkins, 1996.

15. Field TM. Massage therapy effects. Am Psychol 1998; 53(12):1270–1281.

16. Mair P, Kornberger E, Schwarz B, et al. Forward blood flow during cardiopulmonary resuscitation in patients with severe accidental hypothermia. An echocardiographic study. Acta Anaesthesiol Scand 1998;42(10):1139–1144.

17. Boczar ME, Howard MA, Rivers EP, et al. A technique revisited: hemodynamic comparison of closed- and open-chest cardiac massage during human cardiopulmonary resuscitation. Crit Care Med 1995;23(3):498–503.

18. Redberg RF, Tucker KJ, Cohen TJ, et al. Physiology of blood flow during cardiopulmonary resuscitation. A transesophageal echocardiographic study. Circulation 1993;88(2):534–542.

19. Horiuchi K, Johnson R, Weissman C. Influence of lower limb pneumatic compression on pulmonary artery temperature: effect on cardiac output measurements. Crit Care Med 1999;27(6):1096–1099.

20. Malone MD, Cisek PL, Comerota AJ Jr, et al. High-pressure, rapid-inflation pneumatic compression improves venous hemodynamics in healthy volunteers and patients who are post-thrombotic. J Vasc Surg 1999;29(4):593–599.

21. Liu K, Chen LE, Seaber AV, et al. Intermittent pneumatic compression of legs increases microcirculation in distant skeletal muscle. J Orthop Res 1999;17(1):88–95.

22. Vanek VW. Meta-analysis of effectiveness of intermittent pneumatic compression devices with a comparison of thigh-high to knee-high sleeves. Am Surg 1998;64(11):1050–1058.

23. Ricci MA, Fisk P, Knight S, Case T. Hemodynamic evaluation of foot venous compression devices. J Vasc Surg 1997;26(5):803–808.

24. Valtonen EJ, Lilius HG, Svinhufvud U. The effect of syncardial massage produced without synchronization and with different pressure impulse frequencies. Ann Chir Gynaecol Fenn 1973;62:69–72.

25. McGeown JG, McHale NG, Thornbury KD. The role of external compression and movement in lymph propulsion in the sheep hind limb. J Physiol 1987;387:83–93.

26. McGeown JG, McHale NG, Thornbury KD. Effects of varying patterns of external compression on lymph flow in the hind limb of the anaesthetized sheep. J Physiol 1988;397:449–457.

27. Kisner C, Colby LA. Therapeutic exercise: foundations and techniques. 3rd ed. Philadelphia: FA Davis, 1996.

28. Frownfelter DL, Dean E. Principles and practice of cardiopulmonary physical therapy. 3rd ed. St. Louis: CV Mosby, 1996.

29. Frownfelter D, ed. Chest physical therapy and pulmonary rehabilitation: an interdisciplinary approach. Chicago: Year Book, 1978.

30. Fritz S. Mosby's fundamentals of therapeutic massage. St Louis: Mosby-Lifeline, 2000.

31. Hayes J, Cox C. Immediate effects of a five-minute foot massage on patients in critical care. Intensive Crit Care Nurs 1999;15(2):77–82.

32. Ahles TA, Tope DM, Pinkson B, et al. Massage therapy for patients undergoing autologous bone marrow transplantation. J Pain Symptom Manage 1999;18(3):157–163.

33. Field T, Hernandez-Reif M, Hart S, et al. Pregnant women benefit from massage therapy. J Psychosom Obstet Gynecol 1999;20(1):31–38.

34. Richards KC. Effect of a back massage and relaxation intervention on sleep in critically ill patients. Am J Crit Care 1998;7(4):288–299.

35. MacDonald G. Massage as a respite intervention for primary caregivers. Am J Hospice Palliat Care 1998;15(1):43–47.

36. Field T, Schanberg S, Kuhn C, et al. Bulimic adolescents benefits from massage therapy. Adolescence 1998; 33(131):555–563.

37. Field T, Peck M, Krugman S, et al. Burn injuries benefit from massage therapy. J Burn Care Rehabil 1998;19(3):241–244.

38. Field T, Hernandez-Reif M, Seligman S, et al. Juvenile rheumatoid arthritis: benefits from massage therapy. J Pediatr Psychol 1997;22:607–617.

39. Field T, Ironson G, Pickens I, et al. Massage therapy reduces anxiety and enhances EEG pattern of alertness and math computations. Int J Neurosci 1996;86:197–205.

40. Fraser J, Kerr JR. Psychophysiological effects of back massage on elderly institutionalized patients. J Adv Nurs 1993;18:238–245.

41. Field T, Morrow C, Vaideon C, et al. Massage reduces anxiety in child and adolescent psychiatric patients. J Am Acad Child Adolesc Psychiatry 1992;31:124–131.

42. Field T. Maternal depression effects on infants and early interventions. Prev Med 1998;27(2):200–203.

43. Field T, Grizzle N, Scafidi F, Schanberg S. Massage and relaxation therapies effects on depressed adolescent mothers. Adolescence 1996;31:903–911.

44. Field T, Quintino O, Hernandez-Reif M. Adolescents with attention deficit hyperactivity disorder benefit from massage therapy. Adolescence 1998;33:103–108.

45. Field T, Lasko D, Mundy P, et al. Autistic children's attentiveness and responsivity improved after touch therapy. J Autism Dev Disord 1997;27:329–334.

46. Ironson G, Field T, Scafidi F, et al. Massage therapy is associated with enhancement of the immune system's cytotoxic capacity. Int J Neurosci 1996;84:205–217.

47. Zhao A. Study of effects of traditional Chinese massage. Chin J Sports Med 1982;1(1):46–48, 64.

48. Schachner L, Field T, Hernandez-Reif M, et al. Atopic dermatitis symptoms decreased in children following massage therapy. Pediatr Dermatol 1998;15(5): 390–395.

49. Yates J. A physician's guide to therapeutic massage. Vancouver, British Columbia: Massage Therapists' Association of British Columbia, 1990.

50. Hoehn-Saric R. Psychic and somatic anxiety: worries, somatic symptoms and physiological changes. Acta Psychiatr Scand Suppl 1998;393:32–38.

51. Millensen JR. Mind matters: psychological medicine in holistic practice. Seattle, WA: Eastland Press, 1995.

52. Morelli M, Chapman CE, Sullivan SJ. Do cutaneous receptors contribute to the changes in the amplitude of the H-reflex during massage? Electromyogr Clin Neurophysiol 1999;39(7):441–447.

53. Morelli M, Sullivan SJ, Chapman CE. Inhibitory influence of soleus massage onto the medial gastrocnemius H-reflex. Electromyogr Clin Neurophysiol 1998;38(2): 87–93.

54. Goldberg J, Seaborne DE, Sullivan SI, Leduc BE. The effect of therapeutic massage on H-reflex amplitude in persons with a spinal cord injury. Phys Ther 1994;748(8):728–737.

55. Goldberg J, Sullivan SI, Seaborne DE. The effect of two intensities of massage on H-reflex amplitude. Phys Ther 1992;72(6):449–457.

56. Sullivan SJ, Williams LRT, Seaborne D, Morelli M. Effects of massage on alpha neuron excitability. Phys Ther 1991;71(8):555–560.

57. Morelli M, Seaborne DE, Sullivan SJ. H-reflex modulation during manual muscle massage of human triceps surae. Arch Phys Med Rehabil 1991;72(11):915–919.

58. Morelli M, Seaborne DE, Sullivan SJ. Changes in H-reflex amplitude during massage of triceps surae in healthy subjects. J Orthop Sports Phys Ther 1990;12(2):55–59.

59. Newham DJ, Lederman E. Effect of manual therapy techniques on the stretch reflex in normal human quadriceps. Disabil Rehabil 1997;19(8):326–331.

60. Lederman E. Fundamentals of manual therapy. New York: Churchill Livingstone, 1997.

61. Leivadi S, Hernandez-Reif M, Field T, et al. Massage therapy and relaxation effects on university dance students. J Dance Med Sci 1999;3(3):108–112.

62. Crosman LJ, Chateauvert SR, Weisburg J. The effects of massage to the hamstring muscle group on range of motion. Massage J 1985:59–62.

63. Blackman PG, Simmons LR, Crossley KM. Treatment of chronic exertional anterior compartment syndrome with massage: a pilot study. Clin J Sport Med 1998;8(1): 14–17.

64. Shipman MK, Boniface DR, Tefft ME, McCloghry F. Antenatal perineal massage and subsequent perineal outcomes: a randomised controlled trial. Br J Obstet Gynaecol 1997;104(7):787–791.

65. Field DA, Miller S. Cosmetic breast surgery. Am Fam Phys 1992;45(2):711–719.

66. Hernandez-Reif M, Field T, Krasnegor J, et al. Children with cystic fibrosis benefit from massage therapy. J Pediatr Psychol 1999;24(2):175–181.

67. Beeken JE, Parks D, Cory J, Montopoli G. The effectiveness of neuromuscular release massage therapy in five individuals with chronic obstructive lung disease. Clin Nurs Res 1998;7(3):309–325.

68. Field T, Henteleff T, Hernandez–Reif M, et al. Children with asthma have improved pulmonary functions after massage therapy. J Pediatr 1998;132(5):854–858.

69. Labrecque M, Nouwen A, Bergeron M, Rancourt JF. A randomized controlled trial of nonpharmacologic approaches for relief of low back pain during labor. J Fam Pract 1999;48(4):259–263.

70. Field T, Hernandez-Reif M, Taylor S, et al. Labour pain is reduced by massage therapy. J Psychosom Obstet Gynecol 1997;18:286–291.

71. Nixon N, Teschendorff J, Finney J, Karnilowicz W. Expanding the nursing repertory: the effect of massage on post-operative pain. Aust J Adv Nurs 1997;14(3): 21–26.

72. Ferrell-Tory AT, Glick OJ. The use of therapeutic massage as a nursing intervention to modify anxiety and the perception of cancer pain. Cancer Nurs 1993;16(2): 93–101.

73. Weinrich SP, Weinrich MC. The effect of massage on pain in cancer patients. Appl Nurs Res 1990;3(4):140–145.

74. Puustjarvi K, Airaksinen 0, Pontinen PJ. The effect of massage in patients with chronic tension headache. Int J Acupunct Electrother Res 1990;15:159–162.

75. Danneskiold-Samsoe B, Christiansen E, Anderson RB. Myofascial pain and the role of myoglobin. Scand J Rheumatol (Stockholm) 1986;15:174–178.

76. Ernst E. Massage therapy for low back pain: a systematic review. J Pain Symptom Manage 1999;17:65–69.

77. Carreck A. The effect of massage on pain perception threshold. Manipulative Physiother 1994;26(2):10–16.

78. Day JA, Mason RR, Chesrown SE. Effect of massage on serum level of beta-endorphin and beta-lipotropin in healthy adults. Phys Ther 1987;67(6):926–930.

79. Ernst E, Matrai A, lmagyarosy I, et al. Massages cause changes in blood fluidity. Physiotherapy 1987;73(1): 43–45.

80. Arkko PJ, Pakarinen AJ, Kari-Koskinen O. Effects of whole-body massage on serum protein, electrolyte and hormone concentrations, enzyme activities and hematological parameters. Int J Sports Med 1983;4:265–267.

81. Shoemaker I, Tiduus M, Mader R. Failure of manual massage to alter limb blood flow: measures by Doppler ultrasound. Med Sci Sports Exerc 1997;1:610–614.

82. Linde B. Dissociation of insulin absorption and blood flow during massage of a subcutaneous injection site. Diabetes Care 1986;6:570–574.

83. Wyper DJ, McNiven DR. Effects of some physiotherapeutic agents on skeletal muscle blood flow. Physiotherapy 1976;62(3):83–85.

84. Hovind H, Nielsen SL. Effect of massage on blood flow in skeletal muscle. Scand J Rehabil Med 1974;6:74–77.

85. Hansen TI, Kristensen JH. Effect of massage, shortwave diathermy and ultrasound upon ^{133}Xe disappearance rate from muscle and subcutaneous tissue in the human calf. Scand J Rehabil Med 1973;5(4):179–182.

86. Mortimer PS, Simmonds R, Rezvani M, et al. The measurement of skin lymph flow by isotope clearance—reliability, reproducibility, injection dynamics, and the effect of massage. J Invest Dermatol 1990;95(6):677–682.

87. Yamazaki Z, Idezuki Y, Nemoto T, Togawa T. Clinical experiences using pneumatic massage therapy for edematous limbs over the last 10 years. Angiology 1988;39(2):154–163.

88. Yamazaki Z, Fujimori Y, Wada T, et al. Admittance plethysmographic evaluation of undulatory massage for the edematous limb. Lymphology 1979;12:40–42.

89. Martin NA, Zoeller RF, Robertson RJ, Lephart SM. The comparative effects of sports massage, active recovery, and rest in promoting blood lactate clearance after supramaximal leg exercise. J Athletic Train 1998;33(1):30–35.

90. Gupta S, Goswami A, Sadhukhan AK, Mathur DN. Comparative study of lactate removal in short term massage of extremities, active recovery and a passive recovery period after supramaximal exercise sessions. Int J Sports Med 1996;17(2):106–110.

91. Dolgener FA, Morien A. The effect of massage on lactate disappearance. J Strength Condition Res 1993;7(3):159–162.

92. Bale P, James H. Massage, warmdown and rest as recuperative measures after short term intense exercise. Physiother Sport 1991;13(2):4–7.

93. Tiidus PM. Manual massage and recovery of muscle function following exercise: a literature review. J Orthop Sports Phys Ther 1997;25(2):107–112.

94. Callaghan MJ. The role of massage in the management of athletes: a review. Br J Sports Med 1993;27(1):28–33.

95. Cafarelli E, Flint F. Role of massage in preparation for and recovery from exercise. Physiother Sport 1993;16(1):17–20.

96. Harmer PA. The effect of pre-performance massage on stride frequency in sprinters. Athletic Train 1991;26:55–59.

97. Boone T, Cooper R, Thompson WR. A physiologic evaluation of the sports massage. J Athletic Train 1991;26:51–54.

98. Wiktorsson-Moller M, Oberg B, Ekstrand J, Giliquist J. Effects of warming up, massage, and stretching on range of motion and muscle strength in the lower extremity. Am J Sports Med 1983;11(4):249–252.

99. Ernst E. Does post-exercise massage treatment reduce delayed onset muscle soreness? A systematic review. Br J Sports Med 1998;32(3):212–214.

100. Weber MD, Servedis FJ, Woodall WR. The effects of three modalities on delayed onset muscle soreness. J Orthop Sports Phys Ther 1994;20:236–242.

101. Smith LL, Keating MN, Holbert D, et al. The effects of athletic massage on delayed onset muscle soreness, creatine kinase, and neutrophil count: a preliminary report. J Orthop Sports Phys Ther 1994;19(2):93–99.

102. Rinder AN, Sutherland CJ. An investigation of the effects of massage on quadriceps performance after exercise fatigue. Complement Ther Nurs Midwifery 1995;1(4):99–102.

103. Tiidus PM. Massage and ultrasound as therapeutic modalities in exercise-induced muscle damage. Can J Appl Physiol 1999;24(3):267–278.

104. Rodenburg JB, Steenbeek D, Schiereck P, Bar PR. Warm-up, stretching and massage diminish harmful effects of eccentric exercise. Int J Sports Med 1994;15(7):414–419.

105. Drews T, Kreider B, Drinkard B, et al. Effects of post-event massage therapy on repeated endurance cycling. Int J Sports Med 1990;11:407.

106. Drews T, Kreider RB, Drinkard B, Jackson CW. Effects of post-event massage therapy on psychological profiles of exertion, feeling and mood during a 4-day ultra endurance cycling event. Med Sci Sport Exerc 1991;23:91.

107. Weinberg R, Jackson A, Kolodny K. The relationship of massage and exercise to mood enhancement. Sport Psychol 1988;2:202–211.

108. Gam AN, Warming S, Larsen LH, et al. Treatment of myofascial trigger-points with ultrasound combined with massage and exercise—a randomised controlled trial. Pain 1998;77(1):73–79.

109. Gluck NI. Passive care and active rehabilitation in a patient with failed back surgery syndrome. J Manipulative Physiol Ther 1996;19(1):41–47.

110. Hammill JM, Cook TM, Rosecrance JC. Effectiveness of a physical therapy regimen in the treatment of tension-type headache. Headache 1996;36:149–153.

111. Inoue M, Ohtsu I, Tomioka S, et al. [Effects of pulmonary rehabilitation on vital capacity in patients with chronic pulmonary emphysema.] Nihon Kyobu Shikkan Gakkai Zasshi (Japanese) 1996;34(11):1182–1188. (Abstract)

112. Pope MH, Phillips RB, Haugh LD, et al. A prospective randomized three-week trial of spinal manipulation, transcutaneous muscle stimulation, massage and corset in the treatment of subacute low back pain. Spine 1994;19(22):2571–2577.

113. Waylonis GW, Perkins RH. Post-traumatic fibromyalgia. A long term follow-up. Am J Phys Med Rehabil 1994;73(6):403–412.

114. Levoska S, Keinanen-Kiukaanniemi S. Active or passive physiotherapy for occupational cervico-brachial disorders? A comparison of 2 treatment methods with a 1 year follow-up. Arch Phys Med 1993;74(4):425–430.

115. Aksenova AM, Teslenko OI, Boganskaia OA. [Changes in the immune status of peptic ulcer patients after combined treatment including deep massage]. Vopr Kurortol Fizioter Lech Fiz Kult (Russian) 1999;(2):19–20. (Abstract)

116. Makarova MR, Kuznetsov OF, Markina LP, et al. [The effect of massage on the neuromuscular apparatus and blood coagulating system of patients with chronic salpingo-oophoritis]. Vopr Kurortol Fizioter Lech Fiz Kult (Russian) 1998;(6):45–8. (Abstract)

117. Aksenova AM, Romanova MM. [The effect of reflex muscle massage on the body regulator processes of peptic ulcer patients with concomitant diseases]. Vopr Kurortol Fizioter Lech Fiz Kult (Russian) 1998;(6):24–6. (Abstract)

118. Gusarova SA, Kuznetsov OF, Gorbunov FE, Maslovskaia SG. [The characteristics of the effect of point and classical massage on the hemodynamics of patients with a history of transient ischemic attacks in the vertebrobasilar system]. Vopr Kurortol Fizioter Lech Fiz Kult (Russian) 1998;(5):7–9. (Abstract)

119. Kuznetsov OF, Makarova MR, Markina LP. [The comparative effect of classic massage of different intensities on patients with chronic salpingo-oophritis]. Vopr Kurortol Fizioter Lech Fiz Kult (Russian) 1998;(2):20–23. (Abstract)

120. Aksenova AM. [A new method for deep reflex muscular massage]. Vopr Kurortol Fizioter Lech Fiz Kult (Russian) 1997;(4):30–32. (Abstract)

121. Aksenova AM, Reznikov KM, Andreeva VV. [The effect of deep massage and physical exercises on the cerebral circulation in osteochondrosis of the cervicothoracic spine]. Vopr Kurortol Fizioter Lech Fiz Kult (Russian) 1997;(3):19–21. (Abstract)

122. Gusarova SA, Kuznetsov OF, Maslovskaia SG. [The effect of the massage of different areas of the body on the cerebral hemodynamics in patients with a history of acute disorders of the cerebral circulation]. Vopr Kurortol Fizioter Lech Fiz Kult (Russian) 1996;(1):14–6. (Abstract)

123. Richaud C, Bouchet JY, Bosson JL, et al. [Manual fragmentation of deep vein thrombosis]. J Mal Vasc (French) 1995;20(3):166–71. (Abstract)

124. Eliska O, Eliska M. Are peripheral lymphatics damaged by high pressure manual massage? Lymphology 1995;28:21–30.

125. Lindsay WR, Pitcaithly D, Geelen N, et al. A comparison of the effects of four therapy procedures on concentration and responsiveness in people with profound learning disabilities. J Intellect Disabil Res 1997;41(pt 3):201–207.

126. Brooker DJ, Snape M, Johnson E, et al. Single case evaluation of the effects of aromatherapy and massage on disturbed behaviour in severe dementia. Br J Clin Psychol 1997;36(pt 2):287–296.

127. Travell JG, Simons DG. Myofascial pain and dysfunction. The trigger point manual, vol 1. Baltimore: Williams & Wilkins, 1983.

128. Travell JG, Simons DG. Myofascial pain and dysfunction. The trigger point manual, vol 2. Baltimore: Williams & Wilkins, 1992.

129. Simons DG, Travell JG, Simons LS. Travell and Simons' myofascial pain and dysfunction: the trigger point manual, vol 1: upper half of body. 2nd ed. Baltimore: Williams & Wilkins, 1999.

130. Chaitow L. Modern neuromuscular techniques. New York: Churchill Livingstone, 1996.

131. Mannheim CJ, Lavett DK. The myofascial release manual. Thorofare, NJ: Slack (McGraw Hill), 1989.

132. Murphy GJ. Physical medicine modalities and trigger point injections in the management of temporomandibular disorders and assessing treatment outcome. Oral Surg Oral Med Oral Pathol Oral Radiol Endod 1997;83(1):118–122.

133. Fricton JR. Management of masticatory myofascial pain. Semin Orthod 1995;1(4):229–243.

134. Clark GT, Seligman DA, Solberg WK, Pullinger AG. Guidelines for the treatment of temporomandibular disorders. J Craniomandib Disord 1990;4(2):80–88.

135. Seaman DR, Cleveland C III. Spinal pain syndromes: nociceptive, neuropathic, and psychologic mechanisms. J Manipulative Physiol Ther 1999;22(7):458–472.

136. Kovacs FM, Abraira V, Pozo F, et al. Local and remote sustained trigger point therapy for exacerbations of chronic low back pain. A randomized, double-blind, controlled, multicenter trial. Spine 1997;22(7):786–797.

137. Ingber RS. Iliopsoas myofascial dysfunction: a treatable cause of "failed" low back syndrome. Arch Phys Med Rehabil 1989;70(5):382–386.

138. Morris CE. Chiropractic rehabilitation of a patient with S1 radiculopathy associated with a large lumbar disk herniation. J Manipulative Physiol Ther 1999;22(1):38–44.

139. Hawk C, Long C, Azad A. Chiropractic care for women with chronic pelvic pain: a prospective single-group intervention study. J Manipulative Physiol Ther 1997;20(2):73–79.

140. Hughes KH. Painful rib syndrome. A variant of myofascial pain syndrome. AAOHN J 1998;46(3):115–120.

141. Antonelli MA, Vawter RL. Nonarticular pain syndromes. Differentiating generalized, regional, and localized disorders. Postgrad Med 1992;91(2):95–98, 103–104.

142. Gerwin RD. Myofascial pain syndromes in the upper extremity. J Hand Ther 1997;10(2):130–136.

143. Lew PC, Lewis J, Story I. Inter-therapist reliability in locating latent myofascial trigger points using palpation. Manual Ther 1997;2(2):87–90.

144. Hannon JC. The man who mistook his patient for a chair: a speculation regarding sitting mechanical treatment of lower back pain. J Bodywork Movement Ther 1998;2(2):88–100.

145. Han SC, Harrison P. Myofascial pain syndrome and trigger-point management. Reg Anesth 1997;22(1):89–101.

146. Chaitow L. Positional release techniques. New York: Churchill Livingstone, 1996.

147. Prudden B. Pain erasure: the Bonnie Prudden way. New York: M. Evans, 1980.

148. Prudden B. Myotherapy: Bonnie Prudden's complete guide to pain-free living. New York: Ballantine Books, 1984.

149. Masunaga S, Chashi W. Zen Shiatsu: how to harmonize yin and yang for better health. Tokyo: Japan Publishers, 1977.

150. Yamamoto S, McCarty P. The shiatsu handbook. New York: Avery Publishing Group, 1996.

151. Tappan F. Finger pressure to acupuncture points. In: Tappan FM, Benjamin PJ, eds. Tappan's handbook of healing massage techniques. Stamford, CT: Appleton & Lange, 1998:243–268.

152. Wolf JE, Teegarden IM. Jin shin do. In: Tappan FM, Benjamin PJ, eds. Tappan's handbook of healing massage techniques. Stamford, CT: Appleton & Lange, 1998: 295–308.

153. O'Sullivan SB. Strategies to improve motor control. In: O'Sullivan SB, Schmitz J, eds. Physical rehabilitation, assessment and treatment. 2nd ed. Philadelphia: FA Davis, 1988.

154. Leone JA, Kukulka CG. Effects of tendon pressure on alpha motoneuron excitability in patients with stroke. Phys Ther 1988;68(4):475–480.

155. Kukulka CG, Haberichter PA, Mueksch AE, Rohrberg MG. Muscle pressure effects on motoneuron excitability. A special communication. Phys Ther 1987;67(11):1720–1722.

156. Kukulka CG, Beckman SM, Holte JB, Hoppenworth PK. Effects of intermittent tendon pressure on alpha motoneuron excitability. Phys Ther 1986;66(7):1091–1094.

157. Kukulka CG, Fellows WA, Oehlertz JE, Vanderwilt SG. Effect of tendon pressure on alpha motoneuron excitability. Phys Ther 1985;65(5):595–600.

158. Dougans I. The complete illustrated guide to foot reflexology. Boston: Element Books, 1996.

159. Byers DC. Better health with foot reflexology: the original Ingham method. St. Petersburg, FL: Ingham Publishing, 1996.

160. Herskovitz S, Strauch B, Gordon MJV. Shiatsu-induced injury of the median recurrent motor branch. Muscle Nerve 1992;Oct:1215. (Letter)

161. Andrade C, Randall T, Swift T, Brescia N. The effect of a self-managed manual trigger point pressure program with a hand-held massage device on trigger point sensitivity, perceived pain levels, and frequency of self-care in adults with chronic myofascial neck pain. Project report, Samuel Merritt College, Oakland, CA, 1997.

162. Stephenson NL, Weinrich SP, Tavakoli AS. The effects of foot reflexology on anxiety and pain in patients with breast and lung cancer. Oncol Nurs Forum 2000;27(1): 67–72.

163. Kesselring A. [Foot reflexology massage: a clinical study]. Forsch Komplementarmed (German) 1999;6(suppl 1): 38–40. (Abstract)

164. Sudmeier I, Bodner G, Egger I, et al. [Changes of renal blood flow during organ-associated foot reflexology measured by color Doppler sonography]. Forsch Komplementarmed (German) 1999;6(3):129–134. (Abstract)

165. Baerheim A, Algroy R, Skogedal KR, et al. [Feet—a diagnostic tool?] Tidsskr Nor Laegeforen (Norwegian) 1998;118(5):753–755. (Abstract)

166. Kesselring A, Spichiger E, Muller M. [Foot reflexology: an intervention study]. Pflege (German) 1998;11(4):213–218. (Abstract)

167. Kristof O, Schlumpf M, Saller R. [Foot reflex zone massage—a review]. Wien Med Wochenschr (German) 1997;147(18):418–422. (Abstract)

168. Omura Y. Accurate localization of organ representation areas on the feet & hands using the bi-digital O-ring test resonance phenomenon: its clinical implication in diagnosis & treatment—part I. Acupunct Electrother Res 1994;19(2–3):153–190.

169. Kesselring A. [Foot reflex zone massage]. Schweiz Med Wochenschr Suppl (German) 1994;62:88–93. (Abstract)

170. Oleson T, Flocco W. Randomized controlled study of premenstrual symptoms treated with ear, hand, and foot reflexology. Obstet Gynecol 1993;82(6):906–911.

171. Petersen LN, Faurschou P, Olsen OT. [Foot zone therapy and bronchial asthma—a controlled clinical trial]. Ugeskr Laeger (Danish) 1992;154(30):2065–2068. (Abstract)

172. Helms JM. Acupuncture energetics. A clinical approach for physicians. Berkeley, CA: Medical Acupuncture Publishers, 1995.

173. Porkert M, Hempen C-H, The China Academy. Classical acupuncture—the standard textbook. Dinkelscherben, Germany: Phainon Editions and Media GmbH, 1995.

174. Kielkowska A. Your health in your hands. Gdansk, Poland: Kolmio, 1995.

175. Melzack R. Myofascial trigger points: relation to acupuncture and mechanisms of pain. Arch Phys Med Rehabil 1981;62:114–117.

176. Melzack R, Stilwell DN, Fox EJ. Trigger points and acupuncture points for pain: correlations and implications. Pain 1977;3:23.

177. Shenkman Z, Holzman RS, Kim C, et al. Acupressure—acupuncture antiemetic prophylaxis in children undergoing tonsillectomy. Anesthesiology 1999;90(5):1311–1316.

178. Harmon D, Gardiner J, Harrison R, Kelly A. Acupressure and the prevention of nausea and vomiting after laparoscopy. Br J Anaesth 1999;82(3):387–390.

179. Aikins, Murphy P. Alternative therapies for nausea and vomiting of pregnancy. Obstet Gynecol 1998;91(1): 149–155.

180. Stein DJ, Birnbach DJ, Danzer BI, et al. Acupressure versus intravenous metoclopramide to prevent nausea and vomiting during spinal anesthesia for cesarean section. Anesth Analg 1997;84(2):342–345.

181. Ho CM, Hseu SS, Tsai SK, Lee TY. Effect of P-6 acupressure on prevention of nausea and vomiting after epidural morphine for post–cesarean section pain relief. Acta Anaesthesiol Scand 1996;40(3):372–375.

182. Beal MW. Acupuncture and acupressure. Applications to women's reproductive health care. J Nurse Midwifery 1999;44(3):217–230.

183. Chen ML, Lin LC, Wu SC, Lin JG. The effectiveness of acupressure in improving the quality of sleep of institutionalized residents. J Gerontol A Biol Sci Med Sci 1999;54(8):M389–394.

184. Maa SH, Gauthier D, Turner M. Acupressure as an adjunct to a pulmonary rehabilitation program. J Cardiopulm Rehabil 1997;17(4):268–276.

185. Miller L H, Smith AD, Mehler BL. Stress audit. Brookline, MA: Biobehavioral Associates, 1987.

186. Kisner C, Colby L. Therapeutic exercise: foundations and techniques. 3rd ed. Philadelphia: FA Davis, 1990.

Suggested Readings

Airaksinen O, Partanen K, Kolari PJ, Soimalkallio S. Intermittent pneumatic compression therapy in post-traumatic lower limb edema: computed tomography and clinical measurements. Arch Phys Med Rehabil 1991;72(9):667–670.

Airaksinen O. Changes in post-traumatic ankle joint mobility, pain and oedema following intermittent pneumatic compression therapy. Arch Phys Med Rehabil 1997;70(4):341–344.

Alexander R, Bennet-Clerk HC. Storage of elastic energy in muscles and other tissues. Nature 1977;265:114–117.

Ause-Ellias KL, Richard R, Miller SF, Finley RK Jr. The effect of mechanical compression on chronic hand edema after burn injury: a preliminary report. J Burn Care Rehabil 1994;15(1):29–33.

Balke B, Anthony J, Wyatt F. The effects of massage treatment on exercise fatigue. Clin Sports Med 1991;12:184–207.

Balla JI. The late whiplash syndrome. Aust NZ J Surg 1980;50:610–614.

Barr JS, Taslitz N. The influence of back massage on autonomic functions. Phys Ther 1970;50:1679–1691.

Bell GW. Aquatic sports massage therapy. Clin Sports Med 1999;18(2):427–435,ix.

Birukov AA, Peisahov NM. [Changes in the psycho-physiological indices using different techniques of sports massage.] Teoriya i Praktika Fizicheskoi Kult (Russian) 1979;8:21–24. Translated in: Yessis M, ed. Sov Sports Rev 1986;21(1):29.

Birukov AA, Pogosyan NM. [Special means of restoration of work capacity of wrestlers in the periods between bouts.] Teoriya i Praktika Fizicheskoi Kult (Russian) 1983;3:49–50. Translated in: Yessis M, ed. Sov Sports Rev 1983;19(4):191–192.

Bodian M. Use of massage following lid surgery. Eye, Ear, Nose Throat Monthly 1969;48:542–545.

Bonica JJ. Management of myofascial pain syndromes in general practice. JAMA 1957;164:732–738.

Bork K, Korting GW, Faust G. [Serum enzyme levels after a whole body massage.] Arch Dermatol Forsch (German) 1971;240:342–348.

Braverman DL, Schulman RA. Massage techniques in rehabilitation medicine. Phys Med Rehabil Clin N Am 1999;10(3):631–49,ix.

Brown BR. Myofascial syndrome. In: Warfield CA, ed. Principles and practice of pain management. New York: McGraw Hill, 1993:259–264.

Burovych AA, Samtsova IA, Manilov IA. An investigation of the effects of individual variants of sports massage on muscle blood circulation. Sov Sports Sci Rev 1989;24:197–200.

Cady SH, Jones CE. Massage therapy as a workplace intervention for reduction of stress. Percept Motor Skills 1997;84:157–158.

Cailliet R. Soft tissue pain and disability. Philadelphia: FA Davis, 1996.

Carrier EB. Studies on the physiology of capillaries: reaction of human skin capillaries to drugs and other stimuli. Am J Physiol 1922;11:528–547.

Cawley N. A critique of the methodology of research studies evaluating massage. Eur J Cancer Care (Engl). 1997;6(1):23–31.

Chor H, Cleveland D, Davenport HA, et al. Atrophy and regeneration of the gastrocnemius-soleus muscles: effects of physical therapy in monkeys following section and suture of sciatic nerve. JAMA 1939;113:1029–1033.

Chor H, Dolkart RE. A study of simple disuse atrophy in the monkey. Am J Physiol 1936;117:4.

Curties, D. Could massage therapy promote cancer metastasis? Journal of Soft Tissue Manipulation 1994(April–May);3–7.

Danneskiold-Samsoe B, Christiansen E, Lund B, Anderson RB. Regional muscle tension and pain ('fibrositis'): effect of massage on myoglobin in plasma. Scand J Rehabil Med 1982;15:17–20.

Dejung B. [Manual trigger point treatment in chronic lumbosacral pain.] Schweiz Med Wochenschr Suppl (German) 1994;62:82–87.

Delaney GA, McKee AC. Inter- and intra-rater reliability of the pressure threshold meter in measurement of myofascial trigger point sensitivity. Am J Phys Med Rehab 1993;72:136–139.

Dubrovsky, VI. [Changes in muscle and venous flow after massage.] Teoriya i Praktika Fizicheskoi Kult (Russian) 1982;4:56–57. Translated in: M Yessis, ed. Sov Sports Rev 1980;18(3):134–135.

Dunn C, Sleep J, Collett D. Sensing an improvement: an experimental study to evaluate the use of aromatherapy, massage and periods of rest in an intensive care unit. J Adv Nurs 1995;21(1):34–40.

Eason E, Labrecque M, Wells G, Feldman P. Preventing perineal trauma during childbirth: a systematic review. Obstet Gynecol 2000;95(3):464–471.

Edgecombe W, Bain W. The effect of baths, massage and exercise on the blood-pressure. Lancet. 1899;1:1552.

Elkins EC, Herrick JF, Grindlay JH, et al. Effects of various procedures on the flow of lymph. Arch Phys Med 1953;34:31.

Evans RW. Some observations on whiplash injuries. Neurol Clin 1992;10:975–997.

Felhendler D, Lisander B. Effects of non-invasive stimulation of acupoints on the cardiovascular system. Complement Ther Med. 1999;7(4):231–234.

Field T, Hernandez-Reif M, Shaw KH, et al. Glucose levels decreased after giving massage therapy to children with diabetes mellitus. Diabetes Spectrum 1997;10:23–25.

Field T, Quintino O, Henteleff T, et al. Job stress reduction therapies. Altern Ther Health Med 1997;3(4):54–56.

Field T, Seligman S, Scafidi F, Schanberg S. Alleviating posttraumatic stress in children following Hurricane Andrew. J Appl Dev Psychol 1996;17:37–50.

Field T, Sunshine W, Hernandez-Reif M, et al. Chronic fatigue syndrome: massage therapy effects on depression and somatic symptoms in chronic fatigue. J Chron Fatigue Syndrome 1997;3:43–51.

Fire M. Providing massage therapy in a psychiatric hospital. Int J Altern Complement Med 1984;June:24–25.

Fischer AA. Documentation of myofascial trigger points. Arch Phys Med 1988:69:286–291.

Fishbain DA, Goldberg M, Steele R, et al. DSM-III diagnoses of patients with myofascial pain syndrome (fibrositis). Arch Phys Med Rehab 1989;70:433–438.

Fricton J, Kroening R, Haley D. Myofascial pain syndrome: a review of 168 cases. Oral surf 1982;60:615–623.

Fricton JR. Clinical care for myofascial pain. Dent Clin North Am 1991;35(1):1–26.

Gardener AMN, Fox RH, Lawrence C, et al. Reduction of post-traumatic swelling and compartment pressure by impulse compression of the foot. J Bone Joint Surg 1990:72:810–815.

Goats GC. Massage—the scientific basis of an ancient art: part 1. The techniques. Br J Sports Med 1994;28(3):149–152.

Goats GC. Massage—the scientific basis of an ancient art: part 2. Physiological and therapeutic effects. Br J Sports Med 1994;28(3):153–156.

Goldman LB, Rosenberg NL. Myofascial pain syndrome and fibromyalgia. Semin Neurol 1991;11:274–280.

Graff-Radford SB, Reeves JL, Baker RL, Chiu D. Effects of transcutaneous electrical nerve stimulation on myofascial pain and trigger point sensitivity. Pain 1989;37:1–5.

Grimsby D, Grimsby K. Electromyographic and range of motion evaluation to compare the results of two treatment approaches: soft tissue massage versus a segmental manipulation off the cervical spine. Ned Tijdschr Manuele Ther 1993;12(1):2–7.

Guan Z, Zheng G. The effects of massage on the left heart functions in patients of coronary heart disease. J Tradit Chin Med 1995;15(1):59–62.

Gulla J, Singer AJ. Use of alternative therapies among emergency department patients. Ann Emerg Med. 2000; 35(3):226–228.

Gunn CC. Treating myofascial pain: intramuscular stimulation for myofascial pain syndromes of neuropathic origin. Seattle: University of Washington, 1989.

Gusarova SA, Kuznetsov OF, Gorbunov FE, Maslovskaia SG. [The use of point massage in patients with circulatory encephalopathy.] Vopr Kurortol Fizioter Lech Fiz Kult (Russian) 1997;(6):11–13.

Hack GD, Robinson WL, Koritzer RT. Previously undescribed relation between muscle and dura. Proceedings of the Congress of Neurological Surgeons. Phoenix, AZ, Feb 14–18, 1995.

Hartman PS. Management of myofascial dysfunction of the shoulder. In: Donatelli RA, ed. Physical therapy of the shoulder. New York: Churchill Livingstone, 1991.

Hemmings B, Smith M, Graydon J, Dyson R. Effects of massage on physiological restoration, perceived recovery, and repeated sports performance. Br J Sports Med. 2000;34(2): 109–114; discussion 115.

Hemphill L, Kemp J. Implementing a therapeutic massage program in a tertiary and ambulatory care VA setting: the healing power of touch. Nurs Clin North Am. 2000;35(2): 489–497.

Hernandez-Reif M, Field T, Hart S. Smoking cravings are reduced by self-massage. Prev Med. 1999;28(1):28–32.

Hernandez-Reif M, Field T, Theakson J, Field T. Multiple sclerosis patients benefit from massage therapy. J Bodywork Move Ther 1998;2:168–174.

Hernandez-Reif M, Martinez A, Field T, Quintero O, Hart S, Burman I. Premenstrual symptoms are relieved by massage therapy. J Psychosom Obstet Gynaecol. 2000;21(1):9–15.

Hey LR, Helewa A. Myofascial pain syndrome: a critical review of the literature. Physiol Can 1994;46(1):28–36.

Hobbs S, Davies PD. Critical review of how nurses research massage therapy: are they using the best methods? Complementary Therapies in Nursing and Midwifery. 1998;4(2):35–40.

Holmes MH, Lai WM, Mow VC. Compression effects on cartilage permeability. In: Hargens AR, ed. Tissue nutrition and viability. New York: Springer-Verlag, 1986.

Hondras MA, Linde K, Jones AP. Manual therapy for asthma. Cochrane Database Syst Rev. 2000;(2):CD001002.

Huang FY, Huang LM. Effect of local massage on vaccination: DTP and DTPa. Chung Hua Min Kuo Hsiao Erh Ko I Hsueh Hui Tsa Chih 1999;40(3):166–170.

Hulme J, Waterman H, Hillier VF. The effect of foot massage on patients' perception of care following laparoscopic sterilization as day case patients. J Adv Nurs 1999;30(2):460–468.

Jacobs M. Massage for the relief of pain: anatomical and physiological considerations. Phys Ther Rev 1960;40(2): 93–98.

Jami L. Golgi tendon organs in mammalian skeletal muscle: functional properties and central actions. Physiol Rev 1992;73(3):623–666.

Janda, V. On t he concept of postural muscles and posture in man. Aust J Physiother 1983;20(3):83–84.

Jimenez AC, Lane ME. Serial determinations of pressure threshold tolerance in chronic pain patients. Arch Phys Med Rehab 1985;66:545–546.

Jones NA, Field T. Massage and music therapies attenuate frontal EEG asymmetry in depressed adolescents. Adolescence. 1999;34(135):529–534.

Jones DA, Round JM. Skeletal muscle in health and disease. Manchester: Manchester University Press, 1990.

Jordan KD, Jessup D. The recuperative effects of sports massage as compared to rest. Massage Ther J 1990;Winter:57–67.

Katz J, Wowk A, Culp D, Wakeling BA. A randomized, controlled study of the pain- and tension-reducing effects of 15 min workplace massage treatments versus seated rest for nurses in a large teaching hospital. Pain Res Manage 1999;4(2):81–88.

Katz J, Wowk A, Culp D, Wakeling H. Pain and tension are reduced among hospital nurses after on-site massage treatments: a pilot study. J Perianaesth Nurs 1999;14: 128–133.

Kinney BM. External fatty tissue massage (the "endermologie" and "silhouette" procedures). Plast Reconstr Surg 1997; 100(7):1903–1904.

Kolich M, Taboun SM, Mohamed AI. Low back muscle activity in an automobile seat with a lumbar massage system. Int J Occup Saf Ergon 2000;6(1):113–128.

Kraus H, ed. Diagnosis and treatment of muscle pain. Chicago: Quintessence, 1988.

Krilov VN, Talishev FM, Burovikh AN. The use of restorative massage in the training of high level basketball players. Sov Sci Rev 1985;20:7–9.

Ladd MP, Kottke FJ, Blanchard RS. Studies of the effect of massage on the flow of lymph from the foreleg of the dog. ArchPhys Med 1952;33(10):604–612.

Le-Vu B, Dumortier A, Guillaume MV, et al. [Efficacy of massage and mobilization of the upper limb after surgical treatment of breast cancer.] Bull Cancer (French) 1997; 84(10):957–961.

Li Z, Liu J, Wu Y, et al. Effect of massotherapy on the in vivo free radical metabolism in patients with prolapse of lumbar intervertebral disc and cervical spondylopathy. J Tradit Chin Med 1995;15(1):53–58.

Linde B, Philip A. Massage-enhanced insulin-absorption— increased distribution or dissociation of insulin? Diabetes Res 1989;11(4):191–194.

Lipton SA. Prevention of classic migraine headache by digital massage of the superficial temporal arteries during visual aura. Ann Neurol 1986;19(5):515–516. (Letter)

Losito JM, O'Neil J. Rehabilitation of foot and ankle injuries. Clin Podiatr Med Surg 1997;14(3):533–557.

Lowe JC, Honeyman-Lowe G. Facilitating the decrease in fibromyalgic pain during metabolic rehabilitation: an essential role for soft tissue therapies. J Bodywork Move Ther 1998;2(4):208–217.

Lund I, Lundeberg T, Kurosawa M, Uvnas-Moberg K. Sensory stimulation (massage) reduces blood pressure in unanaesthetized rats. J Auton Nerv Syst 1999;78(1):30–37.

Lynn J. Using complementary therapies: reflexology. Prof Nurse 1996;11(5):321–322.

Manyam BV, Sanchez-Ramos JR. Traditional and complementary therapies in Parkinson's disease. Adv Neurol 1999;80: 565–574.

McCain GA. Treatment of fibromyalgia and myofascial pain syndromes. In: Rachlin ES, ed. Myofascial pain and fibromyalgia. St. Louis: Mosby Year Book, 1994:31–44.

McCain GA, Scudds RA. The concept of primary fibromyalgia (fibrositis): clinical value, relation and significance to other chronic musculoskeletal pain syndromes. Pain 1988;33: 273–287.

Molea D, Mucek B, Blanken C, et al. Evaluation of two manipulative techniques in the treatment of post exercise muscle soreness. J Am Osteopath Assoc 1987;87(7): 477–483.

Morelli M, Chapman CE, Sullivan SJ. Do cutaneous receptors contribute to the changes in the amplitude of the H-reflex during massgae? Electromyogr Clin Neurophysiol. 1999;39 (7):441–447.

Morhenn VB. Firm stroking of human skin leads to vasodilatation possibly due to the release of substance P. J Dermatol Sci 2000;22(2):138–144.

Nguyen HP, Le DL, Tran QM, et al. CHROMASSI: a therapy advice system based on chrono-massage and acupression using the method of ZiWuLiuZhu. Medinfo 1995;8(pt 2):998.

Nordschow M, Bierman W. The influence of manual massage on muscle relaxation: effect on trunk flexion. J Am Phys Ther Assoc 1962;42(10):653–657.

Nussbaum EL, Downes L. Reliability of clinical pressure-pain algometric measurements obtained on consecutive days. Phys Ther 1998;78(2):160–169.

Ortego, NE. Acupressure: an alternative approach to mental health counselling through bodymind awareness. Nurse Pract Forum 1994;5(2):72–76.

Paikov, VB. Means of restoration in the training of speed skaters. Sov Sports Rev 1988;20:7–12.

Partsch H, Mostbeck A, Leitner G. [Experimental studies on the efficacy of pressure wave massage (Lymphapress) in lymphedema.] Z Lymphol (German) 1981;5(1):35–39.

Petermans J, Zicot M. [Musculo-venous pump in the elderly.] J Mal Vasc (French) 994;19(2):115–118.

Pfaffenrath V, Rehm M. Migraine in pregnancy: what are the safest treatment options? Drug Safety 1998;19(5):383–388.

Potapov IA, Abisheva TM. [The action of massage on lymph formation and transport.] Vopr Kurortol Fizioter Lech Fiz Kult (Russian) 1989;(5):44–47.

Poznick-Patewitz E. Cephalic spasm of head and neck muscles. Headache 1976;15:261–266.

Rachlin ES. Musculofascial pain syndromes. Med Times Jan 1984:34–47.

Rachlin ES. Trigger point management. In: Rachlin ES, ed. Myofascial pain and fibromyalgia. St. Louis: Mosby Year Book, 1994:173–195.

Rachlin I. Therapeutic massage in the treatment of myofascial pain syndromes and fibromyalgia. In: Raclin ES, ed. Myofascial pain and fibromyalgia. Baltimore: Mosby, 1994.

Reeves JL, Jaeger B, Graff-Radford SB. Reliability of the pressure algometer as a measure of myofascial trigger point sensitivity. Pain 1986;24:313–321.

Rubin D. Myofascial trigger point syndromes: an approach to management. Arch Phys Med Rehabil 1981;62(3): 107–110.

Sander M, Siegert R, Gundlach KK. [Results of physiotherapy for patients with myofacial dysfunction.] Dtsch Zahnarztl Z (German) 1989;44(11 Spec No):S12–14.

Schneider W, Dvorak J. [Functional treatment of diseases and injuries of the cervical spine.] Orthopade (German) 1996;25(6):519–523.

Scudds RA, Trachsel LCE, Luckhurst BJ, Percy JS. A comparative study of pain, sleep quality and pain responsiveness in fibrositis and myofascial pain syndrome. J Rheum 1989; 16(suppl 19):120–126.

Severini V, Venerando A. The physiological effects of massage on the cardiovascular system. Eur Medicophys 1967;3: 165–183.

Simons DG. Muscular pain syndromes. In: Fricton JR, Awad EA, eds. Advances in pain research and therapy, vol 17. New York: Raven Press, 1990.

Simons DG, Simons LS. Chronic myofascial pain syndrome. In: Tollison CD, ed. Handbook of chronic pain management. Baltimore: Williams & Wilkins, 1989:509–529.

Sinyakov AF, Belov ES. Restoration of work capacity of gymnasts. Gymnastika 1982;1:48–51.

Snyder-Mackler LS, Bork C, Bourbon B, Trumbore D. Effect of helium-neon laser on musculoskeletal trigger points. Phys Ther 1986;66:1087–1090.

Sola AE. Trigger point therapy. In: Robers JR, Hooges JR, eds: Clinical procedures in emergency medicine. Philadelphia: WB Saunders, 1985.

Sola AE, Rodenberger MS, Gettys BB. Incidence of hypersensitive areas in posterior shoulder muscles: a survey of two hundred young adults. Am J Phys Med 1955;34:585–590.

Sullivan SJ, Blumberger J, Lachowicz C, Raymond D. Does massage decrease laryngeal tension in a subject with complete tetraplegia. Percept Mot Skills 1997;84(1):169–170.

Sunshine W, Field T, Schanberg S, et al. Massage therapy and transcutaneous electrical stimulation effects on fibromyalgia. J Clin Rheumatol 1997;2:18–22.

Suskind MI, Hajek NA, Hines HM. Effects of massage on denervated skeletal muscle. Arch Phys Med 1946;27: 133–135.

Takeuchi H, Jawad MS, Eccles R. The effects of nasal massage of the "yingxiang" acupuncture point on nasal airway resistance and sensation of nasal airflow in patients with nasal congestion associated with acute upper respiratory tract infection. Am J Rhinol 1999;13(2):77–79.

Travell J. Pain mechanisms in connective tissue. In: Ragan C, ed. Connective tissues, transactions of the second conference, 1951. New York: Josiah Macy Jr Foundation, 1952:90, 92–94, 105, 119, 121.

Travell JG, Rinzler SH. The myofascial genesis of pain. Postgrad Med 1952;11:425–434.

Tunnell PW. Protocol for visual assessment: postural evaluation of the muscular system through visual inspection. J Bodywork Move Ther 1996;1(1):21–27.

Urba SG. Non-pharmacologic pain management in terminal care. Clin Geri Med 1996;12(2):301–311.

Valtonen EJ. Syncardial massage for treating extremities swollen by traumata, vein diseases or idiopathic lymphedema. Acta Chir Scand 1967;133:363–367.

Wakim KG, Martin GM, Krusen FH. Influence of centripetal rhythmic compression on localized edema of an extremity. Arch Phys Med 1955;36:98.

Wakim KG, Martin GM, Terrier JC, et al. Effects of massage on the circulation in normal and paralyzed extremities. Arch Phys Med 1949;30:135–144.

Watson S, Watson S. The effects of massage: an holistic approach to care. Nurs Stand 1997;11(47):45–47.

Wilkinson S, Aldridge J, Salmon I, Cain E, Wilson B. An evaluation of aromatherapy massage in palliative care. Palliat Med. 1999;13(5):409–417.

Williams PE, Goldspink G. Changes in sarcomere length and physiological properties of immobilised muscle. J Anat 1978;127:459–468.

Yunus MB. Fibromyalgia syndrome and myofascial pain syndrome: clinical features, laboratory tests, diagnosis, and pathophysiologic mechanisms. In: Rachlin ES, ed. Myofascial pain and fibromyalgia. St. Louis: Mosby Year Book, 1994:3–29.

Yunus MB, Kalyan-Raman UP, Kalyan-Raman K. Primary fibromyalgia syndrome and myofascial pain syndrome: clinical features and muscle pathology. Arch Phys Med Rehab 1988;69:451–454.

Yunus MB, Masi AT, Aldag JC. A controlled study of primary fibromyalgia syndrome: clinical features and association with other functional syndromes. J Rheumatol 1989;16(suppl 19):62–71.

Zalessky M. [Coaching, medico-biological and psychological means of restoration]. Legkaya Atletika (Russian) 1979;2: 20–22.

Zalessky M. [Restoration for middle, long-distance, steeplechase and marathon runners and speed walkers]. Legkaya Atletika (Russian) 1980;3:10–13.

Zeitlin D, Keller SE, Shiflett SC, Schleifer SJ, Bartlett JA. Immunological effects of massage therapy during academic stress. Psychosom Med 2000;62(1):83–84.

8

Connective Tissue Techniques

*C*onnective tissue techniques are those massage techniques that palpate, lengthen, and promote remodeling of connective tissue. These techniques include skin rolling, myofascial release, direct fascial technique, and friction. This chapter describes each of these techniques, how to perform the technique, and how to apply it in a practice sequence. It also includes a discussion of the indications, contraindications, cautions, outcomes, and postintervention care associated with each technique.

Summary of Impairment-Level Outcome of Care for Connective Tissue Techniques

Impairment-Level Outcome of Care	*Technique*			
	Skin Rolling	*Myofascial Release*	*Direct Fascial Technique*	*Friction*
Decreased resting muscle tension or neuromuscular tone	–	P	P	–
Separation/lengthening of fascia	P	✓	P	P
Promotion of dense connective tissue remodeling	–	P	P	P
Increased muscle extensibility	–	✓	P	P
Increased joint range of motion	P	✓	✓	✓
Systemic sedation/decreased anxiety	–	P	✓	–
Increased rib cage mobility	–	P	P	–
Decreased TrP activity	–	P	P	–
Pain reduction	P	✓	✓	✓
Normalized structural alignment	–	P	✓	–
Balance of agonist/antagonist function	–	P	✓	–
Improved quality and quantity of movement	–	P	✓	–
Enhanced muscle performance	–	P	✓	–

✓, the outcome is supported by research summarized in this chapter; P, the outcome is probable; –, nonexistent, negligible, or improbable effects.

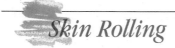

Skin Rolling

OTHER NAMES USED FOR THIS TECHNIQUE

"Rolling," "tissue rolling."[1–3]

DEFINITION

Skin rolling: A gliding stroke in which tissue superficial to the investing layer of deep fascia is grasped, continuously lifted, and rolled over underlying tissues in a wavelike motion.[1–3]

NOTES

1. This unusual technique is often classified as a form of petrissage because it grasps and lifts the tissues (see Chapter 7, Neuromuscular Techniques). Skin rolling is, however, fundamentally different from petrissage in that it is not applied to muscle, but rather to the more superficial subcutaneous tissues.[1–8] The resistance to stretch that can be palpated during the application of this technique is due to tightness in the skin and superficial fascia, which may in turn be related to underlying tension in deep fascia and muscle. When skin rolling is applied slowly, it produces a viscoelastic stretch of the superficial fascia that results in clinical effects and a feel on palpation that is similar to that of other connective tissue techniques described below in this chapter (see Box 8-4).

2. "Subcutaneous tissue rolling" would be a more accurate name for this technique; however, the term skin rolling is used consistently in the literature.[1,2,4–10]

CLINICAL INDICATIONS AND IMPAIRMENT-LEVEL OUTCOMES OF CARE

Skin rolling is a useful technique for both client examination and treatment. The clinician can use skin rolling to assess restrictions in the mobility of the client's skin and superficial fascia that may be the chronic-stage sequelae of burns, wounds, surgery, and orthopedic injuries.[3,4,9] In addition, eliciting complaints of pain or palpating tissue resistance during the application of skin rolling may indicate an underlying chronic elevation of muscle tension, segmental vertebral dysfunction, or organic pathology.[9–11]

As a treatment technique, the clinician can use repetitive applications of skin rolling to improve the mobility of skin and subcutaneous connective tissues and thus increase joint range of motion.[1–9,12] When the clinician applies skin rolling slowly and with a greater force, the anatomical continuity of fascial layers may result in the mechanical lengthening effects of this technique penetrating to deeper fascial layers. Finally, a common (side) effect of skin rolling is the production of a significant reactive hyperemia.[12]

CAUTIONS AND CONTRAINDICATIONS

Clinical training and supervised practice are critical for the proper application of skin rolling. Advanced training may be advisable in certain situations, particularly when dealing with pathological conditions. All of the general and local contraindications noted for massage techniques apply to the use of skin rolling (see Chapter 2, The Clinical Decision-Making Process).[4,5,7,13] As for all of the connective tissue techniques, there are several absolute contraindications to the local application of skin rolling: acute hyperemia or inflammation of the client's tissues, hypermobile or unstable joints, or skin that is fragile because of age or drug use.[4] The clinician may apply skin rolling with reduced force if the client's tissues are in the subacute (fibroblastic) phase of the inflammatory response, provided that any swelling has resolved and the client can tolerate treatment. The technique should be used with caution in the presence of systemic connective tissue disorders. In addition, in the osteopathic tradition, the presence of persistently or recurrently immobile skin overlying a particular spinal segment is thought to indicate underlying functional/organic imbalance or pathology in the viscera supplied by that segment.[9,12] In areas of fascial binding, this technique can be painful and must be applied with due regard for the client's pain tolerance.

Prerequisite Skills for Skin Rolling

Before applying skin rolling, students should be able to

Assess variations in skin elasticity and resistance to drag

Use standing and seated aligned postures

Palpate the thickness of superficial fat and fascia

Locate the investing layer of deep fascia

Describe how skin attaches to underlying fascia and the variations in skin–fascial connections that normally occur throughout the body

---

Manual Technique begins on page 240

MANUAL TECHNIQUE

Skin Rolling

In the following figures (Figs. 8-1 to 8-6), skin rolling is applied to the various regions of the body. Figures are ordered from head to foot in supine and then prone. Each figure illustrates most of the guidelines for manual technique outlined below.

1. No oil is required. The clinician removes all previously applied oil from the client's skin. The technique can be reasonably well applied through fabric.

2. The hands grasp the client's skin, superficial fascia, and associated fat between the thumb(s) and fingertip(s). They then lift these tissues in a direction that is perpendicular to the surface of the client's skin.

3. The clinician uses as broad a contact surface as possible, except with small body segments (Fig. 8-1), to minimize the likelihood of the client experiencing a pinching sensation. The contact surface includes all the distal phalanges and the entire heel of the hand for areas where the client's skin is looser or where there is more fat (Fig. 8-5).

4. The hands simultaneously maintain the stretch on the client's tissues and roll the superficial tissues along the surface in a slow wave. There are two concurrent stretching forces: one perpendicular to the skin and the other parallel to the skin. A gliding motion occurs as the clinician simultaneously gathers and releases the client's tissues while maintaining the grasping and lifting motion. This gliding motion can be maintained until the tissue is rolled away from the clinician. The hands do not release the roll of the client's tissues until the end of the stroke.

5. Two-handed or single-handed skin rolling are both possible; however, skin rolling is easier to perform two-handed, with the hands positioned close together and working in concert.

6. Skin rolling can be performed in a variety of different directions. Since skin attaches to superficial fascia differently in the various parts of the body, it may be consistently easier to perform skin rolling in a particular direction in a given region (Figs. 8-3, 8-4, and 8-6).

7. In an intervention, the clinician performs skin rolling over an entire region once, then returns to adherent or sensitive spots for additional passes, performing the technique in different directions, until the client's subcutaneous tissues lift easily and any reported sensitivity has decreased.

8. When applied at a slow rate (<1 cm/sec) and with moderate lifting force, skin rolling can produce a "creep" of the client's superficial fascia—an effect that can affect the underlying investing layer of the deep fascia.

9. Even with the broadest hand contact, the force of skin rolling is delivered to a relatively small area, and clients may not be able to tolerate this technique. If clients are very sensitive to the pressure of skin rolling, the clinician can use either a superficial myofascial release across the client's skin or a direct fascial technique applied with a light pressure and a broad contact surface to obtain similar results.

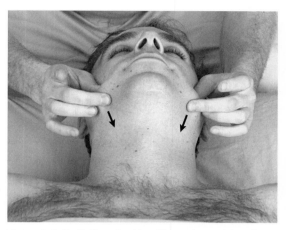

Figure 8-1. Gentle fingertip skin rolling makes an interesting beginning or ending to a complete face massage.

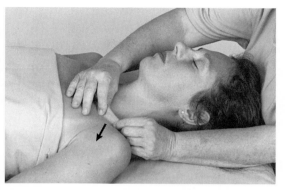

Figure 8-2. Skin rolling over the clavicle and anterior neck engages the superficial fascia with its embedded platysma muscle.

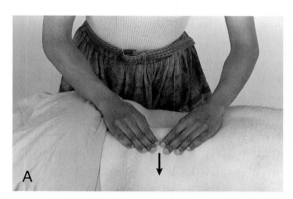

A

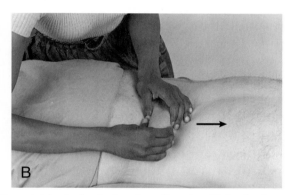

B

Figure 8-3. **A, B.** Tissue response in the lower back is affected by the underlying lumbar fascia and usually varies with the direction of the strokes.

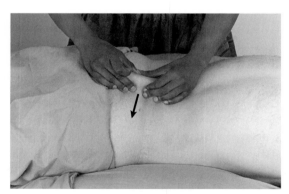

Figure 8-4. Skin and superficial fascia in the region of the sacrum lie over dense fascial attachments and lift less easily.

Manual Technique Figures continue on next page

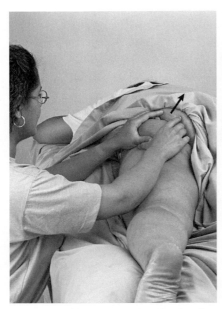

Figure 8-5. In fatty areas, such as the gluteals, a heel-and-fingers contact will include more tissue.

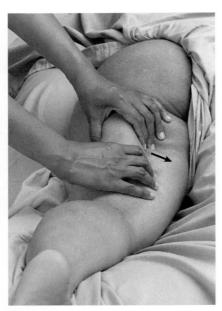

Figure 8-6. It is usually easier to perform skin rolling around, rather than along, the limbs.

Components of Skin Rolling

Contact: Distal phalanges of finger(s) plus the thumb, thenar eminence, or heel of the hand

Pressure: Sufficient to allow lifting of the superficial tissues

Tissues engaged: Skin, superficial fascia, fat; indirectly engages deeper layers of fascia

Amplitude/length: Variable, at the discretion of the clinician

Rate: Slow, less than 1 to 4 cm/sec

Duration: 30 sec or longer

Intergrades with:[a] Direct fascial technique, petrissage

Context: Apply alone to mobilize surface connective tissue restrictions, such as scars; apply before and after direct fascial technique or myofascial release to evaluate tissue mobility

---

[a]To merge gradually one into another.

CLINICIAN'S POSITION AND MOVEMENT

1. The basic positions used by the clinician are described in Chapter 4, Preparation and Positioning for Treatment, in the sections on upright standing or upright sitting positions.
2. Since the force of skin rolling is produced entirely by the hands, any comfortable upright standing or upright sitting position can be used.
3. Use of a sitting position will reduce hyperextension of the wrists if the clinician is grasping the client's tissues between the fingers and the heels of the hands (Fig. 8-5).

PALPATE

As he performs the technique, the clinician palpates the client's skin and tissues for the following:

1. Temperature and texture of the skin
2. Texture and thickness of superficial fat; lipomas and fibrositic deposits are common on the back and around the pelvic girdle.
3. Tightness of the superficial fascia, which is palpated as a resistance to stretching the client's tissues perpendicular to the skin surface, resistance to stretching the tissues parallel to the skin surface, or resistance to ease of rolling the tissues during the stroke
4. Viscoelastic stretch of the tissues; if the clinician performs skin rolling slowly, it may be possible for him to palpate a slow viscoelastic stretch or creep of the client's superficial tissues.

OBSERVE

As he performs the technique, the clinician observes the client for the signs listed below.

1. General appearance of skin, specifically circulatory or trophic changes
2. Visible chronic tension in muscles, which can be associated with tightness of the overlying superficial fascia

3. Reactive hyperemia; skin rolling often quickly produces a reactive hyperemia that can last for minutes

COMMUNICATION WITH THE CLIENT

The clinician uses communication to solicit feedback on the client's level of comfort and concerns about the effects of the technique. Some examples of statements that the clinician can use are listed below.

1. "Let me know if you feel a burning sensation as I roll your skin." Initially, skin rolling produces an unpleasant "burning" sensation as the client's tight superficial fascia is stretched. This sensation cannot be completely avoided; therefore, the clinician should moderate the degree of lift he uses in response to the client's feedback or change to a broader connective tissue technique.
2. Reassure the client that skin rolling will neither produce stretch marks nor temporarily or permanently slacken healthy skin in any visible way.
3. No massage techniques—including skin rolling—have been shown to reduce "cellulite."

OTHER APPROPRIATE TECHNIQUES

There are several modalities that the clinician can use in a complementary manner when using skin rolling. In particular, myofascial release or direct fascial technique applied with a light force can be used to achieve similar effects.

POSTINTERVENTION SELF-CARE

1. The clinician can teach the client how to perform self-administered skin rolling in accessible areas.
2. The client can use muscle stretches that specifically target the area being treated. These stretch positions are to be sustained for 30 sec or longer to assist in mobilizing restrictions in the superficial fascia.

A Practice Sequence for Skin Rolling

Practice time: 30 min per person

Prone: Undrape half of the client's posterior torso, from the shoulder down to the gluteal fold. Ensure that spinous processes are accessible.

1. Beginning at the shoulder: Lift the client's skin and as much of the subcutaneous fat as possible and roll the tissue down the back and buttock in one long uninterrupted movement (if possible).

2. Return to the shoulder: Move laterally or medially, and make successive passes in the same direction until all of the exposed area has been treated. During application, mentally note where tissue restrictions occur.

3. Cover the same area with similar long parallel strokes, this time working in a superior direction. Again, mentally note where tissue restrictions occur.

4. Cover the same area with shorter parallel strokes, this time working from medial to lateral and then lateral to medial. Note the difference in the response of the tissue.

5. Return to the areas that appeared to exhibit greater restriction. Apply the technique repeatedly in a variety of directions. Reassess the quality of the tissue restrictions. You may wish to have the client stand, actively move, and compare the two sides of the body.

Perform a comparable sequence on the other side of the client's body.

At the end, investigate how skin rolling can be applied to other areas of the body, such as the scalp, hands, feet, and around joints.

Home study: Devise and apply comparable routines for other regions.

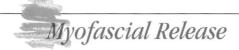

Myofascial Release

OTHER NAMES USED FOR THIS TECHNIQUE

"Myofascial stretching."[14]

DEFINITION

Myofascial release: A technique that combines a nongliding fascial traction with varying amounts of orthopedic stretch to produce a moderate, sustained tensional force on the muscle and its associated fascia, which results in palpable viscoelastic lengthening (creep) and plastic deformation of the fascia.[1,3,14–15]

NOTES

1. Myofascial release is sometimes used as part of a wider system of treatment—known by the same name—which may incorporate a variety of craniosacral, osteopathic, and other soft-tissue techniques.[14,15]

2. Some authors[11] describe both "direct" and "indirect" applications of myofascial release. "Direct" here means that the force of the technique is directed toward, and then through, the primary tissue restriction; in other words, the motion is applied through and beyond the restrictive fascial barrier. This is in contrast to indirect techniques in which the force is applied, or the client moved, away from the fascial barrier or restriction of motion.[11,39] Indirect applications of myofascial release are not covered in this book.

CLINICAL INDICATIONS AND IMPAIRMENT-LEVEL OUTCOMES OF CARE

Myofascial release is indicated to lengthen fascial layers, to restore mobility between fascial layers, and to decrease the effects of adhesions on the locomotor system. Myofascial release is therefore indicated in a wide variety of conditions in which chronic fascial shortening results in limited joint range and ease of movement, such as postural conditions (kyphosis, lordosis, scoliosis, elevated shoulders, and anterior head posture), chronic aftereffects of trauma, chronic fascial compartment syndromes, and neurological or circulatory compression syndromes, such as thoracic outlet syndrome.[15–23] In these situations, myofascial release contributes to normalized structural alignment, balance of agonist/antagonist muscle function, improved quality and quantity of movement between and across body segments, and pain reduction through primary treatment of dysfunction.[11,14,15] This technique may also assist in resolving chronic trigger point (TrP) syndromes, in counteracting the effects of prolonged stress, and in facilitating athletic performance through enhanced muscle performance secondary to the increase of extensibility.

CAUTIONS AND CONTRAINDICATIONS

Clinical training and supervised practice are critical for the proper application of myofascial release. Advanced training may be advisable in certain situations, particularly when dealing with pathological conditions. All of the general and local contraindications noted for massage techniques apply to the use of myofascial release (see Chapter 2, The Clinical Decision-Making Process).[4,5,7,13] As for all of the connective tissue techniques, there are several cautions and contraindications to the use of myofascial release; these include malignancy, cellulitis, fever, systemic or local infection, acute circulatory conditions, osteomyelitis, aneurysm, obstructive edema, acute rheumatoid arthritis, open wounds, sutures, hematomas, healing fractures, osteoporosis, anticoagulant therapy, advanced diabetes, and hypersensitivity of the skin.[15] In addition, the clinician should use extreme caution when performing myofascial release in the area of flaccid paralysis, lax or unstable

---

Prerequisite Skills for Myofascial Release

Before applying myofascial release, students should be able to

- Assess the mobility of superficial fascia and the investing layer of deep fascia
- Assess standing alignment and gait for postural and structural imbalances
- Assess the length of myofascial units
- Apply body weight efficiently for extended periods using standing and seated aligned postures
- Describe the orientation of skeletal muscle fibers
- Describe the relationship between muscle and its associated fascia
- Describe and palpate major fascial structures and sheathes that are directly associated with skeletal muscle

---

How Connective Tissue Responds to Tensile Stress

There is extensive research on the behavior of dense connective tissue in response to mechanical loads.[24–32] Some relevant concepts are

Tension/tensile force: Any force that is so oriented that its effect is to lengthen a structure.

Elastic: Behaving like a spring. Elastic stretch is recoverable in the sense that the length that is gained during the stretch will disappear once the tensile force is released.

Plastic: Behaving like putty. Plastic stretch is nonrecoverable in the sense that the length that is gained during the stretch will remain once the tensile force is released.

Viscoelastic: Showing both plastic and elastic behavior. Viscoelastic stretch is partially recoverable in the sense that some of the length that is gained during the stretch will remain once the tensile force is released.

"Creep" (viscoelastic "creep"): Gradual lengthening of connective tissue that occurs with sustained tensile force and that corresponds to the viscous or plastic behavior of dense connective tissue. Creep can be palpated during manipulations that place connective tissue under sustained tension.

The elastic and plastic response of connective tissue to tensile forces can vary with the rate and duration of the force that is applied. The best way to permanently lengthen connective tissue structures, without compromising their structural integrity, is to apply prolonged low-intensity forces.

---

joints, or diseased joints that are supported by fascial "splinting." In addition, myofascial release should be used with caution and only in the nonacute stages of systemic connective tissue disorders.

The clinician needs to appreciate the broader impact of myofascial release on the client's system as a whole. Although the force with which the clinician performs myofascial release is not particularly great, significant changes in the client's myofascial balance can occur quickly. Since the client's interwoven fascial system demonstrates "whole-system" behavior,[15,33,34] the mechanical effects of myofascial release are not just local or even always predominantly local. Furthermore, this technique can produce strong autonomic effects, reflex effects, and somatoemotional release, particularly when it is used for long periods.[14] This necessitates a conservative approach and careful observation and communication with the client.

In light of the effects of myofascial release, the clinician should ensure that he is able to accurately perform a basic visual postural analysis before he begins to apply myofascial release during an intervention.[33,34] Furthermore, clinicians learning to perform myofascial release techniques should initially limit their applications of this technique to less than 10 min in any given session and periodically conduct at least a visual reassessment. Care must be taken to ensure that the client looks and feels "balanced" at the end of a session, especially if there has been unilateral work around the legs or pelvis. The clinician must strive to maintain balanced function of the client's agonist, antagonist, and synergist muscle groups and to use a rigorous analysis of possible treatment effects.

Manual Technique begins on next page

MANUAL TECHNIQUE[14,15]

Myofascial Release

In the following figures (Figs. 8-7 to 8-14), myofascial release is applied to the various regions of the body. Figures are ordered from head to foot in supine and then prone. Each figure illustrates most of the guidelines for manual technique outlined below. *Arrows* indicate the direction of the applied force. No glide occurs between the clinician's hands and the client's skin.

1. The tissues to be treated (e.g., a muscle, part of a muscle, a myotatic unit, or an entire limb) are placed in a position of stretch that is just short of tautness or at the point of tautness.

2. The chosen contact surfaces are placed at opposite ends of the target tissues that are to be stretched (Figs. 8-7, 8-9, and 8-14). Contact surfaces commonly chosen by the clinician are the entire palmar surface of the hand, the heel of the hand, or the forearm. The clinician compresses the client's tissues enough to engage the investing layer of deep fascia (or deeper), and then exerts a light-to-moderate horizontal drag or traction force in opposite directions. This motion stretches the tissues between the hands in a direction parallel to the line of the muscle fibers. The contact surfaces should not glide over the client's skin.

   If one end of the target tissues is stabilized by the weight of the body, then the clinician may execute the stretch with both hands positioned at the other end, e.g., Figures 8-8, 8-11, 8-12.

3. The clinician sustains the horizontal drag or stretching force at a constant level as the client's tissues begins to lengthen slowly. If no palpable or visible stretch is observed after 90 sec, the clinician should ask the client to consciously "breathe into" the area being stretched or to cough.[15] The clinician may also adjust the angle of stretch slightly, lighten the pressure, or change the target tissue entirely to produce an effective release.

4. The clinician takes up the slack as the client's tissues lengthen. For example, if the hands have been placed at opposite ends of a muscle, they spread apart very slowly without gliding over the skin (Figs. 8-7, 8-9, 8-10, 8-13A and B, and 8-14). Both hands will stretch away from the point of proximal stabilization when one end of the stretch is stabilized by the client's body weight (Figs. 8-8, 8-11, and 8-12). One author suggests that a minimum of 90 sec is necessary for a myofascial release and advises clinicians to hold initial releases for 3 to 5 min so that lengthening can proceed through a succession of fascial barriers.[15]

5. For interventions of shorter duration, crossed-hand positions permit more comfortable leverage, especially with large muscles (Figs. 8-9, 8-10, and 8-13A and B). However, when used for a prolonged time these may be stressful on the clinician's wrists.

6. The clinician can exert variable amounts of compression into the client's tissues prior to initiating the lengthening traction; however, it is advisable to begin with a light compression to ensure contact with the investing layer of the deep fascia that overlies the superficial layer of muscle. This is necessary because hand contact that initially appears to engage only superficial tissue layers may affect deeper fascial layers once the hands sustain the horizontal traction force and the myofascial release occurs. It is not primarily the amount of force applied but also the duration of the sustained application of force that results in a stretch of connective tissue (see Box 8-4). In addition, the use of greater force is more likely to result in the client experiencing pain, guarding, and apprehension. Consequently, the clinician should not use more than moderate force.

Manual Technique continues on page 248

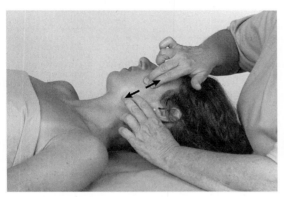

Figure 8-7. Fingertip contact is used to stretch small muscles, such as the masseter.

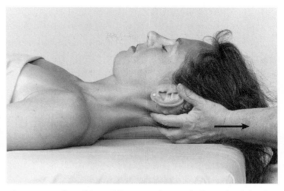

Figure 8-8. Stretching of the posterior cervical myofascial units in supine.

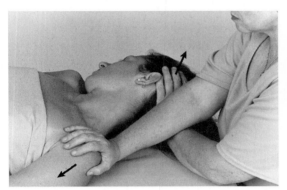

Figure 8-9. Unilateral stretching of upper trapezius from a superior position using crossed hands.

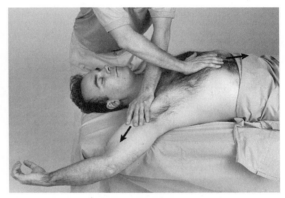

Figure 8-10. Crossed-hand stretching of the lower fibers of the pectoralis major.

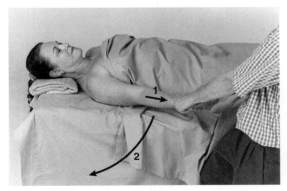

Figure 8-11. Sustained traction can be performed with the client's arm (or leg) in almost any position. The clinician maintains traction and moves the client's arm slowly and progressively into full abduction. This maneuver can be done with the humerus positioned in varying degrees of internal or external rotation.

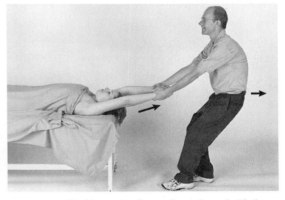

Figure 8-12. Double-arm traction can be performed with the client in prone or supine. Starting from this basic position, the clinician can use small shifts in position to direct the lengthening force to virtually any long muscle group in the upper body. A second clinician can simultaneously provide double-leg traction and thus further expand the effects of the technique.

Manual Technique Figures continue on page 249

7. The clinician can sustain the force of the stretch for 3 to 5 min or longer while the client's tissues move and release through a series of fascial barriers. Alternatively, the clinician can maintain the stretch for a shorter period, then reposition the client's body segment in a position of greater stretch and repeat the procedure until the client's muscle and associated tissues are adequately elongated. With the latter approach, the compressive force may be altered on successive stretches to engage different layers of muscle and fascia, and the angle of stretch adjusted so that the lengthening force is applied to different muscle fibers.

8. Apply and release pressure gradually.

Components for Myofascial Release

Contact: All or part of both hands are used

Pressure: Light to moderate

Tissues engaged: Fascia; although associated muscle is also engaged, the fascial response is the primary focus of palpation

Direction: Typically, the force of application is oriented in a direction that is parallel to the long axis of muscles and the muscle fibers; the resulting stretch will occur in the same direction

Amplitude/length: Length increase for a sustained stretch in a long myofascial unit may approach 3 cm

Rate: Rate of creep is very slow and is determined by the region, amount, and health of tissues under stretch

Duration: 90 sec to 5 min or longer

Intergrades with: Static contact, direct fascial technique, and conventional orthopedic stretching

Combined with: May be combined with specific compression to treat trigger points

Context: Commonly applied alone or alternated with direct fascial technique; broad myofascial releases can be used to precede or follow more-specific muscular or connective tissue techniques

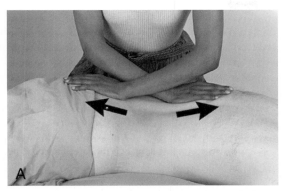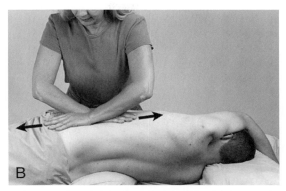

Figure 8-13. **A.** Unilateral crossed-hand stretching of the lumbar region in prone. Extended gentle application of the technique can be required to address the barriers within the dense, many-layered lumbosacral fascia. Hands can also be positioned centrally and oriented across the body to cover the paraspinal musculature on both sides of the client's spine and produce a bilateral stretch. **B.** Unilateral crossed-hand stretching of the lumbar region in sidelying. The clinician may facilitate a stretch of the quadratus lumborum by positioning the client's arm over his head and placing a pillow under his opposite side.

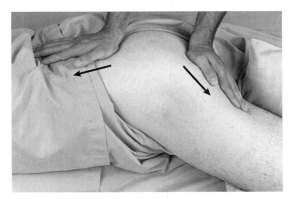

Figure 8-14. Myofascial release of the gluteus maximus.

CLINICIAN'S POSITION AND MOVEMENT

1. The basic positions used by the clinician are described in Chapter 4, Preparation and Positioning for Treatment, in the sections on standing aligned, seated aligned, and other postures.

2. The clinician selects a posture that is both efficient and comfortable, as the position may need to be sustained for several minutes. By using forearm or hand and forearm contacts, the clinician can improve body mechanics and avoid prolonged stress to the wrists.

3. The ergonomic load on the clinician's body can be altered by using small shifts in foot position and center of gravity as the release progresses.

4. Whole-limb and full-body releases can be performed with the assistance of a second (or even a third) clinician.[14]

5. The clinician uses diaphragmatic breathing when the technique requires sustaining a position for a long period with relatively little body movement.

PALPATE

As he performs the technique, the clinician palpates the client's tissues for the following:

1. Viscoelastic stretch or creep of the tissues. This is relatively easy to palpate during correct performance of myofascial release because the clinician's hand is not moving on the client's skin. Once the clinician achieves the stretch position and carries the initial elastic stretch of the tissues to its end point, gradual separation of the hands will reflect creep. Creep has a slow, soft, "hydraulic" feel (like pulling taffy or putty), which may be due in part to the constrained movement of fluid out of the extracellular matrix under the pressure exerted by the release.

2. Location of layers of fascia. The clinician attempts to engage the same fascial layer with both hands, so that the hands "communicate," and each hand senses small changes in the amount and direction of the force being exerted by the other, as though they were pulling on opposite ends of a connected sheet. The ability to isolate and palpate layers of fascia is a skill that requires practice.

3. Rhythm and motion of the stretch. Successful application of myofascial release depends on the clinician noting the inherent rhythm and motion of each stretch as it progresses. Closing the eyes can help to focus attention on the hands and the results

of palpation; this is especially useful when learning the technique.

4. Cranial rhythm. Small, palpable shifts in the orientation of the stretch force that seem to occur on their own may reflect the client's cranial rhythm or the untwisting of asymmetrically shortened fascial sheaths. In its simplest form, myofascial release can be performed without reference to the cranial rhythm. Clinicians who wish to refine the technique of attending to the cranial rhythm during myofascial release are referred to the work of Upledger.[35] Even at earlier stages of learning to perform myofascial releases, however, the clinician should endeavour to palpate the small, three-dimensional movements that can accompany the developing release.

OBSERVE

As he performs the technique, the clinician observes the client for changes in muscle tension and tissue lengthening. The signs listed below may signal this.

1. Local lengthening. During the release, the clinician can observe small amounts (millimeters to 1 or 2 cm) of local tissue lengthening, depending on the size of the area under stretch.

2. Lowered muscle resting tension. After the clinician releases the force of the stretch, local tissue contours may soften and flatten, reflecting lowered muscle resting tension.

3. Thixotrophic rehydration. The thixotropic rehydration of the ground substance of tissues may contribute to a further softening of local tissue contours after the force of the stretch is released.

4. Changes in other body segments. Lengthening and positional shifts may appear in proximal, distal, or adjacent segments during the application of myofascial release. The clinician must cultivate the habit of continually evaluating adjacent body segments for changes with the client on and off the table.

5. Structural alignment. Changes in structural relationships of the client's body segments are best assessed by inspection of standing static alignment and gait, both during and at the end of the session.

COMMUNICATION WITH THE CLIENT

The clinician uses communication that may encourage general relaxation and facilitate tissue lengthening. Some examples of statements that the clinician can use are listed below.

1. "Deepen your breathing without forcing it in any way." Conscious deep diaphragmatic breathing facilitates release, while lack of it impedes release. Occasionally, coughing can also facilitate release.
2. "Close your eyes and let your awareness move to . . ." The clinician asks the client to close the eyes to focus better on the sensation of tissue lengthening.
3. "Let me know if you begin to feel uncomfortable." Both the pressure and the sensation of lengthening usually feel pleasant and at all times should be tolerable.
4. The clinician asks the client to compare areas that have been treated with those that haven't (for example, comparing the left side with the right side). Clients may find changes more apparent when they are sitting or walking. Clinicians may find that providing clients with sufficient time for them to observe and report the ongoing effects of the technique is an indispensable teaching tool, particularly in the case of clients whose poor habits of muscular use contribute to their dysfunction.
5. "Does anything feel out of place?" "Do your left and right sides match?" "Can you describe the difference between the left and the right sides of your body?" The clinician must ensure that the client feels balanced at the end of a session.
6. "It's normal to feel uncoordinated for a day or so after the treatment." Clients are often aware of altered proprioception and biomechanics for a day or two after undergoing a substantial release. While these changes are not painful, the client may find them uncomfortable. Consequently, the clinician should advise clients that this discomfort may occur and that it can be reduced by simple daily activities, such as walking.
7. "Please phone if you experience anything unusual after the treatment, especially if you have persistent pain." When a significant shift in agonist/ antagonist balance occurs, the client may experience transient muscle soreness in areas other than those that were treated. This occurs because of an increased loading of antagonists, synergists, or other muscles in the kinetic chain. The clinician should, therefore, advise the client to report any postintervention soreness that is more than mild or that lasts longer than 2 days.

OTHER APPROPRIATE TECHNIQUES

There are several modalities that the clinician can use in a complementary manner with myofascial release.

1. In controlled laboratory conditions the precise heating of tissue facilitates a greater elongation of collagenous structures without resulting in structural damage.[29,32,36] In clinical practice, however, the application of heat prior to any sustained loading of connective tissue can increase the risk of collagenous rupture. Consequently, the clinician should avoid the application of either heat or cold before performing connective tissue techniques, unless his aim is specifically to rupture or denature collagen.[36] Heat applied after the use of myofascial release can enhance the temporary increase in the pliability of myofascial tissue.
2. Myofascial release can be applied with specific reference to the craniosacral rhythm and be integrated with craniosacral technique and direct fascial technique.[1,14,15]
3. Also of benefit are neuromuscular or muscle energy techniques, joint mobilization and manipulation, and spinal traction performed from the head or pelvis.[15]
4. Chronic conditions may require correction for bony asymmetry.
5. When the client experiences significant shifts in posture, postural awareness training, neuromuscular education, and movement awareness training may be of benefit.[8] Systems of comprehensive postural awareness and movement training, such as the Alexander technique,[37] may be used in these situations. Ergonomic retraining related to the client's work environment may be required.
6. Stretching.
7. Strengthening.
8. Electrotherapeutic modalities such as biofeedback, electrical muscle stimulation, and transcutaneous electrical nerve stimulation (TENS).[8]

POSTINTERVENTION SELF-CARE

1. The clinician can teach the client how to perform precise self-stretching exercises using moderate force and a longer-than-typical duration.
2. The client can perform postural, movement awareness, and strengthening exercises as required.

A Practice Sequence for Myofascial Release

Practice time: 40 min per person

The following sequence for the more superficial lumbar and pelvic muscles can be extended by allowing each stretch to develop for longer than a minute and by pausing more often to take up the slack in the tissues. It is advisable to allocate a comparable amount of time for each of the stretches (90 or more), so that a balanced intervention results. Before practice, review the fiber directions for the myofascial units to be treated, and review static alignment and gait.

Before initiating the intervention, scan the client for static alignment and gait. In particular, pay attention to the relationship between the client's lumbar vertebrae and pelvis.

1. Begin with the client in prone over an abdominal pillow. Apply several crossed-hand stretches across the lumbar portion of the latissimus dorsi.
2. Turn the client to sidelying. Stretch the ipsilateral leg and open the space between the 12th rib and the iliac crest (the lateral fascial portion of the obliques).
3. With the client's leg in the same position, apply myofascial releases between origins and insertions of gluteus medius and minimus.
4. Have the client draw the legs up into a semifetal position. In this position, lengthen the lower portion of the erector spinae and then the gluteus maximus.
5. Turn the client to the other side, and repeat steps 2, 3, and 4.
6. Turn the client to supine. Apply myofascial releases to the tensor fascia lata and rectus femoris on both sides. Allow the leg to hang over the side of the table if necessary.
7. Apply a conventional psoas stretch to both sides.
8. To finish, apply gentle sustained traction to each leg. Then apply a gentle sustained spinal traction from the neck and then from the sacrum.

Direct Fascial Technique

OTHER NAMES USED FOR THIS TECHNIQUE

"Connective tissue technique," "connective tissue massage," "myofascial massage," "deep tissue massage," "deep stroking," "strumming," "ironing," "myofascial manipulation," "soft-tissue mobilization."[1,3–6,8,15,38]

DEFINITION

Direct fascial technique: A slow, gliding technique that applies a moderate, sustained tensional force to the superficial fascia or to the deep fascia and associated muscle. It results in viscoelastic lengthening (creep) and plastic deformation of the fascia.[1,3–6,15,38]

NOTES

1. *Direct* used in relation to fascial technique means that the force of the technique is directed toward, and then through, the tissue restriction; in other words, the motion is applied through and beyond the restrictive fascial barrier. This is in contrast to indirect techniques, such as counterstrain or positional release, in which the force is applied, or the client moved, away from the fascial barrier or restriction of motion.[11,39] Indirect techniques are not covered in this book.

2. Direct fascial technique is one of the most influential massage innovations of this century, popularized initially through the work of Ida Rolf in the United States and Elizabeth Dicke in Germany, who developed and elaborated on the technique for two distinctly different purposes.[34,40,41] Practitioners of the various Structural Integration schools, who seek to comprehensively realign client's bodies and reeducate them in the use of their bodies, apply direct fascial techniques to superficial and deep fascial layers and throughout the musculature within the framework of a 10-session series. These schools include Rolfing® and its various descendants: Hellerwork℠, Soma Neuromuscular Integration™, Neuromuscular Integration and Structural Alignment (NISA), The Guild for Structural Integration, and Postural Integration.[4,6,34,42] In Dicke's Bindegewebsmassage (Connective Tissue Massage [CTM]), direct fascial technique is applied in precise sequences to the skin and superficial fascial layers to elicit specific physiological reflex effects.[1,40] The CTM system also uses skin rolling and short strokes, which do not glide but nonetheless exert specific subdermal traction to fascia.[1] This system has a much larger following in Europe than in North America.

3. At a glance, direct fascial technique sometimes resembles modern neuromuscular techniques, such as stripping, that engage muscle while producing a sustained unidirectional drag in one plane (see previous chapter). When applied over the muscle belly, direct fascial technique may achieve some of the effects of neuromuscular techniques. It differs substantially from neuromuscular techniques, however, in terms of the focus during palpation, location of application, intention, and effect on connective tissue.

CLINICAL INDICATIONS AND IMPAIRMENT-LEVEL OUTCOMES OF CARE

Direct fascial technique has general clinical effects that are similar to those of myofascial release, that is, lengthening and restoring mobility between fascial layers. Additionally, direct fascial technique can be used within comprehensive systems of treatment, such as Structural Integration or CTM, to address different outcomes. Like myofascial release, direct fascial technique can be used in the treatment of conditions in which chronic fascial shortening results in limited joint range and ease of movement, such as postural conditions (kyphosis, lordosis, scoliosis, elevated shoulders, and anterior head posture), chronic aftereffects of trauma, chronic fascial compartment syndromes, neurological or circulatory compression syndromes such as thoracic outlet syndrome, chronic low back dysfunction, and mild spasticity.[15,34,40–44] In these situations, direct fascial technique contributes to normalized structural alignment, balance of agonist/antagonist muscle function, improved quality and quantity of movement between and across body segments, and improved energy consumption.[41,42,44–46] These effects and enhanced muscle performance secondary to the increased muscle extensibility may make the technique useful for athletic performance. Direct fascial technique has complex direct and indirect effects on pain through endorphin-mediated analgesia, the restoration of mobility, and the reduction of anxiety.[46–56] The technique also often results in a local reactive hyperemia and may indirectly affect local circulation.[1,40]

Within the context of Structural Integration regimens, direct fascial technique has other clinical effects. First, it appears to produce an increase in parasympathetic tone,[46,47] and when applied during a series of sessions, it can result in a lasting reduction in anxiety states.[48–50] Studies on the use of direct fascial technique in CTM interventions, however, have reported less consistent autonomic effects, although the texts on CTM suggest that it is useful for treating autonomic imbalance.[40,51,52]

When direct fascial technique (or any other massage technique) affects autonomic activity, it can produce generalized indirect visceral effects. CTM, however, takes this notion further to suggest that the clinician can exert a direct regulating effect on a client's organ function via somatovisceral reflexes, by detecting and freeing tightness in somatic connective tissue.[57–64] The scientific basis for this theory is uncertain. The literature states that the skin can develop predictable areas of hypersensitivity (Head's zones) and that muscles and related fascia can exhibit predictable areas of increased tone (MacKenzie's zones) in response to specific visceral pathology.[40,57] Unfortunately, there is a lack of English-language research to support the existence of direct somatovisceral paths of influence on organ function. Since little of the potentially substantiating German and Russian literature has been translated into English, even in abstract form,[65,66] review articles in English-language journals suggest that there is no empirical evidence for the concept of somatovisceral reflexes.[67] Consequently, advocates of CTM have recently acknowledged that the scientific basis for somatovisceral reflexes requires clarification and research.[57,58] Perhaps, clinicians may look forward to receiving greater clarity on the basic notions about the psyche-soma-viscera relationship in the future.

CAUTIONS AND CONTRAINDICATIONS

Clinical training and supervised practice are critical for the proper application of direct fascial technique. Advanced training may be advisable in certain situations, particularly when dealing with pathological conditions. All of the general and local contraindications noted for massage techniques apply to the use of direct fascial technique (see Chapter 2, The Clinical Decision-Making Process).[4,5,7,13] As for all of the connective tissue techniques, there are several cautions and contraindications to the use of direct fascial technique; these include malignancy, cellulitis, fever, systemic or local infection, acute circulatory conditions, osteomyelitis, aneurysm, obstructive edema, acute rheumatoid arthritis, open wounds, sutures, hematomas, healing fractures, osteoporosis, anticoagulant therapy, advanced diabetes, and hypersensitivity of the skin.[15] In addition, the clinician should use extreme caution when performing direct fascial technique in areas of flaccid paralysis, lax or unstable joints, or diseased joints that are supported by fascial "splinting." In addition, direct fascial technique should be used with caution and only in the nonacute stages of systemic connective tissue disorders.

The clinician needs to appreciate the broader impact of direct fascial technique on the client's system as a whole. Although the force with which the clinician performs direct fascial technique is not particularly great, significant changes in the client's myofascial balance can occur very quickly—within one or two strokes. Since the client's interwoven fascial system demonstrates "whole-system" behavior,[15,33,34] the mechanical effects of direct fascial technique are not just local or even always predominantly local. Furthermore, this technique can produce strong autonomic effects, reflex effects, and somatoemotional release, particularly when it is used for long periods in one intervention.[14] This necessitates a conservative approach and careful observation and communication with the client.

In light of the effects of direct fascial technique, the clinician should ensure that he is able to accurately perform a basic visual postural analysis before he begins to apply direct fascial techniques during an intervention.[33,34] Furthermore, clinicians learning to perform direct fascial technique should initially limit their applications of this technique to less than 10 min in any given session and periodically conduct at least a visual reassessment. Care must be taken to maintain communication with the client and to ensure that the client looks and feels balanced at the end of a session, especially if there has been unilateral work around the legs or pelvis. The clinician must strive to maintain balanced function of

the client's agonist, antagonist, and synergist muscle groups and to use a rigorous analysis of possible treatment effects.

Prerequisite Skills for Direct Fascial Technique

Before applying direct fascial technique, students should be able to

Assess the mobility of superficial fascia and the investing layer of deep fascia

Assess standing alignment and gait for postural and structural imbalances

Assess the length of myofascial units

Use lunge and lean, and standing and seated controlled leans to apply body weight efficiently

Describe the anatomical relationship between fascia and muscle

Describe and palpate all major fascial structures including retinacula, fascia around joints, and intermuscular septa

---

Manual Technique begins on page 256

MANUAL TECHNIQUE

Direct Fascial Technique

In the following figures (Figs. 8-15 to 8-23), direct fascial technique is applied to the various regions of the body. Figures are ordered from head to foot in supine and then prone. Each figure illustrates most of the guidelines for manual technique outlined below.

1. Fascia is most accessible for treatment at locations where it is exposed and has the least associated muscle bulk: at joints, on retinacula, and around bony prominences, such as the sacrum and the occipital ridge (Figs. 8-15 to 8-18, 8-22, 8-23). These areas often receive less attention during "classical" massage because they have less muscle bulk, yet they are of the utmost importance when using direct fascial technique. Most systems that use direct fascial technique emphasize the importance of working on the dense lumbosacral fascia at each session, either at the beginning of the session, as in CTM, or the conclusion of the session, as in Structural Integration[40,41,47] (Fig. 8-21, *lower arrow*).

2. No oil is required. The clinician removes all oil previously applied to the client's skin.

3. There are two basic steps to directing the force. First, the hands compress into the client's tissues to engage the most superficial layer of restriction. Then they slowly glide horizontally along the client's skin, while maintaining the same compressive force, to exert traction on a fascial layer. The clinician moves over the client's skin at a rate of approximately 5 to 15 cm/sec, while producing strokes that freely cross joint lines to follow continuous fascial layers (Fig. 8-18).

4. The clinician can produce strokes of any length. At the end of the stroke, the hands break contact and pause for several seconds. There is no return stroke. Shorter strokes may be more tolerable in hairy areas.

5. The hands may direct a horizontal force in any direction in relation to the client's muscle fibers. On the torso, they may move with greater ease and more effectively in a superior direction on the ventral surface and in an inferior direction on the dorsal surface ("up the front, down the back"). The clinician may produce strokes in the direction in which it seems easiest to move the skin and subcutaneous tissues, or in the other direction. These two directions for strokes can be described as the "less direct" approach and "more direct" approach, respectively. These guidelines are not inviolable; the clinician can experiment with a variety of directions and evaluate the results of each stroke continuously by inspection and palpation, bearing in mind that the goal of the technique is to achieve an overall increase in tissue length and pliability.

6. The hands must remain on the chosen layer, as far as possible. Since this layer may not always be readily palpable, the clinician can attempt to maintain the same compressive force throughout a given stroke and can stay on the layer of tissue that feels equal in hardness, density, or resistance.

7. The clinician repeats the stroke again, returns to focus on a less mobile portion of the client's tissues, or covers the original area from a different direction. If the superficial layer of fascia can be dragged horizontally in all directions with relative ease, then compression can be increased to engage a deeper layer of fascia prior to repeating the stroke.

8. The order in which treatment proceeds is important. The clinician should free superficial layers of fascia before the deeper layers (at least regionally) and initially work with broad surfaces and a general approach. The benefits of direct fascial technique accumulate incrementally and the side effects are minimized when the fascial layers are freed in an orderly succession from superficial to deep.[41] As a

Manual Technique continues on page 258

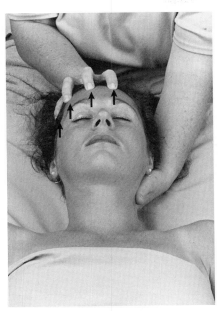

Figure 8-15. Lifting the scalp aponeurosis with the fingertips. Slow strokes begin at the brow and cross the forehead to the hairline. On the scalp, short interconnected strokes can reduce pulling of the hair. The clinician attempts to generate an equal amount of force with all fingers.

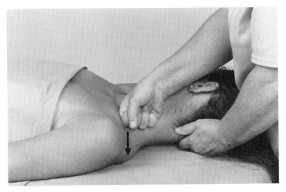

Figure 8-16. A fist usually fits well into the space above the clavicle. Strokes in a posterolateral direction that follow the clavicle can release the scalenes.

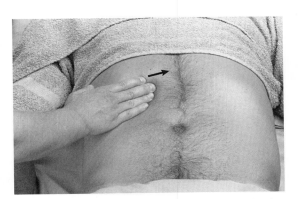

Figure 8-17. The entire anterior costal margin is an anchor for fascia from above and below. This costal margin must be treated when lengthening the front of the torso. Avoid the xiphoid process.

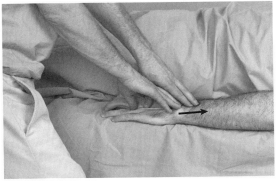

Figure 8-18. Direct fascial technique applied to the retinacula of the wrist (or ankle) can have a lengthening effect throughout the related girdle. Note the desired neutral position of the clinician's joints.

Manual Technique Figures continue on page 259

result, it is incorrect to attempt to use greater pressure to move deeper layers of fascia before ensuring that the superficial layers of fascia are thoroughly mobile. This is the case whether the treatment is general or localized.

9. After two or three strokes, change the location of application, regardless of whether or not there is palpable or visible tissue response. If the client's contracted tissues do not seem to respond, the clinician can change the stroke direction; work on the same layer proximally, distally, or across the midline; or work on a different area before returning to the area of the unresponsive tissue. It is valuable for the clinician to cultivate the habit of thinking about presenting problems in a global manner; since the fascial system is interconnected, what is perceived to be a local problem may be a more generalized issue.

10. The hands are positioned in a manner that avoids hyperextension of any of the joints of the fingers (Figs. 8-17 and 8-18). An arched hand position in which the metacarpophalangeal and interphalangeal joints are slightly flexed is acceptable for pushing strokes that require the use of the fingers.

Components of Direct Fascial Technique

Contact: Fingers (adducted together, may be reinforced) knuckles, fist, elbow, ulnar border of the forearm

Pressure: Light to heavy

Tissues engaged: Fascia; although associated muscle is also engaged, the fascial response is the primary focus of palpation

Direction: Varies; the force of application is often, but not necessarily, oriented in a direction that is parallel to the long axis of the myofascial units

Amplitude/length: Less than 5 to 50 cm

Rate: Slow, less than 5 to 15 cm/sec

Duration: 5 sec or longer

Intergrades with: Stripping, frictions, myofascial release

Combines with: The lengthening effects of this technique can be dramatically enhanced by simultaneous slow active movement by the client of the body segment being treated

Context: Commonly applied alone or alternated with myofascial release by experienced clinicians; it is advisable for the less-experienced clinician to precede or follow direct fascial technique with regional broad-contact petrissage (see Chapter 7, Neuromuscular Techniques)

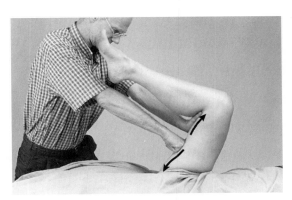

Figure 8-19. Lengthening the fascial sheathes over and between the hamstrings can be done in supine or prone. Individual knuckles can be inserted into the intermuscular septa. On heavier clients, the technique illustrated may require the use of the clinician's elbow.

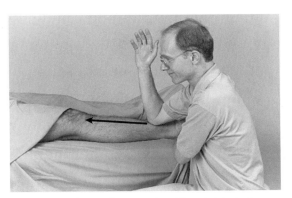

Figure 8-20. The anterior compartment is surprisingly dense and requires use of body weight. Here the clinician applies body weight in a controlled kneeling posture.

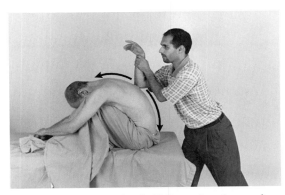

Figure 8-21. Fascia associated with the erector spinae can be treated with the client's back in many positions, from neutral to fully flexed; in prone, seated, or sidelying. Here, the clinician slides in the spinal groove along the medial surface of longissimus, taking care to avoid the spinous processes.

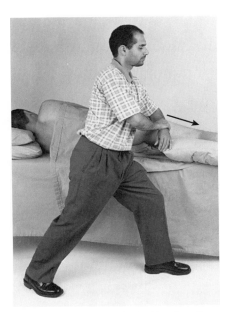

Figure 8-22. The dense iliotibial band requires a forearm or elbow with judicious use of body weight. Include the superior iliac attachments.

Manual Technique Figures continue on next page

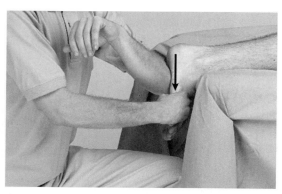

Figure 8-23. The olecranon or the fist are easily tolerated contact surfaces for applying direct fascial technique to the plantar fascia. The client's foot should be dorsiflexed to at least neutral; further increasing dorsiflexion will expose the fascia to more pressure.

CLINICIAN'S POSITION AND MOVEMENT

1. The basic positions used by the clinician are described in Chapter 4, Preparation and Positioning for Treatment. Since little body movement occurs during the slow strokes, any position that is efficient, stable, and comfortable is appropriate. Lunge and lean positions as well as standing, seated, and kneeling controlled lean positions are all useful because they enable the clinician to use body weight in a controlled manner to engage deeper fascial layers. Figures 8-19, 8-20, 8-22, and 8-23 show good body mechanics in some of these positions.

2. Especially when using body weight to augment the force of the technique, the clinician must use slow, controlled movements. Furthermore, use of body weight must not obstruct the clinician's ability to palpate subtle lengthening in the client's fascial sheaths.

3. The treatment of chronic restrictions in soft tissue may require the use of a fair amount of body weight; nevertheless, the clinician must always be relaxed, poised, and alert to signs of overexertion. Common signs of physical and mental overexertion include elevated shoulders, excessive hand and forearm tension, and uncontrolled leaning. The clinician's posture in Figure 8-21 shows the beginning of an uncontrolled lean.

PALPATE

As he performs the technique, the clinician palpates the client's tissues for the following:

1. Fascial structures. The palpation of the major fascial structures, such as the iliotibial tract, retinacula, occiptofrontal aponeurosis, clavipectoral fascia, and large intermuscular septa, can be relatively easy.[33,40] By contrast, it can be virtually impossible to palpate minor fascial sheaths in areas where there is associated muscle bulk. Similarly, although surgical scarring or consolidated edema resulting from a major trauma can produce obvious palpable fascial thickening and restriction, it requires considerable practice to detect less obvious restrictions in connective tissue. With the application of direct fascial technique, discrete connective tissue structures can become palpably softer, and hard, fibrous areas may feel fuller, softer, hydrated, and less fibrous.

2. Fascial layers. Although clinicians may on occasion clearly palpate the movement of an entire fascial sheath from the point of contact, they are wise not to take the term layer literally. In many ways, layer is a metaphor that is used to help clinicians focus their attention on a useful object of palpation. The clinician must develop the ability to palpate the behavior of an entire layer of connective tissue while

it is under sustained horizontal traction and while the contact surface is gliding (an extremely refined skill). In addition, a shift to more-generalized palpation may be difficult for clinicians who are accustomed to using classical neuromuscular techniques, such as petrissage, in which their attention is focused on the qualities of the tissues that are immediately under hand.

3. Resistance to sustained lengthening. The resistance to a sustained lengthening force may arise from any location in the fascial layer that is under traction. With practice, the clinician may be able to identify resistance to lengthening that originates from a point distant from the local point of contact.

4. Viscoelastic stretch or creep. Creep occurs during direct fascial technique, although it is more difficult to identify than when it occurs during myofascial release, since the glide of the contact surface occurs simultaneously with the creep of the tissue that is under traction.

5. Adhesions or trigger points. During treatment the clinician's hands may glide over adhesions or trigger points that may soften with continued application of regional direct fascial technique. If this does not occur, then he may choose to change to a more specific technique, such as specific compression or friction.

OBSERVE

As he performs the technique, the clinician observes the client for changes in tissue quality and lengthening. The signs listed below may signal this.

1. Hyperemia. A reactive hyperemia may accompany the application of this technique.

2. Local tissue contours. Observe areas that are drawn in, flattened or elevated areas, atrophy, or hypertrophy.[40] Tissue contours may change following the application of direct fascial technique.

3. Thixotrophic rehydration. The thixotropic rehydration of the ground substance of tissues may contribute to a further softening of local tissue contours after the force of the technique is released.

4. Changes in other body segments. Lengthening and positional shifts may appear in proximal, distal, or adjacent segments during the application of myofascial release. The clinician must cultivate the habit of continually evaluating adjacent body segments for changes, with the client on and off the table.

5. Structural alignment. Changes in structural relationships of the client's body segments are best assessed by inspection of standing static alignment and gait, both during and at the end of the session.

COMMUNICATION WITH THE CLIENT

The clinician uses communication that may encourage general relaxation and facilitate tissue lengthening. Some examples of statements that the clinician can use are listed below.

1. "Let me know if you begin to feel uncomfortable." In general, once a client overcomes the initial strangeness of direct fascial technique, it should feel pleasant. The clinician needs to inform the client about the different types of sensations that may arise. Clients frequently experience a burning sensation when superficial fascial layers are first stretched. When the clinician uses specific contact surfaces, such as his fingers, a cutting or scratching sensation may occur.[40] The client may experience local discomfort when there is a significant local fascial restriction. In general, the clinician must ensure that the client understands that the amount of pressure used must be tolerable and is under control of the client, not the clinician.

2. "Notice what's occurring in your body . . . it's not unusual to experience sensations some distance from the location of my hands." Clients frequently report sensations that occur some distance from the clinician's hands and may need to be reassured that this is normal. These are generally of two types: a transient referral from a latent trigger point that the clinician's hands pass over or direct mechanical pulling of some distant part of the fascial layer that is currently under traction.

3. "Deepen your breathing without forcing it in any way." Conscious diaphragmatic breathing facilitates fascial release, and lack of it impedes release. "As you breathe in, imagine the breath flowing into your . . ." It can be beneficial to have clients imagine their breath flowing into and out of the area that is being treated.

4. "Can you describe the difference between the left and the right sides of your body?" The clinician asks the client to compare areas that have been treated with those areas that haven't (for example, comparing the left side with the right side). Clients may find changes more apparent when they are sitting or walking. Clinicians may find that providing clients with sufficient time for them to observe and report the ongoing effects of the technique is an indispensable teaching tool, particularly in the case of clients whose poor habits of muscular use contribute to their dysfunction.

5. "Does anything feel out-of-place?" "Do your left and right sides match?" "Can you live with this until your next session?" The clinician must ensure that the client feels balanced at the end of a session.

6. "It's normal to feel uncoordinated for a day or so after the treatment." Clients are often aware of altered proprioception and biomechanics for a day or two after undergoing a substantial release. While these changes are not painful, the client may find them uncomfortable. Consequently the clinician should advise clients that this discomfort may occur and that it can be reduced by simple daily activities, such as walking.

7. "Please phone if you experience anything unusual after the treatment, especially if you have persistent pain." When a significant shift in agonist/antagonist balance occurs, the client may experience transient muscle soreness in areas other than those that were treated. This occurs because of an increased loading of antagonists, synergists, or other muscles in the kinetic chain. The clinician should, therefore, advise the client to report any postintervention soreness that is more than mild or that lasts longer than 2 days.

8. When the client presents with a history of past physical or emotional trauma, it is possible, although uncommon, for spontaneous autonomic rebalancing to be accompanied by somatoemotional release. The facilitation of somatoemotional release requires sensitivity and presence on the part of the clinician. This is discussed further in Chapter 2, The Clinical Decision-Making Process.

OTHER APPROPRIATE TECHNIQUES

There are several modalities that the clinician can use in a complementary manner with direct fascial technique.

1. In controlled laboratory conditions, the precise heating of tissue facilitates greater elongation of collagenous structures without resulting in structural damage.[29,32,36] In clinical practice, however, the application of heat prior to any sustained loading of connective tissue can increase the risk of collagenous rupture. Consequently, the clinician should avoid the application of either heat or cold before performing connective tissue techniques, unless his

---

A Practice Sequence for Direct Fascial Technique

Practice time: 45 min per person

The shoulder girdle, with a focus on the arms, is a good place to begin learning direct fascial technique. Since individuals' forearms and hands are often tense, length changes are easily observed. In addition, these changes will not affect the dynamics of the weight-bearing lower kinetic chain.

Several factors are important to keep in mind throughout the intervention. Contact connective tissue and apply traction to tissue layers in a horizontal direction. Work with a slow rate of glide, pause between strokes, and get frequent feedback from your client. Observe tissues for lengthening in addition to using palpation.

Visually inspect the client's upper body structure.

Supine:

1. Apply short fingertip strokes in several directions: over the retinacula of the wrist; repeatedly over the palmar fascia and both thenar and hypothenar eminences; and around the joints and bones of the fingers. Observe the effect that this has on the entire shoulder girdle.

2. Use a broader contact surface, such as your forearm, palm, or fist, on both ventral and dorsal surfaces of the client's forearm. Using more-specific finger or thumb contact, try to enter the space between the muscles to work on the intermuscular fascial layers. Again, observe the results.

3. In the same manner as for the forearms, use broad and then more-specific contact to treat the client's upper arms. Include the fascia over the deltoid, and the lateral and medial intermuscular septa.

Reassess.

4. Give equal treatment to the client's other arm.

To finish, apply each of the following strokes several times.

5. Supine. Reach under the client to the midthoracic level and then drag the tips of your flexed fingers up the erector spinae on either side of the client's spine from the midthorax to the occiput.

6. Head turned. Use a broad surface like the heel of the hand moving anterior to posterior across the scalenes. Treat one side at a time.

7. Seated with trunk flexion. Apply long, descending strokes along the erector spinae with the elbow or forearm.

Visually reassess.

aim is specifically to rupture or denature collagen.[36] Heat applied after the use of myofascial release can enhance the temporary increase in the pliability of myofascial tissue.

2. Also of benefit are neuromuscular or muscle energy techniques, joint mobilization and manipulation, and spinal traction performed from the head or pelvis.[15]

3. Chronic conditions may require correction for bony asymmetry.

4. When the client experiences significant shifts in posture, postural awareness training, neuromuscular education, and movement awareness training may be of benefit,[8] Systems of comprehensive postural awareness and movement training, such as the Alexander technique,[37] may be used in these situations. Ergonomic retraining related to the client's work environment may be required.

5. Stretching.

6. Strengthening.

7. Electrotherapeutic modalities such as biofeedback, electrical muscle stimulation, and TENS.[8]

POSTINTERVENTION SELF-CARE

1. The clinician can teach the client how to perform precise self-stretching exercises using moderate force and a longer duration than usual.

2. The client can perform postural, movement awareness, or strengthening exercises as required.

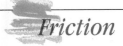

Friction

OTHER NAMES USED FOR THIS TECHNIQUE

"Circular friction," "transverse friction," "deep friction," "deep transverse friction," "cross-fiber friction," "Cyriax friction."[1–8]

DEFINITION

Friction: A repetitive, specific, nongliding technique that produces movement between the fibers of dense connective tissue, increasing tissue extensibility, and promoting ordered alignment of collagen within the tissues.[1–8]

NOTES

1. Various forms of this connective tissue technique differ in the direction and the amount of force that is applied. Nevertheless, the treatment aims, clinical effects, focus of palpation, and many aspects of the manual technique are similar, whether the force is directed across or parallel to the fiber direction of well-defined structures, such as tendons or ligaments, or to less-well-defined dense connective tissue formations, such as adhesions and fibroses.

2. Historically, the term friction has a broad, ambiguous usage that has embraced virtually any manner of rubbing between two surfaces. Tappan describes a "superficial friction" that is a fast chafing of the body's surface.[5] Other authors have used the term friction to refer to nongliding techniques that repetitively move one layer of muscle over another, which are similar to petrissage in terms of their shearing forces and clinical effects (see Chapter 7, Neuromuscular Techniques).[4,8] In this text, the term friction is reserved for the specific connective tissue technique described in the sections below.

3. An extremely attenuated version of the technique described below may be applied to clients with subacute orthopedic injuries.

CLINICAL INDICATIONS AND IMPAIRMENT-LEVEL OUTCOME OF CARE

Friction maintains, or increases, the extensibility of connective tissue by promoting the realignment and remodeling of its constituent collagen fibers.[68] Consequently, friction can be used to treat any condition in which mobility may be compromised by irregular tissue remodeling that occurred during the consolidation and maturation stages of connective tissue healing. It is indicated in the rehabilitation of virtually all chronic orthopedic injuries, including sprains (with one dissenting opinion[75]), strains, and fractures.[68–76] In these situations, friction may result in maintained or increased joint range, capsular mobility, and accessory movement.[68,69,75,77,78] Opinions differ, however, regarding the effectiveness of friction in increasing the extensibility of hypertrophic scar tissue.[79–80] Friction is also an effective intervention—often the manual intervention of choice—for repetitive strain injuries such as tendinitis, tenosynovitis, bursitis, and plantar fasciitis, in which there is ongoing microtrauma, low-grade inflammation, and tissue remodeling.[68,69,81–85] Finally, like many other massage techniques, friction may result in analgesia and a significant postintervention transient reactive hyperemia.[68–74]

How Connective Tissue Responds to Immobility

Immobilization of connective tissue produces a succession of important biochemical changes;[86-90] these include:

Decreased concentration of hyaluronic acid in the matrix

Decreased water-bonding capacity of the matrix

Decreased water content of the matrix

Approximation of collagen fibers

Increased collagen cross-linking

These in turn may contribute to the clinical impairments of:

Increased tissue stiffness

Decreased tissue mobility

Restrictions of joint capsule and ligaments

Impaired joint mobility

Pain

Damaged tissue that is carefully stressed during the healing process, by appropriate movement or massage, will show improved hydration of the extracellular matrix and more-orderly deposition of collagen. This will result in stronger, more distensible, and more functional scar tissue.

CAUTIONS AND CONTRAINDICATIONS

Clinical training and supervised practice are critical for the proper application of friction. Advanced training may be advisable in certain situations, particularly when dealing with pathological conditions. All of the general and local contraindications noted for massage techniques apply to the use of friction (see Chapter 2, The Clinical Decision-Making Process).[13] As for all of the connective tissue techniques, there are several cautions and contraindications to the use of friction; these include the following: hemophilia, thrombus, malignancy, vascular insufficiency, cellulitis, phlebitis, fever, systemic or local infection, acute circulatory conditions, osteomyelitis, aneurysm, obstructive edema, acute rheumatoid arthritis, open wounds, sutures, hematomas, healing fractures, osteoporosis, client's use of local or systemic analgesic, anti-inflammatory, or anticoagulant drugs, advanced diabetes, and hypersensitivity of the skin (see Chapter 2, The Clinical Decision-Making Process).[4,5,7,13,15] All signs of acute inflammation, such as spasm, pain at rest, heat, redness, and unconsolidated edema, must be absent prior to the use of friction.[68] Friction should not be performed in the area of hematomas, calcifications, peripheral nerves, or fragile skin.[69] The clinician should use extreme caution when applying friction around hypermobile or unstable joints, such as those that result from recurrent sprains or dislocations, systemic connective tissue disorders, and osteoporosis. Finally, the clinician should use care when applying friction in hypotonic regions or in the vicinity of active trigger points.

Prerequisite Skills for Friction

Before applying friction, students should be able to

Distinguish between the edema associated with acute and chronic orthopedic conditions

Recognize normal and poorly modeled connective tissue, using palpation

Assess the key signs for contractile and noncontractile tissues

Describe, locate, and palpate accessible ligaments and tendons

Use a variety of reinforced contact surfaces to deliver high levels of specific pressure

Use a standing controlled lean to transfer body weight

Negotiate an acceptable level of discomfort with the client

Use key signs and client feedback to determine the duration of friction

Recognize overtreatment, and minimize its effects

Manual Technique begins on page 266

MANUAL TECHNIQUE

Friction

In the following figures (Figs. 8-24 to 8-31), friction is applied to the various regions of the body. Figures are ordered from head to foot in supine and then prone. Each figure illustrates most of the guidelines for manual technique outlined below.[68–70,72,74]

1. Prior to performing friction, the clinician clips or files the nails so that they are very short.

2. No oil is required. If oil has been applied, it is removed from the client's skin with alcohol, to prevent slippage.

3. The clinician positions the body segment to be treated so that there is sufficient tension for the force of the friction to be effectively isolated to the target tissues without affecting the surrounding normal tissues.[68–70,72,74] If the target tissues are slack, the contact surface will tend to slide over them, and the force of the friction will dissipate in the adjacent healthy tissue and cause inflammation. On the other hand, if the target tissues are too stretched, they become difficult to penetrate at all. A useful rule of thumb is that the more superficial the tissue, the more stretch should be exerted on the body segment. For example, if the lesion is confined to a synovial sheath or is between the sheath and its tendon, that tendon is placed on the fullest tolerable stretch. For ligaments, a position between neutral and a full stretch will suffice, depending on the desired depth for the friction. For lesions within a tendon, some manual stretch must be maintained while the friction is performed; however, if the lesion is deep in the muscle, the superficial tissues must be slackened to allow access to the lesion. Finally, the degree of stretch that is most effective can also vary with the hardness of the target tissue.

4. The hands use focused and specific contact. Usually some combination of the first three digits is held tightly together and reinforced. The third digit can reinforce on the index, or the index may be reinforced between the thumb and third digits (see Figs. 8-24 to 8-29 and Fig. 8-31). When the lesion is deep or large and requires the use of body weight to access it, the olecranon process can be substituted for the fingers (Fig. 8-30). When the target tissues are very dense and hard, a wooden or plastic "T-bar" may be necessary (Fig. 7-61). Regardless of the contact surface that the clinician uses, frequent change of contact surfaces will minimize the likelihood of repetitive strain.

5. The hands do not glide over the client's skin. Furthermore, there is minimal movement of the hand in relation to any of the tissues that are superficial to the target tissue; that is, all of the tissues that are superficial to the target tissue should move with the hand. The aim of friction is to increase the extensibility of immobile connective tissue by mobilizing one area of the target tissue in relation to another by producing small movements within the immobile connective tissue. Good palpation skills and unerring control of pressure are essential to achieving this aim.

6. The clinician initially sets the depth of friction at a level that engages the most superficial layer of the connective tissue that is in need of remodeling. If the lesion is superficial, this may require little pressure; however, if the lesion is located beneath several layers of muscle, considerable force may be required, even when the clinician adequately prepares the intervening tissues (Figs. 8-24, 8-29, and 8-30).

7. The clinician uses short strokes (<2 cm) to move the superficial portion of the target tissues back and forth over the deeper portion. It is important to avoid

Manual Technique continues on page 268

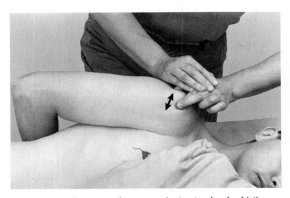

Figure 8-24. To expose the supraspinatus tendon for friction, the client's arm is extended, adducted, and internally rotated. The insertions of the tendons of the rotator cuff muscles lie beneath the thick, coarse-fibered deltoid muscle. Lesions in the rotator cuff muscles are precisely located using the client's response to deep palpation.

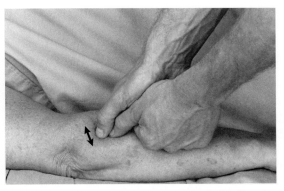

Figure 8-25. Lesions in the common extensor tendon ("tennis elbow") can develop anywhere between the tenoperiosteal and musculotendinous junctions. The clinician must pretreat local trigger points and avoid damaging the radial nerve with the friction.

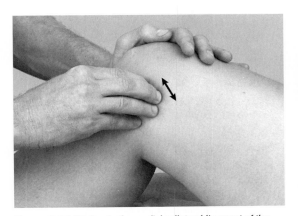

Figure 8-26. Friction to the medial collateral ligament of the knee. The knee is positioned to exert a moderate stretch on the ligament. Friction for sprains should be given at the maximum allowable flexion and extension.[69]

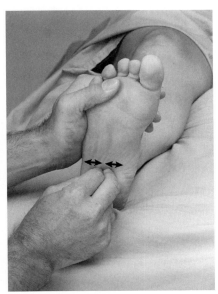

Figure 8-27. The foot must be dorsiflexed when applying friction to the dense plantar fascia, particularly when treating plantar fasciitis. If digital contact is difficult for the client to tolerate, precede the use of friction with a more general stroke, such as kneading.

Manual Technique Figures continue on page 269

slipping off, or bumping over, the target tissues, since this increases the likelihood that adjacent healthy tissue will be damaged. Although Cyriax[72,74] suggests that friction should be applied with "sufficient sweep," it is acceptable, and it is more controlled, to use short strokes, unless the target tissue is quite narrow and easily traversed with one stroke (Figs. 8-24 to 8-26). In this case, the clinician can ensure coverage of the entire breadth of the lesion by applying friction to adjacent areas with shorter strokes.

8. The direction of the stroke is specifically across fibers when treating ligament or tendon. When treating fascia or scar tissue in which the collagen has a less regular organization, directions may be alternated or a circular stroke produced.

9. Friction is typically applied at a rate of 2 to 3 cycles per second.[68] Three cycles per second represents the maximum rate for an experienced clinician working on a superficial lesion. A more modest rate of 1 to 2 cycles per second can be effective and, at the same time, facilitates palpation and reduces the possibility of overtreatment.

10. The hands maintain contact with the same tissue layer while the friction is performed until palpable softening of that tissue occurs or for 2 min, whichever comes first.

11. The clinician should take frequent breaks of several seconds to change contact surfaces, taking care to accurately relocate the lesion and to reestablish a similar depth of friction.

12. If the client gives positive feedback (see "Communication with the Client," on page 270), the clinician can increase pressure to engage a deeper layer of the target tissue or shift very slightly to an adjacent area and then perform another cycle of friction.

13. If the lesion is located on a limb, the clinician may use an easier approach to achieving the required depth and control for the technique. This involves maintaining static specific compression on the target tissue with one hand, while moving the client's limb with the other to produce the required motion between the target tissue and the clinician's hand (Figs. 8-30 and 8-31). This technique is often also more tolerable to the client.

14. Depending on the client's feedback about level of comfort, the maximum time for the application of friction in the first intervention is 6 min.[68] The duration of application can increase by increments of 2 or 3 min per session,[68] with an upper limit (virtually never required) of 15 to 20 min.[68,69]

Components of Friction

Contact: Reinforced finger(s), thumb, knuckle, olecranon

Pressure: Light to heavy, depending on location of lesion

Tissues engaged: Dense connective tissue (ligament, tendon, fascia, extraneous deep connective tissue, scar tissue, or fibrosis in muscle)

Direction: Varies depending on the fiber orientation of the structure; currently, transverse friction is most commonly used, although circular friction may be useful, and parallel friction has been advocated in the past

Amplitude/length: Short, less than 1 to 2 cm

Rate: Slow, less than 1 to 3 cycles per second is recommended, with a 3-cycle per second maximum

Duration: 30 sec to 15 min

Intergrades with: Petrissage, specific compression, direct fascial technique

Context: May be performed alone; another option is to precede friction with regional petrissage, myofascial release, or direct fascial technique; one can follow friction with superficial effleurage and passive or active stretches

A cold pack is applied afterward, if overtreatment has occurred.

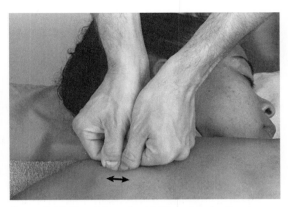

Figure 8-28. The clinician should differentiate the fibrosis commonly found at the lower attachment of the levator scapulae from a trigger point before treating it with friction.

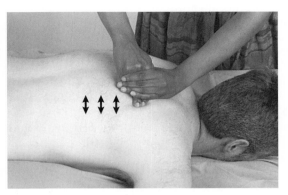

Figure 8-29. The tendinous slips of iliocostalis thoracis are prone to become "ropy" or "stringy" due to chronic inflammation, especially if a client is hyperkyphotic. This local lack of tissue resilience can be improved with friction.

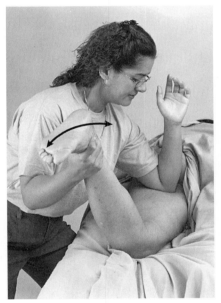

Figure 8-30. This friction of the hamstring just distal to its attachment on the ischial tuberosity begins with deep specific compression on the tendon using the clinician's body weight and the elbow. The clinician then uses the client's lower leg to internally and externally rotate the femur to control the cross-fiber movement between the contact surface and the target tissue.

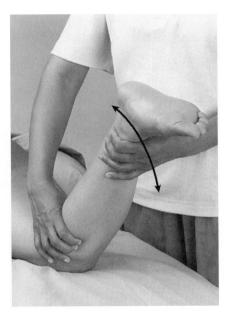

Figure 8-31. The first two fingers of the clinician's right hand contact the pes anserinus. Controlled movement of the contact surface over the bursa or tendinous insertions can be accomplished easily by flexing and extending the client's knee while holding the contact hand steady.

CLINICIAN'S POSITION AND MOVEMENT

1. The basic positions used by the clinician are described in Chapter 4, Preparation and Positioning for Treatment.
2. Effective application of friction demands a judicious use of the clinician's body weight. It may be hard to achieve appropriate results by relying on hand and arm strength alone, except when treating small, superficial lesions. In a standing or seated controlled lean position, the clinician can hold the hand and arm stable and use a slight rocking of the body to produce sufficient force of friction and the required movement of the contact surface.
3. Use of the elbow in standing or seated controlled lean demands skilled proprioceptive palpation (Fig. 8-30).

PALPATE

As he performs the technique, the clinician palpates the client's skin and tissues for the following:

1. Contours. Chronic orthopedic injuries often appear to be "swollen" or enlarged; however, palpable extravasated fluid must not be present when friction is applied.
2. Density or hardness of the target tissue. The clinician needs to compare the target tissues with adjacent uninvolved tissue or comparable tissues on the client's opposite side, to form an impression of what normal bulk and texture are for that individual.
3. Fiber direction. The clinician notes the fiber direction of discrete structures, such as tendon or ligament, prior to treatment.
4. Location of target tissue. The clinician must accurately locate the desired target tissue throughout the application of friction.
5. Softening of tissue. Taut bands or hardened slabs of tissue may soften as a result of rehydration of the ground substance or rupture of collagen fibrils. This palpable softening should be accompanied by a reduction of tenderness and improvement of the client's key symptoms.
6. Reduction of hypertrophy. Hypertrophied structures may be reduced during even one session of friction.
7. Resistance to stretch. The resistance to stretch of contractile tissue should decline as treatment progresses.

OBSERVE

While performing the technique, the clinician observes the quality of the target tissue and signs of the client's comfort. The signs listed below may signal this.

1. Surface contours reflect the bulk, tautness, and hardness of the target tissues.

2. Reactive hyperemia. Rapid reddening of the client's skin may indicate an abrasion caused by nails that are too long.
3. The client's facial expression should reflect relaxation and comfort.

COMMUNICATION WITH THE CLIENT

Friction presents the highest risk for producing local tissue damage of all the massage techniques, since it involves a strong repetitive force that is localized to a very small area. If the clinician uses proper communication, he can avoid overtreatment and increasing inflammation. Beyond the production of a transient hyperemia, the point of friction is **not** to increase inflammation in already damaged tissue, though this can sometimes result from overzealous application. The following protocol for communication, adapted from Hertling and Kessler,[68] provides guidelines for obtaining frequent feedback and testing the client as a means of minimizing the risk of overtreatment.

1. Immediately before applying friction, the clinician tests the sensitivity of the target tissues in one of two ways: With contractile tissues, he palpates the tissues while performing resisted isometric movements; with inert tissues, he palpates the tissues while performing a passive stretch. He can also ask the client to rate current pain on a 10-point scale to obtain a more objective measure of how sensitive the lesion may be to mechanical stress. This provides an essential baseline for measuring progress and grading the dosage of friction applied during the session.
2. "Where is it most tender to touch?"' The clinician must use orthopedic testing to determine the structure that requires friction. In addition, the clinician can solicit client feedback in response to palpation, to identify the location of the inflammation within the implicated structure.
3. Friction should begin at a level that the client reports is tolerable—no more than level 4 discomfort on a 10-point scale. The client should demonstrate neither signs of pain, such as inhibited breathing or grimacing, nor more-subtle signs of sympathetic arousal. The clinician assures the client that the initial discomfort (if any) usually declines as the friction proceeds and directs the client to speak up immediately if discomfort increases during the friction.
4. Toward the end of the first cycle (up to 2 min), the clinician asks the client if the discomfort caused by the friction is more or less than it was at the beginning of the intervention. If the discomfort has lessened, he can increase the pressure on the basis of the client's level of tolerance and proceed for an additional 2 min.

5. At the end of three cycles (up to 6 min), the clinician retests key signs. If the lesion is less sensitive during testing, he may continue to use friction if it is not the first intervention.

6. If the client reports that the discomfort caused by the friction has increased or if the lesion is more reactive on retesting, the clinician must stop applying friction for that session, use superficial effleurage to drain toward the nearest lymph nodes, and apply ice to the area until visible vasoconstriction (blanching) occurs.

OTHER APPROPRIATE TECHNIQUES

There are several modalities that the clinician can use in a complementary manner with friction.

1. In controlled laboratory conditions, the precise heating of tissue facilitates a greater elongation of collagenous structures without resulting in structural damage.[29,32,36] In clinical practice, however, the application of heat prior to any sustained loading of connective tissue can increase the risk of collagenous rupture. Consequently, the clinician should avoid the application of either heat or cold before performing connective tissue techniques, unless his aim is specifically to rupture or denature collagen.[36] This may be the case when using friction to treat a large adhesion. Heat applied after the use of friction can enhance the temporary increase in the pliability of myofascial tissue.

2. For some conditions, a local application of myofascial release or direct fascial technique prior to the application of friction may reduce the need for extensive or prolonged use of friction. Preapplication of ultrasound has also been recommended.[69]

3. Gentle passive stretch of the target tissues and active movement in the pain-free range of motion can be beneficial following friction.[69]

4. Should overtreatment occur, application of cryotherapy (cold pack) until vasoconstriction (blanching) occurs is indicated.

5. Splints, taping, and ergonomic or neuromuscular retraining may be useful in reducing repetitive strain or preventing recurrence of accident.[8]

POSTINTERVENTION SELF-CARE

1. If the client reports more than a moderate soreness after the application of friction, the clinician can instruct her to apply a cold pack to the area for 10 to 14 min at intervals for the next 24 h.[68,69,72]

2. The client can learn to perform gentle stretches of the target tissue for 30 sec several times a day between interventions.

3. The clinician should instruct the client who has a repetitive strain injury to avoid aggravating activities.

4. The client with a lesion in contractile tissue should avoid resisted exercise or extensive stretching and only perform painless passive or active movements until later in the healing process. At that point, more-aggressive stretching and strengthening may be indicated.

A Practice Sequence for Friction

Practice Time: 30 min per person

To acquire a feel for this technique, practice around large joints where connective tissue is easily accessible. The ankle is a good choice, since it is a common location of sprains and is often the site of residual fibrosis. The client's knees are also an appropriate choice of joints. The joint chosen for practice should show no signs of instability.

Connective tissue is remarkably tough, and a stable, healthy joint can certainly withstand up to 5 min of properly applied friction without showing signs of negative effects. Respect your client's pain tolerance; do not apply friction to any given spot (for practice purposes) for more than a minute, and avoid "endangerment sites," such as the locations of major nerves (the radial nerve at the elbow).

1. Ensure that your nails are very short!

2. Begin by applying 5 min of petrissage to the major muscles that cross the joint (see Chapter 7, Neuromuscular Techniques); this is particularly useful when treating lesions in contractile tissue.

3. Remove residual lubricant completely.

4. Evaluate for (hypothetical) key signs: do passive and/or contractile testing and thoroughly palpate around the joint for tenderness.

5. Beginning superficially, apply friction for a minute to five or six different locations around the client's joint: on the tendon (also paratendon), the ligament, and the retinaculum. A minute of friction is generally long enough to detect a palpable change—the tissue to which friction was applied should feel slightly spongy. If this change is uncertain, do a bilateral comparison. If there is no detectable change, increase the pressure of the stroke slightly, and try a different location for a minute.

6. Retest key signs.

7. Have the client stretch the treated area.

8. Drain toward the regional lymph nodes with superficial effleurage or superficial lymph drainage technique.

9. Ensure that the client shows no signs of overtreatment, although it is unlikely to occur with treatment of this brief a duration.

Home study: Superior gluteal insertions are a common site of fibrosis. Devise a comparable sequence for that area that uses knuckle or elbow contact to deliver the friction. Apply this sequence bilaterally.

Clinical Example	
Client profile	A 40-year-old male computer programmer with right-sided lateral epicondylitis (repetitive strain injury) secondary to keyboarding, poor posture, and poor ergonomics
Summary of clinical findings	*Subjective* 1. Complaints of pain at rest and while keyboarding 2. Complaints of inability to keyboard for more than 10 min without severe pain 3. Complaints of dropping objects held in his right hand during work and self-care activities because of pain and a feeling of weakness 4. Complaints of mild swelling after work 5. Visual analog scale pain rating = 8.5 6. Reports lack of ergonomic modifications to work station 7. Poor knowledge of ergonomics and self-care *Objective* *Impairments* 1. Pain elicited on resisted R wrist and finger extension 2. Grip strength: R grip < L grip on testing with JAMAR 3. Palpation: Fascial shortening in area of R common extensor origin and forearm musculature 4. Posture: kyphotic, forward head posture *Functional Limitations* 1. Unable to keyboard for longer than 10 min or perform job requirements as a computer programmer, secondary to pain 2. Compromised ability to perform work and self-care because of pain and weakness—drops objects held in R. hand 3. Unable to perform recreational activity of racquetball, secondary to pain
Treatment planning	*Treatment rationale* To reduce the pain and inflammation associated with lateral epicondylitis and to provide education on self-care and ergonomics to prevent future exacerbations of this condition.

Impairment	Role of therapeutic massage
Pain	Primary treatment; direct effect since the pain is secondary to inflammation of the tissues at common extensor origin
	Primary treatment; direct effect resulting from counterirritant analgesia
Inflammation	Primary treatment; reduction of signs of inflammation is a direct effect
Abnormal connective tissue density	Primary treatment; promotion of dense connective tissue remodelling is a direct effect
Fascial shortening	Primary treatment; fascial lengthening is a direct effect
General postural dysfunction	Primary treatment, direct effect resulting from fascial lengthening
Decreased strength	Secondary effect since decreased strength is largely due to pain and inflammation

(continued)

Massage techniques	Petrissage, myofascial technique, direct fascial technique applied to shortened muscles of anterior body related to kyphosis and forward head posture. Superficial effleurage, petrissage, myofascial release, direct fascial technique applied to entire forearm, especially muscles of the extensor compartment (some work on the contralateral arm may be required to maintain right-left balance). Friction to common extensor origin.
Other appropriate techniques and interventions	Ice if signs of acute inflammation are present; ice postfriction if signs of overtreatment are present; wrist and hand stretches; wrist- and hand-strengthening exercises; postural stretches; postural education; ergonomic examination; education in ergonomics; and self-care.
Functional outcomes	1. Client will be able to keyboard, with the use of ergonomic modifications, for 1 h with appropriate stretching and rest periods without complaints of pain 2. Client will be able to carry 10-lb weight in R hand 25 feet without complaints of pain or dropping the weight as needed for performing household chores 3. Client will be able to play racquetball for 20 min following the appropriate warm-up, without complaints of pain

References

1. Holey E, Cook E. Therapeutic massage. London, England: WB Saunders, 1997.
2. Hollis M. Massage for therapists. 2nd ed. Oxford, England: Blackwell Science, 1998.
3. Cantu RI, Grodin AJ. Myofascial manipulation: theory and clinical application. Gaithersburg, MD: Aspen, 1992.
4. Fritz S. Fundamentals of therapeutic massage. St Louis: Mosby-Lifeline, 1995.
5. Tappan FM, Benjamin P. Tappan's handbook of healing massage techniques. 3rd ed. Stamford, CT: Appleton & Lange, 1998.
6. Loving J. Massage therapy. Stamford, CT: Appleton & Lange, 1999.
7. de Domenico G, Wood EC. Beard's massage. 4th ed. Philadelphia: WB Saunders, 1997.
8. American Physical Therapy Association. Guide to physical therapist practice. Phys Ther 1997;77(11):1155–1674.
9. Chaitow L. Palpation skills. New York: Churchill Livingstone, 1997.
10. Maigne R. Low back pain of thoracolumbar origin. Arch Phys Med Rehabil 1980;61(9):389–395.
11. Greenman PE. Principles of manual medicine. 2nd ed. Baltimore, MD: Williams & Wilkins, 1996.
12. Chaitow L. Modern neuromuscular techniques. New York: Churchill Livingstone, 1996.
13. Fritz S. Mosby's fundamentals of therapeutic massage. St Louis: Mosby-Lifeline, 2000.
14. Mannheim CJ, Lavett DK. The myofascial release manual. Thorofare, NJ: Slack (McGraw Hill), 1989.
15. Barnes JF. Myofascial release. In: Hammer WI, ed. Functional soft tissue examination and treatment by manual methods. 2nd ed. Gaithersburg, MD: Aspen, 1999:533–548.
16. Sucher BM, Heath DM. Thoracic outlet syndrome—a myofascial variant: part 3. Structural and postural considerations. J Am Osteopath Assoc 1993;93(3):334, 340–345.
17. Sucher BM. Thoracic outlet syndrome—a myofascial variant: part 2. Treatment. J Am Osteopath Assoc 1990; 90(9):810–812, 817–823.
18. Sucher BM. Thoracic outlet syndrome—a myofascial variant: part 1. Pathology and diagnosis. J Am Osteopath Assoc 1990;90(8):686–696, 703–704.
19. Sucher BM. Myofascial manipulative release of carpal tunnel syndrome: documentation with magnetic resonance imaging. J Am Osteopath Assoc 1993;93(12):1273–1278.
20. Sucher BM. Myofascial release of carpal tunnel syndrome. J Am Osteopath Assoc 1993;93(1):92–94, 100–101.
21. Cisler TA. Whiplash as a total-body injury. J Am Osteopath Assoc 1994;94(2):145–148.
22. Hanten WP, Chandler SD. Effects of myofascial release leg pull and sagittal plane isometric contract-relax techniques on passive straight-leg raise angle. J Orthop Sports Phys Ther 1994;20(3):138–144.
23. Radjieski JM, Lumley MA, Cantieri MS. Effect of osteopathic manipulative treatment on length of stay for pancreatitis: a randomized pilot study. J Am Osteopath Assoc 1998;98(5):264–272.
24. Tillman LJ, Chasan NP. Properties of dense connective tissue and wound healing. In: Hertling D, Kessler RM, eds. Management of common musculoskeletal conditions, 3rd ed. Philadelphia: Lippincott-Raven, 1996:8–21.

25. Tillman LJ, Cummings GS. Biologic mechanisms of connective tissue mutability. In: Currier DP, Nelson RM, eds. Dynamics of human biologic tissues. Philadelphia: FA Davis, 1992:1–44.

26. Taylor DC, Dalton JD, Seaber AV, Garret WE. Visco-elastic properties of muscle-tendon units: the biomechanical effects of stretching. Am J Sports Med 1990;18(3):300–309.

27. Frank C, Amiel D, Woo SL, et al. Normal ligament properties and ligament healing. Clin Orthop 1985;196:15–25.

28. Dunn MG, Silver FH. Visco-elastic behavior of human connective tissue: relative contribution of viscous and elastic components. Connect Tissue Res 1983;12:59–70.

29. Sapega AA, Quedenfeld TC. Biophysical factors in range of motion exercise. Physician Sports Med 1981;9(12):57–65.

30. Light KE, Nuzik S, Personius W, Barstrom A. Low load prolonged stretch vs high load brief stretch in treating knee contractures. Phys Ther 1984;64:330–333.

31. Hooley CJ, McCrum NG, Cohen RE. The visco-elastic deformation of tendon. J Biomech 1980;13:521–529.

32. Warren CG, Lehmann JF, Koblanski JN. Heat and stretch procedures: an evaluation using rat tail tendon. Arch Phys Med Rehabil 1976;57:122–126.

33. Schultz RL, Feitis R. Fascial anatomy and physical reality. Berkeley, CA: North Atlantic Books, 1996.

34. Rolf I. Rolfing®: the integration of human structures. New York: Harper & Row, 1977.

35. Upledger J, Vredevoogd JD. Craniosacral therapy. Seattle, WA: Eastland Press, 1983.

36. Cummings GS, Tillman LJ. Remodeling of dense connective tissue in normal adult tissues. In: Currier DP, Nelson RM, eds. Dynamics of human biologic tissues. Philadelphia: FA Davis, 1992:45–73.

37. Barlow W. The Alexander technique. New York: Alfred A Knopf, 1973.

38. Quality Assurance Committee of the College of Massage Therapists of Ontario. Code of ethics and standards of practice. Toronto, Ontario: College of Massage Therapists of Ontario, 1999.

39. DiGiovanna EL, Schiowitz S. An osteopathic approach to diagnosis and treatment. 2nd ed. Philadelphia: Lippincott-Raven, 1997.

40. Ebner M. Connective tissue manipulations: theory and therapeutic application. 3rd ed. Malabar, FL: Krieger, 1985.

41. Rolf I. Rolfing® and physical reality. Rochester, VT: Healing Arts Press, 1990.

42. Stillerman E. The encyclopedia of bodywork. New York: Facts on File, 1996.

43. Cottingham JT, Maitland J. A three-paradigm treatment model using soft tissue mobilization and guided movement-awareness techniques for a patient with chronic low back pain: a case study. J Orthop Sports Phys Ther 1997;26(3):155–167.

44. Perry J, Jones MH, Thomas L. Functional evaluation of Rolfing® in cerebral palsy. Dev Med Child Neurol 1981;23(6):717–729.

45. Hunt VV, Massey W. Electromyographic evaluation of structural integration techniques. Sychoenerg Syst 1977;2:1–12.

46. Cottingham JT, Porges SW, Richmond K. Shifts in pelvic inclination angle and parasympathetic tone produced by Rolfing® soft tissue manipulation. Phys Ther 1988;68(9):1364–1370.

47. Cottingham JT, Porges SW, Lyon T. Effects of soft tissue mobilization (Rolfing® pelvic lift) on parasympathetic tone in two age groups. Phys Ther 1988;68(3):352–356.

48. McKechnie AA, Wilson F, Watson N, Scott D. Anxiety states: a preliminary report on the value of connective tissue massage. J Psychosom Res 1983;27(2):125–129.

49. Weinberg RS, Hunt VV. Effects of structural integration on state-trait anxiety. J Clin Psychol 1979;35(2):319–322.

50. Silverman J, Rappaport M, Hopkins HK, et al. Stress, stimulus intensity control, and the structural integration technique. Confin Psychiatr 1973;16:201–219.

51. Reed BV, Held JM. Effects of sequential connective tissue massage on autonomic nervous system of middle-aged and elderly adults. Phys Ther 1988;68(8):1231–1234.

52. Kisner CD, Taslitz N. Connective tissue massage: influence of the introductory treatment on autonomic functions. Phys Ther 1968;48(2):107–119.

53. Kaada B, Torsteinbo O. Increase of plasma beta-endorphins in connective tissue massage. Gen Pharmacol 1989;20(4):487–489.

54. Kaada B, Torsteinbo O. Vasoactive intestinal polypeptides in connective tissue massage. With a note on VIP in heat pack treatment. Gen Pharmacol 1987;18(4):379–384.

55. Gross D. [Physical therapy and rheumatism of soft tissues]. Schweiz Med Wochenschr (German) 1982;112(35):1214–1218. (Abstract)

56. Frazer FW. Persistent post-sympathetic pain treated by connective tissue massage. Physiotherapy 1978;64(7):211–212.

57. Gifford J, Gifford L. Connective tissue massage. In: Wells PE, Frampton V, Bowsher D, eds. Pain management by physiotherapy. 2nd ed. London: Butterworth-Heinemann, 1994:213–227.

58. Holey LA. Connective tissue zones: an introduction. Physiotherapy 1995;81(7):366–368.

59. Holey LA, Walston MJ. Inter-rater reliability of connective tissue zones recognition. Physiotherapy 1995;81(7):369–372.

60. Holey LA. Connective tissue manipulation: towards a scientific rationale. Physiotherapy 1995;81(12):730–739.

61. Michalsen A, Buhring M. [Connective tissue massage]. Wien Klin Wochenschr (German) 1993;105(8):220–7. (Abstract)

62. Goats GC, Keir KA. Connective tissue massage. Br J Sports Med 1991;25(3):131–133.

63. Palastanga N. Connective tissue massage. In: Grieve GP, ed. Modern manual therapy for the vertebral column. New York: Churchill Livingstone, 1986:827–833.

64. Ebner M. Connective tissue massage. Physiotherapy 1978;64(7):208–210.

65. Gonin M, Gerster JC. [Pigmentation disorders in systemic scleroderma] (French). Schweiz Rundsch Med Prax 1994;83(2):42–45. (Abstract).

66. Predel K. [Physical therapy in gastroenterology]. Z Gesamte Inn Med (German) 1987;42(4):112–114. (Abstract)

67. Nansel D, Szlazak M. Somatic dysfunction and the phenomenon of visceral disease simulation: a probable explanation for the apparent effectiveness of somatic therapy in patients presumed to be suffering from true visceral disease. J Manipulative Physiol Ther 1995;18(6):379–397.

68. Kessler RM, Hertling D. Friction massage. In: Hertling D, Kessler RM, eds. Management of common musculoskeletal conditions. 3rd ed. Philadelphia: Lippincott-Raven, 1996: 133–139.

69. Hammer WI. Friction massage. In: Hammer WI. Functional soft tissue examination and treatment by manual methods. 2nd ed. Gaithersburg, MD: Aspen, 1999:463–478.

70. Palastanga N. The use of transverse frictions for soft tissue lesions. In: Grieve GP, ed. Modern manual therapy for the vertebral column. New York: Churchill Livingstone, 1986:819–825.

71. de Brujin R. Deep transverse friction; its analgesic effect. Int J Sports Med 1984;5(suppl):35–36.

72. Cyriax J, Coldham M. Textbook of orthopedic medicine, vol 2. Treatment by manipulation, massage and injection. 11th ed. London: Bailliere-Tindall, 1984.

73. Chamberlain GJ. Cyriax's friction massage: a review. J Orthop Sports Phys Ther 1982;4(1):16–22.

74. Cyriax J. Deep massage. Physiotherapy 1977;63:60–61.

75. Walker JM. Deep transverse frictions in ligament healing. J Orthop Sports Phys Ther 1984;62:89–94.

76. Bajuk S, Jelnikar T, Ortar M. Rehabilitation of patient with brachial plexus lesion and break in axillary artery. Case study. J Hand Ther 1996;9(4):399–403.

77. Nilsson N, Christensen HW, Hartvigsen J. Lasting changes in passive range motion after spinal manipulation: a randomized, blind, controlled trial. J Manipulative Physiol Ther 1996;19(3):165–168.

78. Nilsson N. A randomized controlled trial of the effect of spinal manipulation in the treatment of cervicogenic headache. J Manipulative Physiol Ther 1995;18(7):435–440.

79. O'Sullivan S, Schmitz T. Physical rehabilitation, assessment and treatment. 2nd ed. Philadelphia: FA Davis, 1988.

80. Patino O, Novick C, Merlo A, Benaim F. Massage in hypertrophic scars. J Burn Care Rehabil 1999;20(3):268–271; discussion 267.

81. Sevier TL, Wilson JK. Treating lateral epicondylitis. Sports Med 1999;28(5):375–380.

82. Hammer WI. The use of friction massage in the management of chronic bursitis of the hip or shoulder. J Manipulative Physiol Ther 1993;16(2):107–111.

83. Fritschy D, de Gautard R. Jumper's knee and ultrasonography. Am J Sports Med 1988;16(6):637–640.

84. Hunter SC, Poole RM. The chronically inflamed tendon. Clin Sports Med 1987;6(2):371–388.

85. Woodman RM, Pare L. Evaluation and treatment of soft tissue lesions of the ankle and forefoot using the Cyriax approach. Phys Ther 1982;62(8):1144–1147.

86. Lagrana NA, Alexander H, Strauchler I, et al. Effect of mechanical load in wound healing. Ann Plast Surg 1983;10:200–208.

87. Magonne T, DeWitt MT, Handeley CJ, et al. In vitro responses of chondrocytes to mechanical loading: the effect of short term mechanical tension. Connect Tissue Res 1984;12:97–109.

88. Arem AJ, Madden JW. Effects of stress on healing wounds. I. Intermittent noncyclical tension. J Surg Res 1976;20: 93–102.

89. Woo S, Matthews JV, Akeson WH, et al. Connective tissue response to immobility. Arthritis Rheum 1975;18: 257–264.

90. Akeson WH, Woo SL-Y, Amiel D, et al. The connective tissue response to immobilization: biochemical changes in periarticular connective tissue of the rabbit knee. Clin Orthop 1973;93:356–362.

Suggested Readings

Akeson WH, Amiel D, LaViolette D, et al. The connective tissue response to immobility: an accelerated aging response. Exp Gerontol 1968;3:289–301.

Barnes JF. Myofascial release for craniomandibular pain and dysfunction. Int J Orofac Myol 1996;22:20–22.

Bernau-Eigen M. Rolfing®: A somatic approach to the integration of human structures. Nurse Pract Forum 1998;9(4): 235–242.

Brattberg G. Connective tissue massage in the treatment of fibromyalgia. Eur J Pain. 1999;3(3):235–244.

Crawford JS, Simpson J, Crawford P. Myofascial release provides symptomatic relief from chest wall tenderness occasionally seen following lumpectomy and radiation in breast cancer patients. Int J Radiat Oncol Biol Phys 1996;34(5):1188–1189. (Letter).

Cummings GS, Crutchfield CA, Barnes MR. Soft tissue changes in contractures. Atlanta, GA: Stokesville, 1995.

Davidson CJ, Ganion LR, Gehlsen GM, et al. Rat tendon morphologic and functional changes resulting from soft tissue mobilization. Med Sci Sports Exerc 1997;29(3): 313–319.

Dicke E. Meine Bindegewebsmassage (German). Stuttgart: Hippokrates, 1953.

Dicke E, Schliack H, Wolff A. A manual of reflexive therapy of connective tissue. Scarsdale, NY: Simon, 1978.

Fung YCB. Elasticity of soft tissues in simple elongation. Am J Physiol 1967;213:1532–1544.

Gehlsen GM, Ganion LR, Helfst R. Fibroblast responses to variation in soft tissue mobilization pressure. Med Sci Sports Exerc. 1999;31(4):531–535.

Giese S. Hentz VR. Posterior interosseous syndrome resulting from deep tissue massage. Plastic and Reconstructive Survery. 1998;102(5):1778–1779. (Letter).

Glaser O, Dalicho AW. Segment massage: Massage Reflektorischer Zonen, Verl (German). Leipzig, Germany: Georg Thieme, 1955.

Hardy MA. The biology of scar formation. Phys Ther 1989;69(12):22–32.

Head H. On disturbance of sensation with special reference to the pain of visceral disease. Brain 1893;16:1–133.

Holey LA, Lawler H. The effects of classical massage and connective tissue manipulation on bowel function. Br J Ther Rehabil 1995;2(11):627–631.

Hunter G. Specific soft tissue mobilization in the treatment of soft-tissue lesions. Physiotherapy 1994;30(1):15–21.

Jamison CE, Marangoni RD, Glaser AA. Visco-elastic properties of soft tissue by discrete model characterization. J Biomech 1968;1:33–46.

Kerr HD. Ureteral stent displacement associated with deep massage. Wisconsin Medical Journal. 1997;96(12):57–58.

King RK. Myofascial massage therapy: towards postural balance. Chicago: self-published training manual by Bobkat Productions, 1996.

LaBan MM. Collagen tissue: implications of its response to stress in vitro. Arch Phys Med Rehabil 1962;43:461–466.

Leahy PM. Improved treatments for carpal tunnel. Chiro Sports Med 1995;9:6–9.

Leahy PM, Mock LE. Myofascial release technique and mechanical compromise of peripheral nerves of the upper extremity. Chiro Sports Med 1992;6:139–150.

Lowther DA. The effect of compression and tension on the behavior of connective tissue. In: Glasgow EF, Twomey LT, Scull ER, et al., eds. Aspects of manipulative therapy. 2nd ed. London: Churchill Livingstone, 1985:16–22.

MacKenzie J. Symptoms and their interpretation. London, England: Shaw and Sons, 1909.

Melham TJ, Sevier TL, Malnofski MJ, Wilson JK, Helfst RH Jr. Chronic ankle pain and fibrosis successfully treated with a new noninvasive augmented soft tissue mobilization technique (ASTM): a case report. Med Sci Sports Exerc. 1998;30(6):801–804.

Nilsson N, Christensen HW, Hartvigsen J. The effect of spinal manipulation in the treatment of cervicogenic headache. J Manipulative Physiol Ther 1997;20(5):326–330.

Pellechia GL, Hamel H, Behnke P. Treatment of infrapatellar tendinitis: a combination of modalities and transverse friction massage versus iontophoresis. J Sport Rehabil 1994;3:135–145.

Rigby BJ. The effect of mechanical extension upon the thermal stability of collagen. Biochim Biophys Acta 1964;79:634–636.

Rigby BJ. The mechanical behavior of rat-tail tendon. J Gen Physiol 1959;43:265–283.

Robertson A, Gilmore K, Frith PA, Antic R. Effects of connective tissue massage in subacute asthma. Med J Aust 1984;140(1):52–53. (Letter)

Stromberg DD, Weiderhielm DA. Visco-elastic description of a collagenous tissue in simple elongation. J Appl Physiol 1969;26:857–862.

9

Passive Movement Techniques

*P*assive movement techniques are those massage techniques that primarily palpate the movement of tissues and other structures and use passive motion to treat restrictions in tissue and other structures. These techniques include shaking, rhythmical mobilization, and rocking. This chapter describes each of these techniques, how to perform the technique, and how to apply it in a practice sequence. It also includes a discussion of the indications, contraindications, cautions, outcomes, and postintervention care associated with each technique.

Table 9-1
Summary of Impairment-Level Outcomes of Care for Passive Movement Techniques

Impairment-Level Outcome of Care	Technique		
	Shaking	*Rhythmical Mobilization*	*Rocking*
Systemic sedation	P	P	P
Decreased perceived anxiety	P	P	P
Increased arousal	P	P	–
Counterirritant analgesia	P	P	P
Increased local resting muscle tension or neuromuscular tone	P	–	–
Decreased resting muscle tension	P	P	P
Increased joint mobility	–	P	P
Increased accessory joint motion	–	P	P
Increased rib cage mobility	–	P	P
Increased airway clearance/mobilization of secretions	–	✓	–
Decreased dyspnea	–	P	–
Stimulated peristalsis	P	P	P
Alteration of movement responses	–	✓	✓
Increased ability to perform movement tasks	–	✓	✓

✓, the outcome is supported by research summarized in this or other chapters; P, the outcome is probable; –, nonexistent, negligible, or improbable effects.

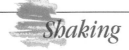
Shaking

OTHER NAMES USED FOR THIS TECHNIQUE

"Muscle shaking," "coarse vibration," "rolling friction," "jostling."[1–8]

DEFINITION

Shaking: Soft tissue—primarily muscle—is repetitively moved back and forth over the underlying bone, with minimal joint movement

NOTES

1. Shaking is sometimes classified as a form of petrissage, since both techniques focus force on skeletal muscle.[3,5] In this book, shaking is presented in a separate chapter from petrissage because the method, effects, and uses differ from those discussed in Chapter 7, Neuromuscular Techniques. In addition, there is a well-established tradition of presenting shaking as a technique in its own right.[6]
2. This book makes a distinction between the shaking of tissue over underlying bone, as defined above, and the shaking of entire structures, such as the rib cage, limbs, and pelvis. The latter technique involves the movement of joints and thus intergrades with more-rigorous joint play techniques (see "Rhythmical Mobilization" and "Rocking" below in this chapter). The manual technique, effects, and uses of these techniques are sufficiently different to justify this distinction.

CLINICAL INDICATIONS AND IMPAIRMENT-LEVEL OUTCOMES OF CARE

Traditionally, the literature has stated that shaking may alter resting muscle tone through the stimulation of complex proprioceptive reflexes.[1,2,4,7] Shaking was thought to have a relaxing effect on skeletal muscle,[1,2,4,7] except for vigorous shaking, which might temporarily and marginally increase muscle tone via the stretch reflex.[6] A recent review of the literature concluded, however, that it may not be possible for any passive technique, such as shaking, to substantially alter muscle tone and that active techniques are far more potent in this regard.[9]

Shaking has a variety of clinical applications. It can be an effective approach to reducing "holding," or psychodynamic tension,[4,7] either as a goal in itself or to prepare for the use of techniques, such as high-grade joint play, in which increased muscular tension may interfere with the execution of the technique. Shaking can be regarded by clients as pleasurable and is useful when the clinician is seeking to achieve fully relaxed skeletal muscle. Shaking is commonly used in precompetition and intercompetition sports massage because of its effects of systemic arousal and enhanced awareness and its possible temporary effect on resting muscle tension.[10–12] Finally, shaking has minor mechanical effects on connective tissue.[7] If applied gently in the fibroplastic stage of connective tissue repair, it may facilitate orderly remodeling of connective tissue. The main impairment-level outcomes of care for shaking are summarized in Table 9-1.

CAUTIONS AND CONTRAINDICATIONS

Clinical training and supervised practice are critical for the proper application of shaking. Advanced training may be advisable in certain situations, particularly when dealing with pathological conditions. All of the general and local contraindications noted for massage techniques apply to the use of shaking (see Chapter 2, The Clinical Decision-Making Process).[13] In particular, the clinician should avoid shaking any muscle that contains an acute injury, even if the hand position is remote from the site of injury. Less-vigorous shaking may be introduced at later stages, provided that it can be performed without causing the client pain. In addition, the use of shaking is contraindicated when the client exhibits spasm, hyperreflexia, or spasticity.

Prerequisite Skills for Shaking

Before shaking tissue over bone, students should be able to

Describe the spatial relationship between bones and major groups of skeletal muscle throughout the body

Specify the fiber direction and spatial relationships of major skeletal muscles

Differentiate by palpation subcutaneous fat and fascia, muscle, tendon, ligament, and bone

Palpate the fiber directions, borders, and tendons of superficial muscles

Assess resting muscle tension

Detect involuntary "holding" of skeletal muscles in response to passive movement

Use all aligned and leaning postures

(See Chapter 3, Review of Client Examination Concepts for Massage, and Chapter 4, Preparation and Positioning for Treatment.)

Manual Technique begins on page 280

MANUAL TECHNIQUE

Shaking

In the following figures (Figs. 9-1 to 9-8), shaking is applied to the various regions of the body. Figures are ordered from head to foot in supine and then prone. Each figure illustrates most of the guidelines for manual technique outlined below.

1. Shaking muscle over underlying bone can have a psychologically sedative or stimulating effect depending on the contact and rate of application the clinician uses when performing the technique.

   A. For sedation: Use an even and relaxed, full palmar contact and a slower rate. Hand contact is flat on flat surfaces of the client's body (Figs. 9-1 and 9-4). In this case, a relaxed hand contact that produces minimal tissue compression will result in the freest tissue excursion. The hand is slightly arched for curved surfaces of the client's body, since this lifts the client's tissues into the palm (Figs. 9-3 and 9-5). The client should perceive the pressure as being evenly distributed over the entire contact surface (not an easy effect to achieve). For each stroke, the hand lifts the client's tissues and then allows them to drop under their own weight. Hand contact is maintained without any break in contact and the strokes are connected. It takes practice to perform this technique with the full, comfortable contact that allows the clinician to apply it for longer periods.

   B. For a stimulating effect: The clinician focuses contact more specifically on the thumb and fingertips (Fig. 9-6), uses more pressure for the stroke, increases the rate, and makes a continuous effort to move the tissues back and forth rather than allowing gravity to perform the return stroke.

2. Wrist(s) remain relaxed as the hand(s) move back and forth rhythmically. On the client's limbs, hands move perpendicular to the long axis of the limb to produce waves of tissue motion that travel along, or parallel to, the long axis of the limb.

3. To achieve movement throughout a region, the hands use a lighter contact and slide along the region as the clinician performs shaking (Figs. 9-6 and 9-7). Alternatively, hand contact can be released every few seconds, the hand moved to a new position in the region, and new hand contact established. Changing hand positions every few seconds can reduce hand strain and results in a stroke that the client may perceive as being more pleasant and less "machine-like."

4. When shaking is performed with two hands, different approaches to coordinating the movement of the hands will produce differing results (Figs. 9-2, 9-5, and 9-8).

5. "Rolling," or "rolling friction,"[2] is a useful two-handed version of shaking that can be performed on the client's limbs. Hands rest on opposite sides of the limb. Both hands work together to roll the client's tissues around the circumference of the long axis of the limb, as one would roll the cylinder of a rolling pin around its core. Hands then simultaneously reverse their direction of movement, rolling the tissue back to, and then past, its original position. The hands repeat these two motions in a rhythmical manner (Figs. 9-2 and 9-8).

6. Shaking can be combined with neuromuscular techniques by compressing into the client's tissues or by gripping and lifting these tissues before beginning the shaking motion.

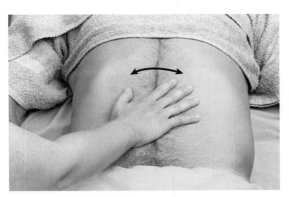

Figure 9-1. This superficial shaking of the abdomen does not cause movement of the pelvis or spine (compare with Figure 9-10.) All types of abdominal shaking can be useful for constipation.

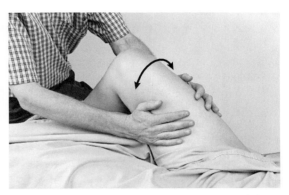

Figure 9-2. Two-handed shaking of the entire thigh with the knee flexed. Hands work together, rolling the tissue around the bone, first one way and then back to, and past, resting position. Varying amounts of compression can be added to produce a more forceful and stimulating stroke.

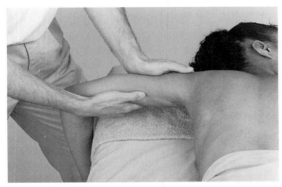

Figure 9-3. When shaking the deltoid, first lift the arm off the table to permit free movement of the client's tissues. If a client involuntary tenses her arm, the clinician draws her awareness to the tension and waits until the shoulder relaxes before beginning the shaking.

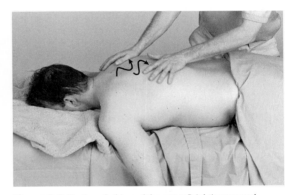

Figure 9-4. During shaking of the superficial tissues and muscles of the back, the two hands can be moved in the same, or in opposite, directions.

Manual Technique Figures continue on page 283

Components of Shaking

Contact: Whole relaxed palmar surface; variable levels of fingertip contact can be used depending on the degree of stimulation desired

Pressure: Light to moderate; constant heavy manual pressure damps the wave of motion that is produced through tissues and should be avoided

Tissues engaged: Hands engage as deep as the superficial muscle layers; the motion produced by the stroke simultaneously engages all the tissues throughout the body segment that is being shaken (for example, muscle, fascia, tendon, ligament, and periosteum)

Direction: Clinician's force is directed around the circumference of the long axis of the body segment; the motion produced by the stroke travels in waves along this long axis

Amplitude: Depends on the region

Rate: 2 to 5 cycles per second

Duration: 5 sec or longer

Intergrades[a] with: Fine vibration

Combined with: Can be combined with broad or specific compression to produce techniques that intergrade with petrissage

Context: Can be alternated with other techniques presented in this chapter in interventions that focus solely on movement; this technique can also be alternated with neuromuscular techniques (see Chapter 7, Neuromuscular Techniques).

[a]To merge gradually one into another.

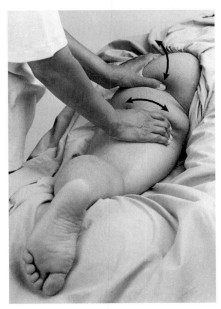

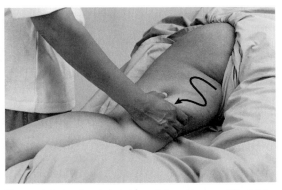

Figure 9-5. Shaking of the gluteals can be done one-handed or two-handed and can simultaneously include the proximal hamstrings. Each hand shakes cross-fiber.

Figure 9-6. One-handed shaking of the adductors of the thigh in prone. The clinician may release and regrasp or may maintain a loose grasp while shaking the client's limb and gliding distally to the knee *(arrow)*.

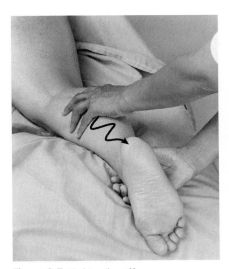

Figure 9-7. Shaking the calf.

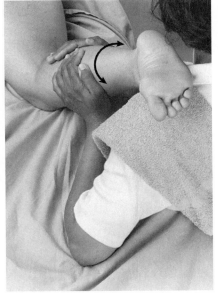

Figure 9-8. This two-handed "rolling" technique for the calf is also possible in supine (position as in Fig. 9-2).

CLINICIAN'S POSITION AND MOVEMENT

1. The basic positions used by the clinician are described in Chapter 4, Preparation and Positioning for Treatment, in the sections on standing aligned posture. The clinician can avoid producing a choppy, irritating stroke by keeping the wrist, elbows, and shoulders relaxed.
2. When the clinician is performing shaking for longer than 30 sec, a relaxed posture can be maintained by periodically standing back to briefly shake out the arms and hands.

PALPATE

While performing the technique, the clinician palpates the client's skin and tissues for the following:

1. The local skin temperature and texture.
2. The tone of the client's superficial muscles and tissues.
3. The excursion of the tissue that is being shaken. The clinician tries to form an impression of how far and how easily the tissues move during the application of the technique. In particular, she identifies how loose, dense, or tight the tissues feel under hand and how this relates to the motion of the tissues.
4. Resistance to tissue movement. The clinician notes whether there is any resistance as the slack is taken out of the tissues. She also notes whether the resistance to movement can be related to a specific tissue or structure that is involved in producing the motion of the stroke. For example, an adhesion at the proximal hamstring attachment can have a visible and palpable effect on the motion of the entire hamstring muscle during shaking.
5. The rhythmic response or cadence of the client's tissue during the stroke. Often, there is a rate and amplitude of shaking that the client finds the most pleasant. This varies with the person, body structure, level of muscle tone, region, and the type of shaking that is being used. It is critical, especially if sedation is the desired effect, to palpate for this optimal cadence and to adjust the rate and amplitude of the stroke to the client's needs.
6. The depth of penetration of the effect of the stroke. As the client's muscles relax and the fluid viscosity of the tissues decreases, the same force will produce effects deeper into and further along the client's tissues. Consequently, as with petrissage, it does not require greater force to achieve a greater penetration of effects, simply the appropriate application of the technique for longer durations.

OBSERVE

As she performs the technique, the clinician observes the client for the degree of muscle movement achieved and to ensure that draping maintains privacy. The signs listed below may signal this.

1. The degree of muscle movement. Movement of the client's muscles will be visibly less within areas of connective tissue hardening and elevated resting muscle tension. Even in normal tissue, movement will vary substantially with different body shapes, proportions of body fat, and levels of conditioning.
2. Inappropriate draping. Since extended shaking can loosen draping, the clinician may need to adjust or retuck a loosened drape to maintain discreet coverage of the client's body.

COMMUNICATION WITH THE CLIENT

The clinician uses communication that ensures the client's comfort during the application of shaking. Some examples of statements that the clinician can use are listed below.

1. "Is this pressure perfectly comfortable?" Or offer the client a choice: "Which feels better: this . . . or this?" The clinician ensures that hand contact is comfortable for the client.
2. "Would it feel more relaxing if I slowed down a bit . . . like this?" Determine whether the rate and rhythm are comfortable for the client.
3. "Is everything OK?" "Are you feeling anything unusual?" When applying shaking continuously for longer than 2 min, the clinician ascertains whether the client is experiencing unpleasant symptoms of sympathetic arousal, such as irritation or nausea.
4. "Is this causing pain anywhere?" The clinician can use this statement to periodically check whether the client perceives that the intervention is causing pain. When the client presents with spasm or inflammation, the application of shaking to a distant area may result in pain by producing small motions at a distance from the point of contact.

OTHER APPROPRIATE TECHNIQUES

There are several modalities that the clinician can use in a complementary manner with shaking. Of note are joint play or passive relaxed movements, since shaking is an excellent precursor to the use of these techniques.

POSTINTERVENTION SELF-CARE

1. The clinician can instruct the client in methods of self-administering shaking to accessible areas of the body, such as the arms and legs.
2. Active shaking movements of the limbs may also

achieve muscle relaxation and facilitate ease of motion.[24]

See the practice sequence for shaking and rhythmical mobilization.

Rhythmical Mobilization

OTHER NAMES USED FOR THIS TECHNIQUE

"Shaking."[6]

DEFINITION

Rhythmical mobilization: Entire structures are repetitively moved, resulting in the movement of soft tissue over bone and the movement of the related joints and internal organs

NOTES

1. Rhythmical mobilization involves the repetitive passive movement of entire structures—usually a limb, a part of a limb, or the limb girdle—and all of the tissues that the treated body segment contains. At times, rhythmical mobilization may resemble passive relaxed movements or joint play/mobilization techniques, both of which are covered extensively in other textbooks. The technique of rhythmical mobilization is, however, less specific than joint play or passive relaxed movements. For example, when treating areas around synovial joints, the movements of rhythmical mobilization are not isolated to anatomical planes, the joint capsule, or even to a single joint; in addition, they are performed in the midrange rather than through the full osteokinematic range of the joint being treated.

CLINICAL INDICATIONS AND IMPAIRMENT-LEVEL OUTCOMES OF CARE

Some of the clinical indications and impairment-level outcomes of care for rhythmical mobilization are similar to those for shaking, described above in this chapter. Like shaking, rhythmical mobilization can be used to reduce holding and muscle tension, to prepare the client for joint play or passive range-of-motion techniques, and in precompetition preparation for athletes. Since rhythmical mobilization results in passive joint motion, it may

produce some of the effects of more-rigorous passive range exercises, such as the mobilization of stiff joints, the stimulation of joint healing, and neuromuscular re-education.[14–19] The repeated approximation and distraction of the joint surfaces that occur during the application of this technique may be used to enhance a client's joint awareness.[20] When it is used in the context of Trager Psychophysical Integration,® rhythmical mobilization may also be of use in the treatment of neurological conditions that alter movement patterns, such as cerebral palsy, muscular dystrophy, and multiple sclerosis.[21–22] Shaking of the rib cage, alternated with rapid repeated compression, percussion ("cupping" or "clapping"), and postural drainage is a standard intervention for mobilizing bronchial secretions in chest physical therapy[6] (see Chapter 10, Percussive Techniques). Finally, rhythmical mobilization may stimulate vestibular reflexes and result in a generalized decrease in postural tone, decreased arousal, and a calming, soothing effect.[9,20]

The main impairment-level outcomes of care for rhythmical mobilization are summarized in Table 9-1.

CAUTIONS AND CONTRAINDICATIONS

Clinical training and supervised practice are critical for the proper application of rhythmical mobilization. Advanced training may be advisable in certain situations, particularly when dealing with pathological conditions. All of the general and local contraindications noted for massage techniques apply to the use of rhythmical mobilization (see Chapter 2, The Clinical Decision-Making Process).[13] These contraindications include metastatic cancer, acute nerve impingement or disk rupture, severe carotid artery disease, use of anticoagulant therapy, and high-risk pregnancies.[21] The clinician should consider a flail chest, fractured or brittle ribs, and recent chest or spinal surgery contraindications to the application of the technique to the rib cage for mobilizing bronchial secretions.[6] Avoid performing rhythmical mobilization on, or adjacent to, the site of acute orthopedic injuries;[21] although the technique may be introduced at later stages of recovery provided that it can be performed without causing the client pain. When clients present with spasm, hyperreflexia, and spasticity, rhythmical mobilization must be applied with reduced force and great sensitivity. Generally, the client's hands and feet can often be moved quite vigorously; elsewhere, however, rhythmical mobilization should be performed at a moderate rate, since it may be intolerably stimulating to the client if it is performed too rapidly. It should not be used when a client suffers from vertigo or motion sickness.[21]

Prerequisite Skills for Rhythmical Mobilization

Before applying rhythmical mobilization, students should be able to

Describe the spatial relationship between bones and major groups of skeletal muscle throughout the body

Describe the agonist, antagonist, and synergist relationships for the joints of the extremities

Describe, measure, and palpate passive osteokinematic movements for all the joints and articulations of the extremities

Detect involuntary "holding" of skeletal muscles in response to passive movement

Use all aligned and leaning postures

(See Chapter 3, Review of Client Examination Concepts for Massage, and Chapter 4, Preparation and Positioning for Treatment.)

Manual Technique begins on page 288

MANUAL TECHNIQUE

Rhythmical Mobilization

In the following figures (Figs. 9-9 to 9-17), rhythmical mobilization is applied to the various regions of the body. Figures are ordered from head to foot in supine and then prone.

1. Hand contact must be comfortable for both the clinician and the client. Hand contact is full and relaxed and uses as much of the hand as possible (Figs. 9-9 to 9-17). Hand position for optimal manual contact will vary with the region of the client's body, the size of the clinician's hands, and the size of the client's body.

2. The clinician strives to maintain an uninterrupted rhythmical flow of movement, even when switching positions and techniques.

3. Rhythmical mobilization has widely distributed mechanical effects and can, therefore, easily become too stimulating for the client. Consequently, the clinician aims to perform the technique with a relaxed tempo that will produce reflex sedation. This requires that the hands maintain contact throughout the motion, while allowing the freest excursion of movement of the body segment being treated. An exception to this is when the clinician is shaking the client's hand or foot briskly for brief periods.

4. The variety of possible rhythmical movements is limited only by the clinician's imagination. Some examples of these variations are listed below.

   A. To mobilize an entire limb from its distal end with the client in prone or supine: the hands assume a very comfortable two-handed grip of the client's wrist or ankle. The clinician simultaneously exerts a gentle traction on the client's limb and lifts it so that it clears the table. Then the clinician immediately performs one or two gentle shaking motions, using the same motion used to initiate vertical waves along a rope. The client's limb will look and feel like a weighted rope during this maneuver, provided that neither too much nor too little traction is used (Fig. 9-10). Traction on the limb is released between repetitions of this technique.

   B. For proximal limb segments, such as the entire shoulder, with the client in prone or supine, or the thigh, with the client in supine: hands are positioned between the client's limb and the table. Hands lift the client's limb segment and let it drop (Figs. 9-13 and 9-15). This maneuver can be repeated as needed.

   C. To roll the upper arm with the client in prone or the thigh with the client in supine: hands roll the client's limb back and forth over the table surface. The clinician may also lift and swing the client's proximal arm (Fig. 9-16) or roll the dependent forearm (Fig. 9-17).

   D. To bounce or swing the proximal limb segment: hands grasp the client's hand with the client in supine or the client's foot with the client in prone. The clinician bends the client's elbow or knee, and bounces the proximal section of the client's limb on the table or swings that limb segment through the air.

   E. To shake or roll the client's entire hand or foot: two hands grasp and briskly shake or roll the client's hand or foot (Figs. 9-11 and 9-14). Individual digits can be shaken or rolled in this manner. These nonspecific mobilizations are useful ways to wake sleeping clients.

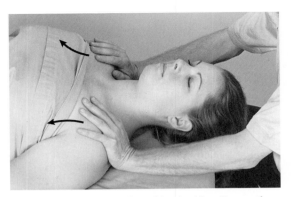

Figure 9-9. Rhythmical settling of the shoulders. Depress the client's shoulder girdle and then allow the shoulders to rebound passively while maintaining hand contact. If the hands depress the shoulders simultaneously, the shoulders bounce up and down. If the hands alternately depress the shoulders, a lateral rocking results.

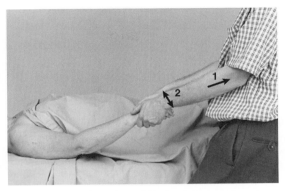

Figure 9-10. Gentle traction, which the clinician produces by leaning backward, precedes longitudinal shaking of the arm. This technique is performed in the same manner as shaking a rope along its length; it must be done gently and not sustained beyond one or two movements before releasing traction, and reapplying. A similar technique can be applied to the leg.

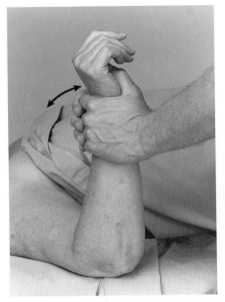

Figure 9-11. Shaking of the entire hand can be vigorous. The illustrated contact allows the clinician to control the flexion/extension movement at the client's wrist.

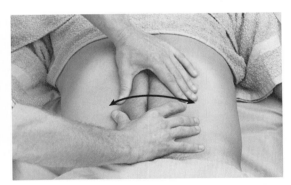

Figure 9-12. Here, the rectus abdominus is gently gathered and lifted off the deeper muscles with a soft, broad contact. The hands maintain this contact, using it to slowly sway the client's abdomen back and forth.

Manual Technique Figures continue on page 291

Components of Rhythmical Mobilization

Contact: Whole palmar surface of one or both hands; hands as relaxed as possible

Pressure: Moderate, enough to securely lift or move the body segment

Tissues engaged: Hands engage at least as deep as the superficial muscle layers

The motion produced by the stroke simultaneously engages all the joint tissues and soft tissues in the region that is being mobilized

Direction: Varies depending on the region being treated; often a body segment is repeatedly lifted or moved and allowed to drop or settle under the force of gravity

Amplitude: Depends on the region

Rate: 0.5 to 2 sec per cycle

Duration: 5 sec or longer

Intergrades with: Shaking, passive range of motion, joint play, and manual traction

Combined with: May be combined with broad-contact compression and muscle squeezing

Context: Can be alternated with other techniques presented in this chapter in interventions that focus solely on movement; this technique often precedes or follows neuromuscular techniques (see Chapter 7, Neuromuscular Techniques).

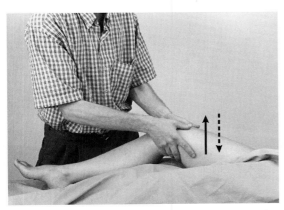

Figure 9-13. The thigh is lifted and then allowed to fall rhythmically *(dotted line)*. The hands can slide distally to deliver the lifting force to the lower leg as well.

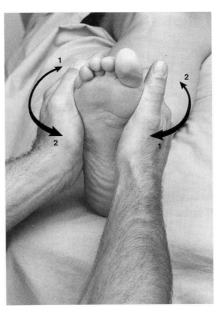

Figure 9-14. Wrists and hands remain loose while rolling the client's entire foot briskly between the hands (two to three cycles per second). This pleasant stroke is a gentle, effective way to rouse sleeping clients.

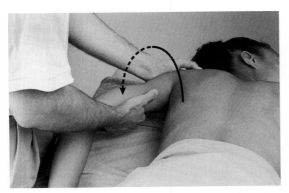

Figure 9-15. "Tossing" the shoulder rhythmically and repetitively. Hands maintain contact as the client's shoulders are allowed to fall back to the table under their own weight *(dotted line)*. Hands may use a gentle force to distract the shoulder as it is being lifted.

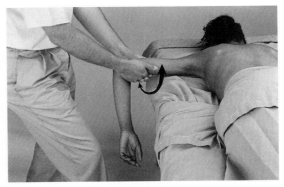

Figure 9-16. Swinging the dependent arm in prone: Rhythmical passive internal and external rotation performed in the midrange of abduction.

Manual Technique Figures continue on next page

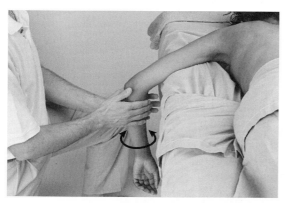

Figure 9-17. Rolling the dependent forearm between the hands. Hand contact slides proximally and distally on the forearm to focus the movement on different areas.

CLINICIAN'S POSITION AND MOVEMENT

1. The basic positions used by the clinician are described throughout Chapter 4, Preparation and Positioning for Treatment.

2. Since a variety of movements are performed during the application of rhythmical mobilization, the clinician must be able to use the full range of mechanically efficient postures.

PALPATE

As she performs the technique, the clinician palpates the client's skin and tissues for the qualities noted below. In doing so, attention is focused primarily on the qualities of the motion she produces with the technique and on the resistance of the client's tissues to movement. The clinician aims to palpate—simultaneously and from a distance—the different tissues and structures that influence the movement produced. Diligent practice on the clinician's part is required to refine awareness of tissue resistance to movement.

1. The local skin temperature and texture.
2. The tone of the client's superficial muscles and tissues.
3. The movement of the joints being shaken. The clinician tries to form an impression of the quality of the motion of the limb or segment as a whole and of the constituent joints. In addition, she notes how the

resistance varies throughout the available range of the induced motion.

4. Resistance to tissue or joint movement. The clinician determines whether the resistance to movement can be related to a specific tissue or structure that is involved in producing the motion of the stroke. For example, hypertonicity in one of the client's scapular stabilizers will have a visible and palpable effect on the manner in which the entire shoulder moves when the upper arm is swung or rolled on the table.

5. The rhythmic response or cadence of the client's tissue during the stroke. Even more so than with shaking, for any given rhythmical movement, the client will have a rate and amplitude that is perceived to be the most pleasant.[23] This varies with the person, body structure, level of muscle tone, region, and the type of rhythmical mobilization that is being used. It is critical, to ensure sedation and avoid the unpleasant effects of sympathetic arousal, to palpate for this optimal cadence and to adjust the rate and amplitude of the stroke to the client's needs.

6. The depth of penetration of the effect of the stroke. As the client's muscles relax and the fluid viscosity of the tissues decreases, the same force will produce effects deeper into, and further along, the client's tissues. Consequently, as with petrissage, it does not require greater force to achieve a greater penetration of effects, simply the appropriate application of the technique for longer periods.

OBSERVE

As she performs the technique, the clinician observes the client for the degree of muscle movement achieved and to maintain privacy. The signs listed below may signal this.

1. How the stroke moves from the points of contact to adjacent areas of the client's body. This observation can provide information about the level of function of intervening tissues and joints; for example, when shaking the client's entire leg with traction, the clinician observes how the lumbar and thoracic spine respond.
2. The degree of muscle movement. Movement of the client's muscles will be visibly less within areas of connective tissue hardening and elevated resting muscle tension. Even in normal tissue, movement will vary substantially with different body shapes and proportions of body fat.
3. Inappropriate draping. Since rhythmical mobilization can loosen draping, the clinician may need to adjust or retuck a loosened drape to maintain discreet coverage of the client's body.

COMMUNICATION WITH THE CLIENT

The clinician uses communication to ensure the client's comfort during the application of rhythmical mobilization. Some examples of statements that the clinician can use are listed below.

1. "Is this hand position comfortable?" Or offer the client a choice: "Which feels better, this . . . or this?" The clinician ensures that hand contact is comfortable for the client.
2. "Would it feel more relaxing if I slowed down a bit . . . like this?" "Is this motion comfortable, or is the movement too great?" Determine whether the rate and amplitude of motion are comfortable for the client.
3. "Is everything OK?" "Are you feeling anything unusual?" When applying rhythmical mobilization continuously for longer than 2 min, the clinician ascertains whether the client is experiencing un-

pleasant symptoms of sympathetic arousal, such as irritation or nausea.
4. "Is this causing pain anywhere?" The clinician can use this statement to periodically check whether the client perceives that the intervention is resulting in pain. When the client presents with spasm or inflammation, the application of rhythmical mobilization to a distant area may result in pain by producing small motions at a distance from the point of contact.

OTHER APPROPRIATE TECHNIQUES

There are several modalities that the clinician can use in a complementary manner with rhythmical mobilization.

1. Rhythmical mobilization is a useful precursor to the use of traction, joint play, or passive relaxed movement techniques. The clinician should match the vigor of the stroke to the level of acuity of the client's condition.
2. When rhythmical mobilization is being used to facilitate the mobilization of bronchial secretions, the clinician can use postural drainage, steam inhalation, forced expiration, and coughing techniques in a complementary manner.
3. Related movement interventions that may be of use are body mechanics and ergonomics training; breathing exercises; gait, locomotion, and balance training; neuromuscular training; and posture-awareness training.[8]

POSTINTERVENTION SELF-CARE:

1. The clinician can instruct the client in methods of self-administering passive relaxed movements to accessible areas of the body, such as the arms and legs (self-mobilization).
2. Active shaking movements of the limbs may also achieve muscle relaxation and facilitate ease of motion.[24]
3. The clinician can instruct the client in the use of postural drainage, steam inhalation, forced expiration, and coughing techniques to facilitate the mobilization of bronchial secretions.

A Practice Sequence for Shaking and Rhythmical Mobilization

Practice time: 15 to 30 min per person or longer

This sequence for anterior and posterior aspects of the legs uses no oil. It can easily be performed through loose clothes or draping, although the techniques are somewhat easier to apply on bare skin.

There are two basic ways of approaching movement sequences. One is to perform each technique in the sequence once for a longer period of time. An alternative, which tends to reduce clinician fatigue and tension, is to introduce all movements quickly, then alternate frequently from one technique to the next, repeating the sequence as time permits.

Strive for smooth continuous motion with no breaks between the various moves. Explore each motion and the infinite number of variations that are possible.

Supine

1. Shake the quadriceps over the femur, then shake the adductors.
2. Flex the client's knee to 90 degrees, sit on the foot, and roll the thigh over the femur before returning the leg to the table.
3. Repeatedly lift the thigh and let it drop while working down the leg to the heel (be careful not to hyperextend the knee).
4. Flex and extend the knee rhythmically in the midrange of the available joint range of motion.
5. With heel-of-hand contacts just proximal to both malleoli shake the whole foot. Gently circumduct the ankle.
6. Grasp the foot, lift it, and apply gentle traction to the leg prior to shaking it.
7. Apply gentle traction to each toe prior to shaking it.

Repeat this sequence two or more times.

Turn client to prone.

8. Shake the gluteals over the pelvis with one or two hands.
9. Flex the client's knee; shake the hamstrings and adductors over the femur; shake the muscles of the posterior compartment.
10. Holding the ankle with two hands, flex knee to 90 degrees, lift the thigh off the table, and swing the entire leg from side to side.
11. Rest the ankle on the clinician's shoulder and roll the muscles of the posterior compartment between two palms.
12. With the knee flexed to 90 degrees, grasp the heel and shake the entire foot.
13. Grasp the foot, lift it, and apply gentle traction to the leg prior to shaking it.
14. Plantarflex and dorsiflex the ankle passively.

Repeat this sequence two or more times.

For home study: Devise a comparable supine and prone sequence for the arm.

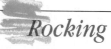

Rocking

OTHER NAMES USED FOR THIS TECHNIQUE

"Pelvic rocking," "rocking vibration."[1–7]

DEFINITION

Rocking: Gentle, repetitive oscillation of the pelvis or torso that is achieved by pushing the pelvis or torso from a midline resting position into lateral deviation and then allowing it to return to resting position. This repetitive movement results in waves of motion that are propagated along the body.

NOTES

1. Rocking is a form of rhythmical mobilization that results in a lateral motion of the body, especially of the pelvis and lumbar spine. The distinctive elements of the manual technique of rocking and the technique's reflex effects merit an independent description.

2. While the effects of this type of motion have been known to every mother (and child) since time immemorial,[25–27] there is little documentation of a rocking technique prior to the latter part of the 20th century.

CLINICAL INDICATIONS AND IMPAIRMENT-LEVEL OUTCOMES OF CARE

Rocking may produce a generalized decrease in postural tone and arousal as a result of stimulation of vestibular reflexes.[20] When it is performed with skill, rocking has a profoundly sedative effect; for that reason alone, this technique is worth mastering.[9,20] As a result of its sedative effect, rocking can be useful in the treatment of stress-related autonomic dysfunction; generalized elevation of skeletal muscle tone; psychodynamic "holding"; insomnia; and mental, physical, or emotional fatigue. Furthermore, rocking motions are often intuitively used to calm infants and can be incorporated into baby massage for this reason.[25–27] It may also be of value in the treatment of a variety of chronic low-back disorders in which clients present with muscular tension, provided that the client is able to tolerate the motion of the technique.[21] Finally, the sedative effect of rocking can also be used to indirectly reduce the client's perception of pain. The main impairment-level outcomes of care for rocking are summarized in Table 9-1.

CAUTIONS AND CONTRAINDICATIONS

Clinical training and supervised practice are critical for the proper application of rocking. Advanced training may be advisable in certain situations, particularly when dealing with pathological conditions. All of the general and local contraindications previously noted for massage techniques and for rhythmical mobilization apply to the use of rocking (see Chapter 2, The Clinical Decision-Making Process).[13] Rocking sets the entire body in motion; therefore, it is contraindicated or should be used with a reduced amplitude of motion for any condition in which pain is exacerbated by movement. The effects of rocking vary with the manner in which the technique is performed and the duration for which it is used. If rocking is performed abruptly or too fast it can quickly produce unpleasant effects like nausea. It should not be used when a client suffers from vertigo or motion sickness.[21] If rocking is used for long periods in the intervention (i.e., more than 10 minutes), it can induce a combination of deep relaxation and mild disorientation in the client that may temporarily reduce competence to perform physical tasks, such as driving. In this situation, the clinician must ensure that the client is capable of functioning before she allows him to leave. If there is any doubt about the client's capabilities, the clinician can return the client to the table; apply some deep, specific petrissage to the soles of the feet; and let him rest for 10 to 20 min before reassessing level of mental function.

Prerequisite Skills for Rocking

Before applying rocking, students should be able to

Describe the movements of the lumbar and thoracic vertebrae

Assess active movement of the spine and pelvis

Assess and track autonomic function

Detect involuntary "holding" of skeletal muscles in response to passive movement

Use standing upright, lunge, and lunge and lean postures

(See Chapter 3, Review of Client Examination Concepts for Massage, and Chapter 4, Preparation and Positioning for Treatment.)

Manual Technique begins on next page

MANUAL TECHNIQUE

Rocking

In the following figures (Figs. 9-18 to 9-24C), rocking is applied to the various regions of the body. Figures are ordered from head to foot in supine and then prone. Each figure illustrates most of the guidelines for manual technique outlined below.

1. If the client can tolerate lying prone without lumbar support, remove the abdominal pillow, since its presence will significantly dampen the motion produced during rocking. Even clients with back pain, who typically require an abdominal pillow when they are prone, may be able to tolerate lying with an increased lordosis as long as the rocking motion continues. The clinician will need to replace the abdominal pillow following application of rocking. A similar situation exists for the use of pillows under the client's knees in supine.

2. Hand contact is relaxed, whole-hand contact with the fingers spread so that pressure is evenly distributed over the contact surface of the hand (Figs. 9-18, 9-19, and 9-22 to 9-23B).

3. The clinician gently pushes the pelvis or torso laterally from the midline resting position in supine (Figs. 9-18 to 9-21) or in prone (Figs. 9-22 to 9-24)—a motion that raises the center of gravity of the client's body. The client's body is then allowed to fall back toward the midline passively; momentum will carry it past the resting position. Precisely at the end of the excursion of the motion of the pelvis or torso, the clinician repeats the application of the same pressure and pushes the client's pelvis or torso past the midline once more. Ideally, rocking consists of a seamlessly interconnected series of pushes and releases (falls) that produce a continuous oscillation of the client's body, with the maximum amplitude of the motion occurring around the client's iliac crest.

4. Although it is preferable to maintain contact during the passive "return stroke," this must be done without impeding the natural "falling" of the body back toward and through the resting position.

5. The clinician times the initiation of each push so that the rocking motion produced is smooth and the client is scarcely aware of the clinician's hand pressure and the point during the motion at which it is applied.

6. Hands change position approximately every 10 sec to avoid producing a motion with a mechanical feel. Hands slide easily from one contact position to another without interrupting the regular rhythm, thus moving the point of contact up and down the client's body.

7. As the application of rocking proceeds and the client relaxes, the clinician will often note an increase in amplitude of the rocking motion and a decreased rate, with little increase in the force applied.

8. Hands may also be positioned where they may alternately push and pull the client's body to generate the rocking motion (Fig. 9-24C). However, since this approach eliminates the passive return of the client's body to its resting position, it is more likely to be inharmonious with the body's natural rhythm and to produce a stroke that is less effective or perceived as unpleasant by the client.

9. It is useful to intersperse rocking with gentle long-axis traction of the legs; this enhances the incremental lengthening of the spine that can result from longer applications of rocking.

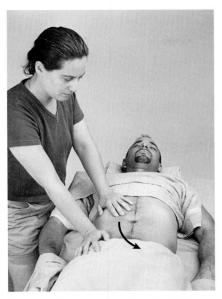

Figure 9-18. Rocking in supine with hand contact on the lower ribs and anterior superior iliac spines.

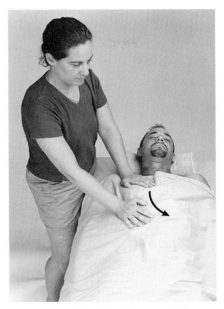

Figure 9-19. As hand contact moves farther from the pelvis, the rocking motion naturally becomes attenuated. In this situation, the rocking motion can be maintained by using upper and lower rib hand contacts.

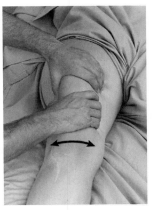

Figure 9-20. Rocking can also be initiated after gently lifting a large muscle mass, such as the quadriceps, hamstrings, or gluteals. The cadence at which rocking can be performed will be dictated by the passive response of the pelvis.

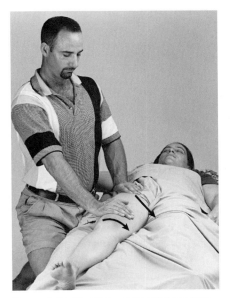

Figure 9-21. The thigh can be rolled into internal rotation while the rocking motion is maintained from the anterior superior iliac spines.

Manual Technique Figures continue on page 299

Components of Rocking

Contact: Entire palmar surface

Pressure: Light to moderate

Tissues engaged: Hands engage as deep as the superficial muscle layers; the motion produced by the stroke simultaneously engages all the tissues throughout the body segments that are being rocked (for example, muscle, fascia, tendon, ligament, and periosteum)

Direction: Clinician's force is directed so that a lateral deviation of the pelvis and or spine from midline is produced; the resulting motion is propagated along the client's body

Amplitude and length: Lateral deviation may reach 10 cm or more from midline, depending on the length of application of the technique and the client's body size and type

Rate: 1 to 2 sec per cycle

Duration: 60 sec to 15+ min

Intergrades with: Passive range of motion and joint play techniques

Combined with: May be combined with compression

Context: May be used alone for sedation; commonly used at the beginning or end of longer sequences that employ other techniques

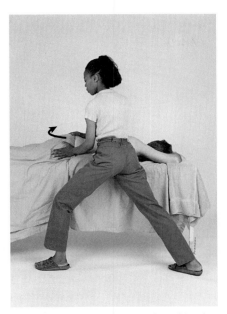

Figure 9-22. Basic hand contact for rocking the back. Hands are placed on the sacrum and the greater trochanter. The clinician directs the force of the motion distally, to produce lumbar traction, and toward the client's contralateral knee. With each stroke, the clinician produces a lateral displacement of the client's pelvis, then allows the pelvis to fall back past the midline without breaking hand contact. The aim is to produce a succession of seamlessly interconnected strokes.

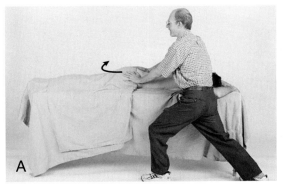

Figure 9-23. A. Hand contact may be varied to different positions as the rocking motion is maintained. Here, the gluteals are gently stretched distally off their superior iliac attachments with the clinician's left hand.

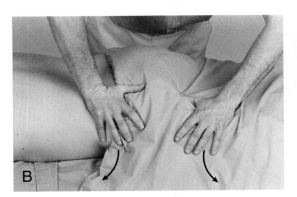

Figure 9-23 (continued). B. Here the gluteals are pushed away from the sacrum with both hands.

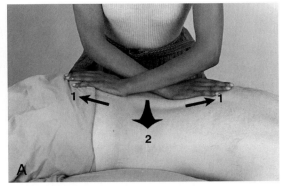

Figure 9-24. A. Techniques for the erector spinae. Crossed-handed contact permits a gentle traction of the erector spinae (1), while simultaneously performing the rocking motion (2). Hand contact is maintained as the pelvis is allowed to fall back past the midline.

Manual Technique Figures continue on next page

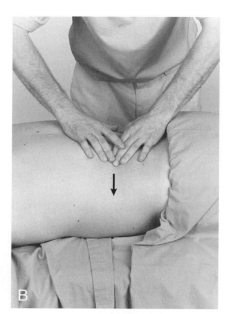

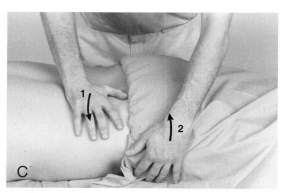

Figure 9-24 (continued). **B.** Techniques for the erector spinae. Two hands gather the erector spinae together while producing the rocking motion. **C.** Alternately, one hand draws the opposite innominate bone toward the clinician, then the other hand gently pushes the erector spinae away from the spinous processes.

CLINICIAN'S POSITION AND MOVEMENT

1. The basic positions used by the clinician are described in Chapter 4, Preparation and Positioning for Treatment, in the sections on standing aligned and lunge postures.

2. The clinician can use a standing upright posture when beginning the application of rocking or when the amplitude of the movement is small.

3. Using a standing lunge-and-lean posture, the clinician can shift body weight backward and forward from the front leg to the back leg in a gentle rocking motion and then transfer this motion through supple arms to the client. This feels much better to the client than a rocking motion that is generated solely through exertion of the clinician's arm and shoulder muscles (Figs. 9-19, 9-22, and 9-23A). As with other massage techniques, using the lower body and pelvis to generate the motion of the stroke, rather than the arms alone, adds a perceptible sureness and evenness to the stroke.

4. Shoulders are relaxed and the arms are outstretched but not stiff during the rhythmical lunge-and-lean movement. In addition, elbows are bent to avoid "straight-arming" (Figs. 9-22 and 9-23).

5. The more rhythmical and relaxed the movement of the clinician's body, the more effective the rocking motion that is produced.

PALPATE

As she performs the technique, the clinician palpates the client's skin and tissues for the qualities noted below. In doing so, her attention is focused primarily on the qualities of the motion she produces with the technique, and on the resistance of the client's tissues to movement.

1. The local skin temperature and texture.

2. The tone of the client's superficial muscles and tissues.

3. The weight of the client's body as it is set into motion by rocking.

4. Resistance to tissue or joint movement. As the client's body is pushed away from its midline resting position, the initial resistance to movement comes from the client's weight. As movement of the client's body continues farther from the midline, additional resistance develops as various tissues are lengthened passively. The goal of rocking is not to achieve the fullest possible passive stretch, but rather to produce a repetitive, pleasurable motion within the inner and midranges of the available range of motion.

5. The inherent rhythm of rocking for the client's body. No two clients' bodies will respond to rocking in the same manner. Several factors can influence the inherent rhythm of the client's body: body type, the amount of body fat, levels of muscular tension, and the client's fascial structure. In general, clients with ectomorphic body types should be rocked at a slightly faster rate and with less movement; conversely, clients with endomorphic body types can tolerate more movement, and the rate will be correspondingly slower. Muscular tension, especially of the low back, can also reduce the amount of movement that the client can tolerate. The clinician must identify the inherent rhythm of each client's body, rather than merely imposing the same motion on every client.

6. Changes in ease of application of the technique. As the application of rocking proceeds and the client relaxes, the clinician will note an increase in amplitude of the rocking motion and a decreased rate, with little increase in the force applied.

OBSERVE

As she performs the technique, the clinician observes the client for the degree of movement achieved and signs of relaxation or sedation. The signs listed below may signal this.

MOVEMENT ACHIEVED

1. Observation of the motion throughout the body during rocking. Careful observation can provide information about the client's body, including patterns of muscular tension, the relationship of body segments, and areas of connective tissue tightness due to past trauma. For example, when rocking the pelvis, the clinician can observe the relative ease of motion of the various spinal segments.

2. Lengthening of the spine, as reflected by a reduction of the client's spinal curves—especially the lumbar lordosis.

RELAXATION OR SEDATION

1. Decrease in rate and depth of breathing
2. Deeper voice tone
3. Changes in skin color, such as flushing; pallor may indicate an undesirable sympathetic response
4. Systemic reduction of muscle tone, as evidenced by softening of the tissue contours or broadening and flattening of body segments
5. Muscle twitches and jerks
6. Increases in peristaltic noises
7. Decreases in heart rate as evidenced by change in pulses that are visible at the neck, wrist, and foot
8. Agitation or sweating, which may indicate an undesirable sympathetic response

COMMUNICATION WITH THE CLIENT

The clinician uses communication to ensure the client's comfort during the application of rocking. Some examples of statements that the clinician can use are listed below.

1. "This technique should make you feel very relaxed, even sleepy . . . it should not feel abrupt." After the clinician establishes a motion that she thinks is consistent with the inherent rhythm of the client's body, she checks that the motion feels comfortable, not forced or excessive in any way.
2. "Do you feel alert enough to drive home?" If rocking is used for long periods during the session or at the end of a session, check to see that the client is sufficiently alert to safely resume daily activities, and observe level of function.
3. The relaxation, sensual pleasure, and motion of rocking may occasionally result in sexual arousal on the part of the client or prompt comments of a sexual nature. The clinician must be prepared to maintain clear verbal and physical boundaries with the client in a mature manner, while neither denigrating nor facilitating the client's sexual response to the technique.

OTHER APPROPRIATE TECHNIQUES

There are several modalities that the clinician can use in a complementary manner with rocking.

1. In particular, to enhance sedative effects, the clinician may make use of diaphragmatic breathing, progressive relaxation, and guided imagery prior to or following rocking.
2. Rocking is a useful precursor to the use of traction, joint play, or passive relaxed movement techniques.
3. Related movement interventions that may be of use are body mechanics and ergonomics training; breathing exercises; gait, locomotion, and balance training; neuromuscular training; and posture awareness training.[8]

POSTINTERVENTION SELF-CARE

1. The clinician instructs the client to rest from 10 to 30 min and to resume activity slowly if experiencing the sedative effects of rocking.
2. The clinician can instruct the client in a form of self-rocking that can be used for relaxation. This is performed on a cushioned floor or firm bed. In supine, the client draws the knees toward the chest with the hands and produces a rocking motion in the sagittal plane by pulling gently on the backs of the knees. During this movement, the client's thighs, pelvis, and lower back flex and extend passively.

A Practice Sequence for Rocking

Allow 30 min per person.

Before attempting a continuous rocking sequence, explore the basic motion on several people, using the following technique. In prone, move the client's pelvis laterally 5 to 10 cm (2 to 4 inches) from the midline, then remove your hands and observe the result. Note how far the body rebounds and how long the motion continues. Try lateral pushes in several places like the ribs, waist, iliac crest, and greater trochanter, observing the motion as before. Repeat this palpation exercise on several people who have different body types. You should start to get a sense of how the response differs from person to person and how rocking can be synchronized to each individual's body.

Continuing in prone, now connect the individual strokes to generate a continuous rocking motion.

Change your hand contacts frequently, alternating between

- Trochanter and sacrum
- Trochanter and superior gluteal insertions
- Crossed-hand lumbar traction position
- Both sides of the iliac crest
- Both sides of the waist
- Pelvis and the erector spinae
- Pelvis and rib cage
- Both sides of the rib cage

Initially, check with the client several times to ensure that the hand contact, rate, and rhythm are comfortable. Experiment with moving your hand contacts as far up and down the body as you can, while still maintaining the basic rocking motion. Notice how the client's body responds differently over time. Use gentle traction of the legs periodically to lengthen the client's back as the muscles there relax. Many people will become drowsy or even fall asleep during this sequence. Continue for 15 min, and give your client 5 min to come back to the present before ending the session.

Home study: Devise and practice a comparable sequence for rocking in supine, using the trochanter, anterior thigh, iliac crest, anterior superior iliac spines, waist, and lower ribs as contact points. Note whether a supine rocking sequence has effects similar to the one described above.

Clinical Example

Client profile	A 25-year-old female professional pentathlete prior to the javelin throw during competition
Summary of clinical findings	*Subjective* 1. No complaints 2. Wants to be physically and mentally prepared to perform optimally during the event *Objective* *Impairments* 1. Likelihood of muscle tear during propulsive motion 2. Less than optimal tissue extensibility 3. Coordination may be less than optimal for peak performance 4. Less than optimal ease of movement through range for peak performance in the javelin throw 5. Less than optimal mental arousal for peak performance Functional limitations Not sufficiently prepared physically and mentally to give peak athletic performance during the competitive javelin event without sustaining an injury
Treatment planning	*Treatment rationale* To prepare the athlete mentally and physically for peak performance during a competitive event

Impairment	Role of Therapeutic Massage
1. Risk of muscle tear	Primary treatment; decreased tissue viscosity and decreased resting level of tension are direct effects
2. Less than optimal tissue extensibility	Primary treatment; increased tissue extensibility is a direct effect
3. Less than optimal coordination	Secondary effect; rhythmical mobilization facilitates neuromuscular patterning
4. Less than optimal ease of movement	Primary treatment, since increased tissue extensibility will facilitate ease of movement
5. Less than optimal mental arousal	Primary treatment; increased arousal is a direct effect of the faster movement techniques

Massage techniques	Rhythmic mobilization and fast shaking, interspersed with repetitive, broad-contact compression and fast petrissage (see Chapter 7, Neuromuscular Techniques)
Other appropriate techniques and interventions	Stretching, passive range of motion, visualization of performance
Functional outcomes	Client will demonstrate peak athletic performance during the javelin event without injury

References

1. Loving J. Massage therapy. Stamford, CT: Appleton & Lange, 1999.
2. Salvo SG. Massage therapy. Philadelphia: WB Saunders, 1999.
3. Hollis M. Massage for therapists. 2nd ed. Oxford, England: Blackwell Science, 1998.
4. Tappan FM, Benjamin P. Tappan's handbook of healing massage techniques. 3rd ed. Stamford, CT: Appleton & Lange, 1998.
5. Holey E, Cook E. Therapeutic massage. London, England: WB Saunders, 1997.

6. de Domenico G, Wood EC. Beard's massage. 4th ed. Philadelphia: WB Saunders, 1997.

7. Fritz, S. Fundamentals of therapeutic massage. St Louis: Mosby-Lifeline, 1995.

8. American Physical Therapy Association. Guide to physical therapist practice. Phys Ther 1997;77(11):1155–1674.

9. Lederman L. Fundamentals of manual therapy. New York: Churchill Livingstone, 1997.

10. Pike G. Sports massage for peak performance. New York: Harper Perennial, 1999.

11. Benjamin PJ, Lamp SP. Understanding sports massage. Champaign, IL: Human Kinetics, 1996.

12. Bob Karcy Productions. A soigneur's sports massage. The massage therapy video library: sports massage series, vol 4. New York: View Video, 1988.

13. Fritz S. Mosby's fundamentals of therapeutic massage. St Louis: Mosby-Lifeline, 2000.

14. Salter RB. The biologic concept of continuous passive motion of synovial joints. The first 18 years of basic research and its clinical application. Clin Orthop 1989;242:12–25.

15. Akeson WH, Amiel D, Woo S-Y. Physiology and therapeutic value of passive motion. In: Helminien JH, Kivaranka I, Rammi M, eds. Joint loading—biology and health of articular structures. Bristol: John Wright, 1987:375–394.

16. Levick JR. Synovial fluid and trans-synovial flow in stationary and moving normal joints. In: Helminien JH, Kivaranka I, Rammi M, eds. Joint loading—biology and health of articular structures. Bristol: John Wright, 1987:149–186.

17. Frank C, Akeson WH, Woo SL-Y, et al. Physiology and therapeutic value of passive joint motion. Clin Orthop 1984;185:113–125.

18. Korcok M. Motion, not immobility, advocated for healing synovial joints. JAMA 1981; 246(18):2005–2006.

19. Gelberman RH, Menon J, Gonsalves M, Akeson WH. The effects of mobilization on vascularisation of healing flexor tendons in dogs. Clin Orthop 1980;153:283–289.

20. O'Sullivan SB. Strategies to improve motor control. In: O'Sullivan SB, Schmitz J. Physical rehabilitation, assessment and treatment. 2nd ed. Philadelphia: FA Davis, 1988.

21. Ramsey SM. Holistic manual therapy techniques. Prim Care 1997;24(4):759–786.

22. Whitt PL, MacKinnon J. Trager psychophysical integration: a method to improve chest mobility of patients with chronic lung disease. Phys Ther 1986;66(2):214–217.

23. Bonnard M, Pailhous J. Contribution of proprioceptive information to preferred versus constrained space-time behavior in rhythmical movements. Exp Brain Res 1999;128(4):568–572.

24. Trager M, Guadagno-Hammond C. Trager mentastics: movement as a way to agelessness. Barrytown, NY: Station Hill Press, 1987.

25. Hill PD, Humenick SS, Tieman B. Maternal activities used to soothe crying of 3-week-old breastfed infants. J Perinat Educ 1997;6(1):13–20.

26. White-Traut RC, Goldman MBC. Pre-mature infant massage: is it safe? Pediatr Nurs 1988;14(4):285–289.

27. White-Traut RC, Nelson MN. Maternally administered tactile, auditory, visual, and vestibular stimulation: relationship to later interactions between mother and premature infants. Res Nurs Health 1988;11(1):31–39.

Suggested Readings

Bauer W, Short CL, Bennett GA. The manner of removal of proteins from normal joints. J Exp Med 1933;5(7):419.

Hendricks T. Effects of immobilisation on connective tissue. J Manual Manipulative Ther 1995;3(3):98–103.

Johnson SK, Frederick J, Kaufman M, Mountjoy B. A controlled investigation of bodywork in multiple sclerosis. J Altern Complement Med 1999;5(3):237–243.

Korner AF, Guilleminault C, Van den Hoed J, Baldwin RB. Reduction of sleep apnea and bradycardia in preterm infants on oscillating water beds: a controlled polygraphic study. Pediatrics 1978;61(4):528–533.

Pederson DR. The soothing effect of rocking as determined by the direction and frequency of movement. Can J Behav Sci 1975;7:237–243.

Rood M. The use of sensory receptors to activate, facilitate, and inhibit motor response, autonomic and somatic, in developmental sequence. In: Sattely C, ed. Approaches to the treatment of patients with neuromuscular dysfunction. Dubuque, IA: William C. Brown, 1962.

Ter Vrugt D, Pederson DR. The effects of vertical rocking frequencies on the arousal level of two-month old infants. Child Dev 1973;44:205–209.

Wyke BD. Articular neurology and manipulative therapy. In: Glasgow EF, Twomey LT, Scull ER, et al., eds. Aspects of manipulative therapy. Edinburgh: Churchill Livingstone, 1987.

10

Percussive Techniques

Percussive techniques are those massage techniques that deform and release tissues quickly through striking of the body in a controlled fashion. These techniques enhance airway clearance and inhibit or enhance neuromuscular tone. This chapter describes the various percussive techniques (clapping, tapping, and others), how to perform them, and how to apply them in a practice sequences. It also includes a discussion of the indications, contraindications, cautions, outcomes of care, and postintervention care associated with percussive techniques.

Table 10-1
Summary of Impairment-Level Outcomes of Care for Percussive Techniques

Impairment-Level Outcome of Care	Technique		
	Clapping	*Tapping*	*Other Forms of Percussion*
Increased airway clearance/mobilization of secretions	✓	–	–
Increased respiration/gaseous exchange	✓	–	–
Decreased dyspnea due to increased airway clearance	✓	–	–
Normalized neuromuscular tone	–	P	P
Alteration of movement responses	–	P	P
Balance of agonist/antagonist function	–	P	P
Pain reduction through counterirritant analgesia	P	P	P
Systemic and sensory arousal and enhanced alertness	P	P	P

✓, the outcome is supported by research summarized in this chapter; P, the outcome is probable; –, nonexistent, negligible, or improbable effects.

Percussion

OTHER NAMES USED FOR THIS TECHNIQUE

"Tapotement."[1–11]

DEFINITION

Percussion: Repeated rhythmical light striking[1–11]

NOTES

While there is unanimous usage of the equivalent terms *percussion* and *tapotement,* there are differences in the names that are applied to some of the forms of percussion. For example, clapping is sometimes known as "cupping."[1,8,10] Alternate names for the forms of percussion are given in the section on manual technique below in this chapter.

CLINICAL INDICATIONS AND IMPAIRMENT-LEVEL OUTCOMES OF CARE

The various forms of percussion have different effects; they can be used for the treatment of airway clearance, as proprioceptive stimulation techniques, for increasing levels of arousal, and for pain relief.

Percussion (specifically, clapping) is used to mechanically loosen secretions in the lungs and facilitate airway clearance, particularly in clinical conditions that are associated with the production of copious or viscous sputum.[1,4,12] In traditional cardiopulmonary physical therapy, percussion is combined with postural drainage and is followed by, or alternated with, vibration of the rib cage or rapid compression and release of the rib cage (called rib "springing" or "shaking").[1,4,12] Postural drainage has its own indications, contraindications, and outcomes.[4] Research suggests that the entire procedure of postural drainage and percussion promotes the movement of sputum in a cephalic direction through the bronchial tree and increases the clearance of sputum,[13–17] with one dissent.[18] The use of postural drainage and percussion may be declining with the advent of many recently developed techniques for airway clearance that use mechanical motion and ventilation.[13–15,19–22]

There are many issues related to whether the measures used in the research on percussion and postural drainage are meaningful and relevant. For example, recent reviews question the use of the volume of sputum cleared by the client as a valid outcome measure in research on bronchial conditions,[13,23] although sputum clearance has been associated with increased client comfort.[14] Other authors consider blood oxygenation to be a more relevant measure of pulmonary function;[12,16,23,24] however, the relationship between improved oxygenation and the clearance of sputum remains unclear.[12,13,25] In addition, the results of research on the effects of postural drainage and percussion on pulmonary function testing are equivocal for several clinical conditions: postsurgically,[26] in critically ill clients with atelectasis,[12,19,27] and in chronic bronchitis and bronchiectasis.[13] Percussion remains valuable in the treatment of cystic fibrosis[14,15,28,29] and some rarer pulmonary conditions.[30]

Several massage texts state that when percussion is applied to muscle belly or tendon, it stimulates stretch reflexes that facilitate the contraction and shortening of muscle.[5,8,10] In addition, traditional physical therapy practice, such as the techniques of Bobath and Rood, has applied various forms of percussion, especially tapping, to muscles or tendons to increase neuromuscular tone

and facilitate normalized movement patterns in clients with neurological conditions such as spasticity.[31] Other sources, however, suggest that tapping tendons or muscles may inhibit contraction both locally and in synergist muscle groups by stimulating cutaneous receptors.[32,33]

Percussion is considered to have a general stimulating effect[1,2,5,6,8–10] that most likely varies with the location, vigor, and duration of its application. This has been the rationale for applying percussion during precompetition sports massage or at the end of sedative massage to increase the client's level of arousal.[2] By contrast, Frownfelter[4] notes that the monotonous rhythm and rate of the application of clapping for extended periods may have a relaxing effect.

Applications of percussion may also have a variety of minor effects. It may produce a local hyperemia.[5,10] As with other massage techniques, percussion produces a transient counterirritant analgesia, which may make it suitable for pain relief in neuralgia or amputation.[1] Finally, mechanical percussion does not facilitate recovery from short-term intense muscular activity.[34] The main impairment-level outcomes of care for percussion are summarized in Table 10-1.

CAUTIONS AND CONTRAINDICATIONS

Clinical training and supervised practice are critical for the proper application of percussive techniques. Advanced training may be advisable, particularly when dealing with pathological conditions. All of the general and local contraindications noted for massage techniques apply to the use of percussion (see Chapter 2, The Clinical Decision-Making Process). The application of percussive techniques should not cause the client pain or discomfort. Posttreatment erythema and client reports of discomfort are undesirable effects that indicate incorrect application of the technique.[4] A thin layer of fabric, such as a sheet or gown, placed between the clinician's hands and the client's skin can reduce skin sensitivity without substantially reducing the force of the technique.[1,4] There are also several specific contraindications to the use of percussion.

Percussion of the thorax is contraindicated in cases of severe rib fracture, untreated tension pneumothorax, confirmed or possible coronary thrombosis or pulmonary embolism, unstable cardiac conditions, conditions that are prone to hemorrhage, after chest or spinal surgery,[1,4] and during an acute episode of asthma.[35] The positional changes required for postural drainage may cause increased oxygen demand, carbon dioxide release, blood pressure, and cardiac output.[1,36] Consequently, the head-down position must be used with caution, particularly if clients are hypertensive or have had a head injury.[1,4,37] Percussion used alone can also increase heart rate and blood pressure.[1,24] Notwithstanding these cautions, postural drainage and percussion can be tolerated by acutely ill clients, provided that the procedure is administered within strict guidelines,[1,4,13,37] such as monitoring critically ill clients for hypoxemia and increasing the administration of oxygen.[17] The procedure should not be applied to clients who have pulmonary conditions that are not associated with increased amounts of sputum.[17] Finally, although neither postural drainage nor percussion exacerbate gastroesophageal reflux,[38] avoid treating clients with these techniques after meals.[4]

There are separate contraindications and cautions for the application of percussion in areas other than the thorax. First of all, even light percussion is locally contraindicated in acute and subacute injuries.[1] Clinicians are advised to avoid muscles with spasm, postexercise cramping, active trigger points, or latent trigger points.[1,10,39] In addition, the application of percussion over bony prominences, such as the clavicles and vertebral spinous processes, is not advisable. Finally, the force of application of percussion should be reduced, or use of this technique avoided, in areas where muscle tone or bulk are less than normal, over the kidneys, around the floating and lower ribs, around the faces of clients with a history of physical or other abuse, and wherever there is hypersensitivity.[1,2,4,8–10]

Prerequisite Skills for Percussion

Before using percussion, students should be able to

Assess level of arousal

Assess muscle tone

Assess pain

Discriminate between superficial subcutaneous tissue and the superficial and deeper layers of muscle

Before using clapping for postural drainage and percussion, students should be able to

Describe the position of the lungs in relation to the ribs, in normal and postural drainage positions

Describe postural drainage positions for the various lobes of the lungs for adults

Within the clinician's scope of practice: Use auscultation, manual chest examination, and analysis of sputum to assess the client's clinical condition

Recognize normal and abnormal chest wall mechanics during the application of broad-contact compression

Apply broad-contact compression, vibration, coarse vibration, rib springing, and rhythmic mobilization to the rib cage

Within the clinician's scope of practice: Give instructions for coughing, breathing, and vocalization to clear sputum

Outline universal precautions for the handling of body fluids

---

Manual Technique begins on next page

Percussion

Figures 10-1 to 10-13 show the hand positions and contact surfaces for the various forms of percussion, as well as applications to several regions of the body. Figures are ordered by the form of percussion.

MANUAL CONTACT SURFACES AND USES OF THE FORMS OF PERCUSSION

The following forms of percussion are organized in terms of the amount of force of application they require—from lesser force to greater force. The amount of stimulation that results from each form of percussion will vary with the force of application, the area of the body being treated, and the rate of application.

Pincement (Figs. 10-1 and 10-2):[2]

The tips of the thumb and index and middle finger are used to gently pinch and lift or pluck the client's tissues lightly. This is the only percussion stroke in which the tissue is lifted off the surface; in all other forms of percussion, the tissues are compressed. Pincement is most often used on the face.

Tapping (Figs. 10-3 and 10-4):[2,6,8–10]

Wrist and forearm remain motionless as the individual fingertips or finger pads, sequentially gently strike the client's tissues, using the same motion as that for keyboarding. In "point hacking," the fingertips strike the client's tissues together as a group with an accompanying wrist motion.[1] Tapping and point hacking are also suitable for use on the face and are commonly used in neuromuscular facilitation.

Hacking (Figs. 10-5 and 10-6):

Fingers and wrists are loose, the palms face each other (in relatively close opposition), and the clinician makes contact with client's skin using the ulnar borders of the 5th finger and the hands (one author suggested making contact with the posterior surface of the three medial fingers[6]). The hands alternate in applying light and rapid strokes.[1] Hacking can be applied to most areas of the body, other than the head, for a mild stimulating effect.

Slapping or "Splatting" ((Figs. 10-7 and 10-8):[2,8,10]

The hand and fingers are loose, and the entire open palmar surface is used. This is suitable for large flat areas,

such as the back or thighs, when a more stimulating effect is desired.

Clapping (Figs. 10-9 and 10-10):[1,2,5,6,8–10]

Few sources[2] distinguish "cupping" from clapping; therefore, in this text the terms are regarded as equivalent. The hand is positioned so that it forms a hollow "cupped" surface that traps air and does not deform on impact.[1,4] To achieve this position, the metacarpophalangeal joints are flexed to about 45 degrees, the interphalangeal joints are in neutral extension, and the fingers and thumb are adducted. The degree to which the hand is cupped varies with the area of the body that the clinician is treating: the hand should be flatter over flat surfaces, such as the posterior chest, and more cupped to fit curved areas, such as the lateral surfaces of the rib cage.[4] The wrist remains as loose as possible during application, and excessive arm movement is avoided, since this can cause rapid fatigue. Clapping is the technique of choice when performing postural drainage to increase airway clearance; it does not have to be particularly forceful or rapid to be effective for this purpose.[4] Clapping can also be used in areas other than the thorax, over large muscle groups.[1]

Beating or "Rapping" (Figs. 10-11 and 10-12):[1,2,8]

The hand is positioned in a loose fist, and the heel of the hand and dorsal surface of the interphalangeal joints are used to percuss larger muscles or even the sacrum. The force of application of this technique is greater than that of clapping, since it is intended to be a more stimulating stroke.[1]

Pounding (Fig. 10-13):[1,2,8,10]

The hand is positioned in a loose fist, and the ulnar surface of the hand is used as the contact surface.[1] During the application of the technique, the elbows are

Manual Technique continues on page 310

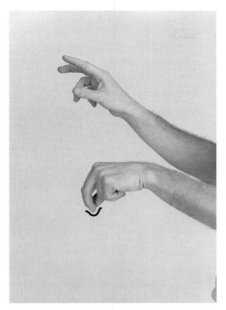

Figure 10-1. Hand position and contact surfaces for pincement. The tissue is lifted or plucked upward.

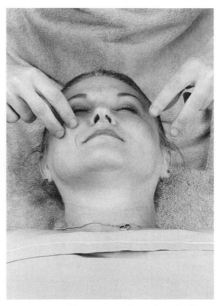

Figure 10-2. Pincement performed on the face.

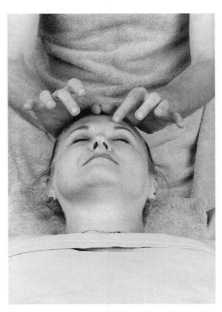

Figure 10-3. Tapping performed one finger at a time on the face.

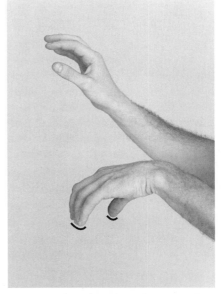

Figure 10-4. Hand position and contact surface for point hacking.

Manual Technique Figures continue on page 311

abducted, the hands are near the clinician's midline, and the strokes are applied in circles that move in the sagittal plane away from the clinician's chest, striking the client and returning toward the clinician's abdomen. This technique is appropriate for the stimulation of large, deep muscle groups.

Note

Some authors consider the compressive vibration and shaking used during postural drainage and percussion to be a form of percussion.[5,6] Compression, coarse vibration, vibration, and shaking are described in Chapter 7, Neuromuscular Techniques, and Chapter 9, Passive Movement Techniques.

MANUAL TECHNIQUE FOR ALL FORMS OF PERCUSSION

1. For all forms of percussion, keep the wrist and hand as relaxed as possible while maintaining the position of the chosen contact surface. Light forms of percussion require only small motions of the fingers or wrist. For the heavier forms, the force of application of the technique is generated through the combined movement of the wrist and forearm, in addition to flexion and extension of the elbow.

2. During the application of percussion, both the contact and release strokes should be quick, light, and even. Both hands are usually used, and they alternate strokes, using a fast, stable rhythm (this can take considerable practice to achieve). An even rate of application is more important to achieve than increased speed. Consequently, the clinician first strives to achieve evenness, and only then increases the tempo of the application. When the technique is performed with both hands, a rate of 3 to 8 Hz is acceptable.

3. The form of percussion and the force with which it is applied must be adjusted to the thickness, type, and sensitivity of the target tissue. Very light force is used over the face and areas of unprotected bone; moderate force is used over thinner muscle groups, as in the forearm, or where there is dense fascia; and the heaviest force is used over large muscles, such as the glutei. The force of application of percussion should also be adjusted to the size, age, and general health of the client.

4. Whenever possible, avoid applying percussion over exactly the same area for more than a few

seconds, since this can become irritating to the client. Instead, move the hands through the region of focus in a consistent pattern, such as a circle, or in parallel lines.[1,4]

5. Apply percussion through a gown, the sheet, or a towel when necessary to reduce irritation.

6. Avoid bony prominences such as the clavicles, and avoid breast tissue. If the client has large breasts, the clinician can, with consent, use one hand to move and hold the breast aside while the other hand performs one-handed percussion.[4]

Components of Percussion

Contact: Fingers, fingertip(s), ulnar border of hands, palms, heels, dorsal surface of interphalangeal joints, in various combinations

Pressure: Light to heavy

Engages: Superficial subcutaneous tissues (lighter forms) to deeper muscle and contained viscera, such as the lungs (heavier forms)

Direction: The contact and release strokes are perpendicular to the surface of the client's body (except for pounding)

Amplitude/length: NA

Rate: 2 to 10 or more cycles per sec (Hz) using both hands

Duration: 30 sec to 20 min or more

Intergrades with:[a] The various forms of percussion intergrade with each other; however, none of these intergrade with other massage techniques

Combines with: None of these forms of percussion combines with other massage techniques

Context: Percussion is commonly used in the following ways: briefly at the end of regional or full-body massage for its stimulating effect; immediately prior to therapeutic exercise to facilitate the performance of exercise; alternating with vibration, rib springing (rapid compression), and rhythmic mobilization of the rib cage, with the client positioned in full or modified postural drainage positions

[a]To merge gradually one into another.

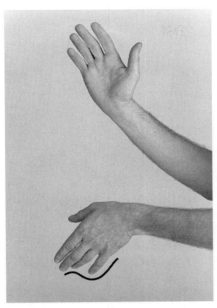

Figure 10-5. Hand position and contact surface for hacking.

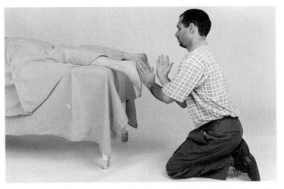

Figure 10-6. Hacking applied to the sole of the foot will gently wake a sleeping client.

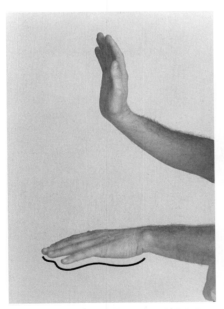

Figure 10-7. Hand position and contact surface for slapping.

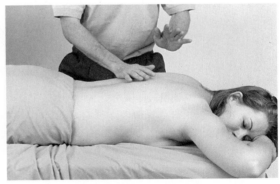

Figure 10-8. Slapping is very stimulating when applied to bare skin. It is suitable for large, flat areas like the back.

Manual Technique Figures continue on next page

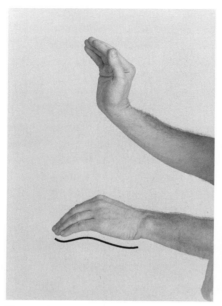

Figure 10-9. Hand position and contact surface for clapping. Contact occurs only around the rim of the hand.

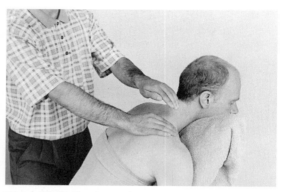

Figure 10-10. Clapping applied to the posterior apical segment of the right lung.

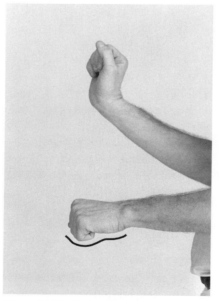

Figure 10-11. Hand position and contact surface for beating.

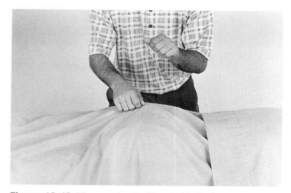

Figure 10-12. Vigorous beating is suitable for large muscles such as the gluteals.

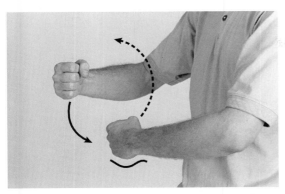

Figure 10-13. Hand position, direction of movement, and contact surface for pounding.

CLINICIAN'S POSITION AND MOVEMENT

1. When treating the limbs and torso, the clinician often stands at a right angle to the long axis of tissues to be treated using a standing upright posture or a wide-stance knee bend (see Chapter 4, Preparation and Positioning for Treatment) (Figs. 10-8 and 10-12). The clinician may incline or lean toward, or over, the target tissues when applying heavier forms of percussion, such as pounding, or to generate a faster rate of application (Fig. 10-6).

2. The elbows are held in moderate flexion, the amount of which will vary with the form of percussion, area, size of client, and working posture chosen (Figs. 10-6, 10-8, 10-12, and 10-13). The power for the strokes of heavier forms of percussion comes from a combination of movements that are performed as the upper arms remain stationary; the primary motion is flexion and extension of the wrist, and the secondary motion is small amounts of elbow flexion and extension.

3. The shoulders, elbows, and wrists must remain loose throughout the applications of all percussive techniques.[1,4]

4. During longer applications of percussion (clapping) that address several lung segments (25 to 40 min), the clinician must change positions frequently to minimize the mechanical strain of performing this physically demanding treatment (Fig. 10-14).

PALPATE

Since the clinician's hands are in contact with the client's tissues for fractions of a second at a time, detailed palpation is impossible. The clinician can, however, form a general impression of the resiliency (springiness) of the tissues being contacted, a factor that will vary with the amount of subcutaneous fat, level of resting muscle tone, and supporting bony structure that is present in the region.

OBSERVE AND LISTEN

While performing the technique, the clinician observes the client and listens for signs of correct application of the technique. The signs listed below may signal this.

1. Each form of percussion makes a characteristic sound on impact. For example, on healthy tissue,

BRONCHIAL DRAINAGE

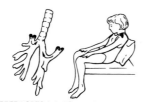

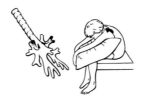

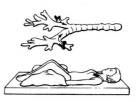

UPPER LOBES Apical Segments

Bed or drainage table flat.

Patient leans back on pillow at 30° angle against therapist.

Therapist claps with markedly cupped hand over area between clavicle and top of scapula on each side.

UPPER LOBES Posterior Segments

Bed or drainage table flat.

Patient leans over folder pillow at 30° angle.

Therapist stands behind and claps over upper back on both sides.

UPPER LOBES Anterior Segments

Bed or drainage table flat.

Patient lies on back with pillow under knees.

Therapist claps between clavicle and nipple on each side.

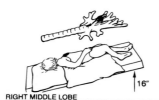

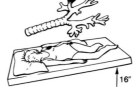

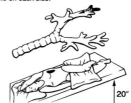

RIGHT MIDDLE LOBE

Foot of table or bed elevated 16 inches.

Patient lies head down on left side and rotates ¼ turn backward. Pillow may be placed behind from shoulder to hip. Knees should be flexed.

Therapist claps over right nipple area. In females with breast development or tenderness, use cupped hand with heel of hand under armpit and fingers extending forward beneath the breast.

LEFT UPPER LOBE Lingular Segments

Foot of table or bed elevated 16 inches.

Patient lies head down on right side and rotates ¼ turn backward. Pillow may be placed behind from shoulder to hip. Knees should be flexed.

Therapist claps with moderately cupped hand over left nipple area. In females with breast development or tenderness, use cupped hand with heel of hand under armpit and fingers extending forward beneath the breast.

LOWER LOBES Anterior Basal Segments

Foot of table or bed elevated 20 inches.

Patient lies on side, head down, pillow under knees.

Therapist claps with slightly cupped hand over lower ribs. (Position shown is for drainage of <u>left</u> anterior basal segment, patient should lie on his left side in same posture).

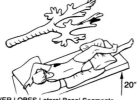

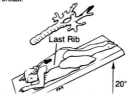

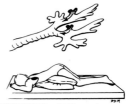

LOWER LOBES Lateral Basal Segments

Foot of table or bed elevated 20 inches.

Patient lies on abdomen, head down, then rotates ¼ turn upward. Upper leg is flexed over a pillow for support.

Therapist claps over uppermost portion of lower ribs. (Position shown is for drainage of right lateral basal segment. To drain the left lateral basal segment, patient should lie on his right side in the same posture).

LOWER LOBES Posterior Basal Segments

Foot of table or bed elevated 20 inches.

Patient lies on abdomen, head down, with pillow under hips. Therapist claps over lower ribs close to spine on each side.

LOWER LOBES Superior Segments

Bed or table flat.

Patient lies on abdomen with two pillows under hips.

Therapist claps over middle of back at tip of scapula on either side of spine.

Figure 10-14. Postural drainage positions for adults. Reprinted from Rothstein J, Roy S, Wolf S. The Rehabilitation Specialist's Handbook. 2nd Edition, 1998: p 534–535 with permission of FA Davis.

cupping makes a hollow resonant sound as the trapped air resonates between the cupped hand and the chest wall. If the hand flattens on impact, this sound will not occur, and more importantly, the effect of the technique may not penetrate as deeply into the lung tissue as needed. The clinician should bear in mind that the sound of cupping on impact—dull, resonant, or hyperresonant—may not be a reliable method of assessing the health of the client's underlying tissues.[40]

2. During the application of postural drainage and percussion, the clinician should listen to, and observe, the client's breathing, coughing, and expectoration.[4]

3. During the application of postural drainage and percussion, the clinician should periodically check the client's face to monitor her comfort level.[4]

4. When applying any percussion stroke for reflex stimulation, the clinician should watch the client for signs of waking, arousal, or irritation.

COMMUNICATION WITH THE CLIENT

The clinician uses communication that prepares the client for treatment and that seeks feedback on the client's level of comfort during the technique. Some examples of statements that the clinician can use are listed below.

IN GENERAL

1. "I'm going to start the percussion now . . . " Since percussive techniques, even when applied gently, often represent an abrupt change in sensation from other massage techniques, the clinician should tell the client when he is going to begin percussion. When the clinician selects cupping or slapping, he should also prepare the client for the noise of the technique.

2. "Do you feel comfortable?" or "Do you need a break?" Since the application of percussion can be extremely stimulating, the clinician should ensure that the client is not feeling irritated by the treatment, especially during longer applications.

3. "Does this cause you pain or discomfort anywhere?" The application of percussion should not cause the client pain or discomfort, regardless of the purpose for which it is being applied.[4]

WHEN CLAPPING IS USED WITH POSTURAL DRAINAGE TO ENHANCE AIRWAY CLEARANCE

1. Clients may start to cough spontaneously during the application of clapping. The clinician should encourage coughing, forced expiration, and expectoration. He should also provide a suitable recepta-

---

A Practice Sequence for Percussion

Allow 20 min per person.

You will not be able to apply percussion continuously throughout this sequence because it is a demanding technique to perform. Use broad-contact compression in between the different forms of percussion to allow your hands and arms to rest.

Prone

A good test area is the back and gluteals. Undrape one side, and let the other remain draped. You will treat both sides to determine the effect of the draping.

To begin, apply a series of broad-contact palmar compression strokes over the entire area for a minute. Apply pincement for a minute. Return to compression for a minute.

Then apply in turn

> Tapping
> Point hacking
> Hacking
> Slapping
> Cupping
> Beating (apply to gluteals only)
> Pounding (apply to gluteals only)

Alternate palmar compression and the progressively more vigorous forms of percussion. Finish with compression. Solicit feedback from your client about how each form of percussion felt and how the application of percussion differed between the draped and undraped sides.

For additional study: Explore the use of lighter forms of percussion on the more densely innervated areas like the face and hands. How much percussive force is tolerable in each of these areas? Which strokes can and cannot be applied?

---

cle for the client's sputum and use appropriate universal precautions in the handling of body fluids.

2. A long sequence of postural drainage and percussion (up to 40 min[4]) can be a strenuous intervention for the client, as well as the clinician. The clinician should frequently check the client's comfort and level of fatigue.

3. Sputum may continue to move for up to an hour following the application of postural drainage and percussion.[4] The clinician should encourage the client to cough and expectorate as required.

OTHER APPROPRIATE TECHNIQUES

There are several modalities that the clinician can use in a complementary manner with percussive techniques.

A Practice Sequence for Postural Drainage and Percussion of an Adult

Allow 30 min per person.

You will need an articulated, tilting treatment table or bed to achieve the elevation required for the various postural drainage positions. If this is not available, you can approximate the positions using eight or more standard pillows.[4,45]

Review any factors in your client's history that would require a reduction in force of application of the percussion (see the contraindications and cautions section above). Note that positioning for pulmonary drainage in tilted positions with the head down in itself will elevate blood pressure, which is a caution for hypertensive clients.[1,4]

Remember to avoid the scapula, clavicle, and breast tissue. If the client has large breasts, the clinician can, with consent, use one hand to move and hold the breast aside while the other hand performs one-handed percussion.[4] Use caution around the floating ribs.

Apply the following cycle of techniques to as many of the segments illustrated in Figure 10-14 as time allows. In a clinical situation, one position should be maintained for 5 or 10 min or even longer. Continuous clapping can then be applied for 3 to 5 min to a small area, followed by vibration and therapeutic breathing exercises. For a practice sequence, these times may be shortened to include a wider selection of positions.

1. Assume a postural drainage position (see Figure 10-14).

2. Apply clapping continuously with a stable rhythm over indicated segment of the lung for 1 or 2 min.

As far as possible, use the cupped hand position and obtain the characteristic resonant sound; this is not always possible for a large-handed clinician; in smaller areas, use only one cupped hand or apply pounding or hacking

3. Compression and coarse vibration are initiated at the peak of each deep inspiration and continued throughout expiration in the following manner: Compress the thorax over the segment as the client begins to exhale. While maintaining this compression, apply coarse vibration throughout the exhalation. Release compression to permit inhalation. The client may also be instructed to forcibly exhale or vocalize "Ahhh."[8] Instruct the client to expectorate as required.

4. Alternatively, apply repeated rapid compression with a rapid partial release between each compression stroke (rib springing[4]); instruct the client to expectorate as required.

5. Intersperse rocking using rib contacts, or rhythmical mobilization of the rib cage, with the application of percussion; this gives both client and clinician a break from more-vigorous technique.

Change positions until several segments of the lung have been treated; at the end of this sequence, position the client in prone and finish with 5 min of sedative massage; instruct your client to sit up, and practice giving instruction for appropriate follow-up care.

FOR POSTURAL DRAINAGE AND PERCUSSION

1. There are several approaches to facilitating the thinning and clearance of sputum. If possible, the clinician should encourage the client to drink water (this should be done 30 to 60 min before the intervention).[4] Steam inhalation (humidification) can reduce the viscosity of the sputum and may also dilate the bronchioles. Aerosol therapy using an ultrasonic nebulizer can assist in liquefying and mobilizing sputum.[4] Prior application of warm moist heat to the client's anterior or posterior thorax may reflexly dilate the bronchioles (if this is appropriate for the client's clinical condition).[41]

2. During postural drainage and percussion, the client is positioned in the sequence of positions for postural drainage (Fig. 10-14). Less rigorous, modified postural drainage positions may be as effective as traditional postural drainage positions.[4,27]

3. Clapping can be interspersed with broad-contact compression and simultaneous vibration of the rib cage.

4. Vibration can be synchronized with forced expiration, coughing, or audible huffing by the client.[1,4,8]

5. The use of suctioning;[13] methods of modifying mechanical ventilator airflow, such as positive expiratory pressure;[15,20,29] and other mechanical devices, such as cyclically inflated pneumatic belts,[20] can be used with clients who have atelectasis or who are critically ill.

FOR FACILITATION AND INHIBITION OF NEUROMUSCULAR TONE

1. Joint traction and approximation, quick stretch, resistance, fine vibration, light touch, and repetitive brushing are techniques that can be used to increase neuromuscular tone and facilitate movement in clients with neurological conditions.[31,42]

2. Specific compression (inhibitory pressure), slow superficial stroking, static contact ("maintained touch"), prolonged cold, and neutral warmth are techniques that can be used to inhibit neuromuscular tone and facilitate movement in clients with neurological conditions.[31,42]

POSTINTERVENTION SELF-CARE

AFTER POSTURAL DRAINAGE AND PERCUSSION

1. The clinician can encourage the clearance of sputum and rest, as required, for the following hour.[4,21,43]
2. The clinician can teach the client techniques for cough stimulation and for effective coughing.[13]
3. The client can benefit from learning exercises for chest-wall mobility, ventilator muscle training, conditioning, reconditioning, neuromuscular relaxation, and postural training.[1,7,15,43]
4. The clinician can instruct the client how to perform autogenic drainage.[20]
5. Although research has not consistently shown that self-administered chest clapping can enhance the rate of sputum clearance or the level of oxygen saturation, clients may find it beneficial.[44]

Clinical Example

Client profile	A 10-year-old boy with cystic fibrosis who was admitted to an acute care setting with acute bronchitis; his clinical condition has responded to medical management, and he is in the later stages of therapy
Summary of clinical findings	*Subjective* Complaints of shortness of breath at rest and during activity; perceived dyspnea measured using the Borg Perceived Exertion Rating Scale[46] *Objective* *Impairments* 1. Increased sputum production 2. Persistent productive cough 3. Impaired/ineffective airway clearance secondary to increased sputum production and ineffective cough and other airway clearance mechanisms 4. Increased anterior-posterior diameter of the chest with decreased lateral costal and diaphragmatic expansion of the rib cage during respiration 5. Sternal respiratory pattern with accessory muscle use and intercostal indrawing during respiration 6. Scattered polyphonic wheezing and crackles throughout the ventilatory cycle audible auscultation 7. Decreased midexpiratory flow rate on spirometric pulmonary function tests 8. Hyperinflation, peribronchiolar thickening, flattening of the diaphragm, and bronchiectasis of the upper lobes apparent on chest x-ray *Functional limitations* 1. Ambulation tolerance 50 feet, secondary to shortness of breath 2. Inability to complete activities of daily living, such as dressing tasks, without frequent rest periods secondary to shortness of breath 3. Decreased levels of oxygen saturation during functional activity
Treatment planning	*Treatment rationale*

Treatment rationale

Impairment	Role of Massage
1. Impaired airway clearance	Primary treatment; direct effect of clapping on the mobilization of sputum, especially when used with postural drainage
2. Decreased rib cage mobility	Primary treatment; direct effect of massage techniques on reducing chronic shortening of intercostal muscles, accessory muscles of breathing, and diaphragm; direct effect of "rib springing" on increasing the mobility of the sternocostal, costovertebral, and costochondral joints

continued

(continued)

	3. Accessory muscle use	Secondary treatment; accessory muscle use reflects an increased work of breathing[3,4] that is not directly affected by the use of massage techniques; effects of massage techniques that can contribute to decreased accessory muscle use include reduction of chronic shortening of accessory muscles, increased perceived relaxation, and decreased perceived anxiety
	4. Dyspnea	Secondary treatment; indirect effect of massage on dyspnea through increased perceived relaxation, decreased perceived anxiety, and increased airway clearance
Massage techniques	· Clapping of the thorax with postural drainage · Rib springing · Coarse vibration combined with broad-contact compression of the rib cage · Petrissage to anterior and posterior thoracic and cervical muscles · Wringing of the rib cage · Stripping of scalene muscles · Direct fascial techniques on the inferior costal margin and along the intercostal spaces	
Other appropriate techniques and interventions[47]	· Effective coughing techniques · Forced expiration or audible huffing to facilitate airway clearance · Use of a Positive Expiratory Pressure Mask · Diaphragmatic breathing exercises · Education in energy conservation techniques during ambulation and activities of daily living · Graded therapeutic exercise program · Encourage fluid replacement · Review of self-administered postural drainage and mechanical percussion for home program	
Functional outcomes of care	1. Client will be able to ambulate 100 feet without a decrease in oxygen saturation and complaints of shortness of breath 2. Client will be able to complete activities of daily living, such as dressing, without frequent complaints of shortness of breath 3. Client will demonstrate the use of appropriate energy-conservation techniques during performance of activities of daily living and ambulation	

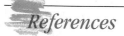

References

1. de Domenico G, Wood EC. Beard's massage. 4th ed. Philadelphia: WB Saunders, 1997.
2. Tappan FM, Benjamin P. Tappan's handbook of healing massage techniques. 3rd ed. Stamford, CT: Appleton & Lange, 1998.
3. Frownfelter DL, Dean E. Principals and practice of cardiopulmonary physical therapy. 3rd ed. St. Louis: CV Mosby, 1996.
4. Frownfelter DL. Chest physical therapy and pulmonary rehabilitation: an interdisciplinary approach. Chicago: Year Book, 1987.
5. Holey E, Cook E. Therapeutic massage. London: WB Saunders, 1997.
6. Hollis M. Massage for therapists. 2nd ed. Oxford, England: Blackwell Science, 1998.
7. American Physical Therapy Association. The guide to physical therapist practice. Phys Ther 1997;77(11):1155–1674.
8. Fritz S. Mosby's fundamentals of therapeutic massage. St. Louis: Mosby-Lifeline, 2000.
9. Loving J. Massage therapy. Stamford, CT: Appleton & Lange, 1999.
10. Salvo SG. Massage therapy. Philadelphia: WB Saunders, 1999.
11. Yates J. A physician's guide to massage therapy; its physiological effects and their application to treatment. British Columbia, Canada: The Massage Therapists Association of British Columbia, 1990.
12. Ciesla ND. Chest physical therapy for patients in the intensive care unit. Phys Ther 1996;76(6):609–625.

13. Jones AP, Rowe BH. Bronchopulmonary hygiene physical therapy in chronic obstructive pulmonary disease and bronchiectasis. Cochrane Library (Oxford) 1998;1–3.

14. Ambrosino N, Callegari G, Galloni C, et al. Clinical evaluation of oscillating positive expiratory pressure for enhancing expectoration in diseases other than cystic fibrosis. Monaldi Arch Chest Dis 1995;50(4): 269–275.

15. Thomas J, Cook DJ, Brooks D. Chest physical therapy management of patients with cystic fibrosis. A meta-analysis. Am J Respir Crit Care Med 1995;151(3 pt 1): 846–850.

16. Gallon A. Evaluation of chest percussion in the treatment of patients with copious sputum production. Respir Med 1991;85(1):45–51.

17. Connors AF Jr, Hammon WE, Martin RJ, Rogers RM. Chest physical therapy. The immediate effect on oxygenation in acutely ill patients. Chest 1980;78(4):559–564.

18. van der Schans CP, Piers DA, Postma DS. Effect of manual percussion on tracheobronchial clearance in patients with chronic airflow obstruction and excessive tracheobronchial secretion. Thorax 1986;41(6):448–452.

19. Raoof S, Chowdhrey N, Raoof S, et al. Effect of combined kinetic therapy and percussion therapy on the resolution of atelectasis in critically ill patients. Chest 1999;115(6):1658–1666.

20. Hardy KA, Anderson BD. Noninvasive clearance of airway secretions. Respir Care Clin North Am 1996;2(2): 323–345.

21. McIlwaine MP, Davidson AG. Airway clearance techniques in the treatment of cystic fibrosis. Curr Opin Pulm Med 1996;2(6):447–451.

22. Thomas J, DeHueck A, Kleiner M, et al. To vibrate or not to vibrate: usefulness of the mechanical vibrator for clearing bronchial secretions. Physiother Can 1995;47(2): 120–125.

23. Dean E. Oxygen transport: a physiologically-based conceptual framework for the practice of cardiopulmonary physiotherapy. Physiotherapy 1994;80(6):347–355.

24. Dallimore K, Jenkins S, Tucker B. Respiratory and cardiovascular responses to manual chest percussion in normal subjects. Aust J Physiother 1998;44(4):267–274.

25. Dall'Alba PT, Burns YR. The relationship between arterial blood gases and removal of airway secretions in neonates. Physiother Theory Pract 1990;6(3):107–116.

26. Eales CJ, Barker M, Cubberley NJ. Evaluation of a single chest physiotherapy treatment to post-operative, mechanically ventilated cardiac surgery patients. Physiother Theory Pract 1995;11(1):23–28.

27. Stiller K, Jenkins S, Grant R, et al. Acute lobar atelectasis: a comparison of five physiotherapy regimens. Physiother Theory Pract 1996;12(4):197–209.

28. Boyd S, Brooks D, Agnew-Coughlin J, Ashwell J. Evaluation of the literature on the effectiveness of physical therapy modalities in the management of children with cystic fibrosis. Pediatr Phys Ther 1994;6(2):70–74.

29. Langenderfer B. Alternatives to percussion and postural drainage: a review of mucus clearance therapies: percussion and postural drainage, autogenic drainage, positive expiratory pressure, flutter valve, intrapulmonary percussive ventilation, and high-frequency chest compression with the ThAIRapy vest. J Cardiopulm Rehabil 1998;18(4): 283–289.

30. Hammon WE, McCaffree DR, Cucchiara AJ. A comparison of manual to mechanical chest percussion for clearance of alveolar material in patients with pulmonary alveolar proteinosis (phospholipidosis). Chest 1993;103(5):1409–1412.

31. Griffin JW. Use of proprioceptive stimuli in therapeutic exercise. Phys Ther 1974;54:1072–1079.

32. Lederman E. Fundamentals of manual therapy. New York: Churchill Livingstone, 1997.

33. Belanger AY, Morin S, Pepin P, et al. Manual muscle tapping decreases H-reflex amplitude in control subjects. Physiother Can 1989;41(4):192–196.

34. Cafarelli E, Sim J, Carolan B, et al. Vibratory massage and term recovery from muscular fatigue. Int J Med 1990;11(6): 474–478.

35. Gameros-Gardea RA. [Inhalation therapy in asthma] (Spanish). Rev Alerg Mex 1996;43(5):109–115. (Abstract)

36. Horiuchi K, Jordan D, Cohen D, et al. Insights into the increased oxygen demand during chest physiotherapy. Crit Care Med 1997;25(8):1347–1351.

37. Imle PC, Mars MP, Ciesla ND, et al. The effect of chest physical therapy on intracranial pressure and cerebral perfusion pressure. Physiother Can 1997;49(1):48–55.

38. Chen HC, Liu CY, Cheng HF, et al. Chest physiotherapy does not exacerbate gastroesophageal reflux in patients with chronic bronchitis and bronchiectasis. Chang Keng I Hsueh Tsa Chih 1998;21(4):409–414.

39. Travell JG, Simons DG. Myofascial pain and dysfunction. The trigger point manual, vol 1. Baltimore: Williams & Wilkins, 1983.

40. Soh TS, Soh SC, Ng LL, et al. Inter-rater reliability of percussion note as a respiratory assessment tool. Physiother Singapore 1998;1(1):9–12.

41. Moor F, Peterson S, Manwell E, et al. Manual of hydrotherapy and massage. Oshawa, Canada: Pacific Press Publishing, 1964.

42. O'Sullivan SB. Strategies to improve motor control. In: O'Sullivan SB, Schmitz J, eds. Physical rehabilitation, assessment and treatment. 2nd ed. Philadelphia: FA Davis, 1988.

43. Kisner C, Colby LA. Therapeutic exercise: foundations and techniques. 3rd ed. Philadelphia: FA Davis, 1996.

44. Carr J, Pryor JA, Hodson ME. Self chest clapping: patients' views and the effects on oxygen saturation. Physiotherapy 1995;81(12):753–757.

45. Wood EC, Becker PD. Beard's massage. 3rd ed. Philadelphia: WB Saunders, 1981.

46. Borg GA. Psychophysical bases of perceived exertion. Med Sci Sport Exerc 1982;14:377–381.

47. Ashwell J, Agnew-Coughlin J, Boyd S, Brooks D. Cystic fibrosis. In: Campbell S, Palisano R, Vander Linden P, eds. Physical therapy for children. Philadelphia: WB Saunders, 1994.

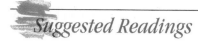

Suggested Readings

Blazey S, Jenkins S, Smith R. Rate and force of application of manual chest percussion by physiotherapists. Aust J Physiother 1998;44(4):257–264.

Chopra SK, Laplin OV, Simmons DH, et al. Effects of hydration and physical therapy on tracheal transport velocity. Am Rev Respir Dis 1977;15:1009–1014.

Clarke SW, Cochrane GM, Webber B. (cited in Chopra et al., 1977.) Effects of sputum on pulmonary function. Thorax 1973;28:262.

Egbert LD, Battit GE, Welch CE, Bartlett MK. Reduction of postoperative pain by encouragement and instruction of patients. N Engl J Med 1964;270:825–827.

Hillegass EA, Sadowsky HS. Essentials of cardiopulmonary physical therapy. Philadelphia: WB Saunders, 1994.

Hussey JM. Effects of chest physiotherapy for children in intensive care after surgery. Physiotherapy 1992;78(2):109–113.

Irwin S, Techlin JS. Cardiopulmonary physical therapy. St. Louis: CV Mosby, 1995.

Mackenzie CG, Imle PC, Ciesla N. Chest physiotherapy in the intensive care unit. 2nd ed. Baltimore: Williams & Wilkins, 1989.

Miller WG. Rehabilitation of patients with chronic obstructive lung disease. Med Clin North Am 1967;5:349.

Nguyen HP, Le DL, Tran QM, et al. CHROMASSI: a therapy advice system based on chrono-massage and acupression using the method of ZiWuLiuZhu. Medinfo 1995;8(pt 2):998.

Petty TL. Chronic obstructive pulmonary disease. New York: Marcel Dekker, 1978.

Pham QT, Peslin R, Puchelle E, et al. (cited in Chopra et al., 1977.) Respiratory function and the rheological status of bronchial secretions collected by spontaneous expectoration and after physiotherapy. Bull Physiopathol Respir (Nancy) 1973;9:292.

Watchie J. Cardiopulmonary physical therapy—a clinical manual. Philadelphia: WB Saunders, 1995.

Webber BA, Pryor JA. Physiotherapy for respiratory and cardiac problems. Edinburgh: Churchill Livingstone, 1993.

11

The Treatment Process and Discharge Planning

*T*his chapter builds on the clinical decision-making model presented in earlier chapters by providing details on how to craft and progress interventions and treatment regimens that use massage techniques. It discusses the steps in the selection of techniques and the design of local or regional massage sequences and reviews the principles on which the progression of techniques and treatment regimens is based. Since there is a variation in the extent to which health care professions use massage within interventions, this chapter focuses on the crafting of a massage sequence or regimen and assumes that readers will modify the relative emphasis on massage techniques versus other treatment techniques according to their professional needs.

Steps in the Design of Massage Sequences

The techniques chapters have introduced a variety of clinically useful massage techniques that can be used in interventions and their scientific bases. In addition, Chapter 2, The Clinical Decision-Making Process, provided a general framework for the examination, treatment, and discharge process. This material will provide the foundation for the current discussion of the principles that underlie the process of crafting individual interventions. This approach will involve the use of five steps: *(a)* summarizing the clinical findings and outcomes of care, *(b)* selecting treatment techniques, *(c)* specifying the scope and duration of the massage, *(d)* choosing a predominant general massage technique, and *(e)* sequencing the chosen massage techniques according to principles. The basis for this discussion comes from the work of a long lineage of influential writers who have proposed principles of practice, from a consideration of the science underlying the individual massage techniques, from the observation of effective clinicians with differing trainings, and from common sense. We suggest that students and novice clinicians take a methodical approach to designing written sequences before applying massage sequences to clients. Although this appears to be a slow process, with repetition the critical thinking inherent to the process of designing massage sequences will eventually become second nature to the clinician. At this point, she will perform much of the design of sequences and regimens mentally during the course of the evaluative and treatment-planning phases of the clinical decision-making process.

The term massage sequence is used in this chapter to refer to a structured, outcome-based series or succession of massage techniques that compose an intervention or a part of an intervention. This term is used instead of the term routine because the latter implies the application of massage techniques without the required assessment of the client's needs. Massage sequences are not random, but are highly structured in their timing and manual technique. The structure of a massage sequence should reflect the clinician's understanding of the purpose of the constituent techniques and of the client's needs. The structure should also be consistent with the principles of massage sequence design that address why massage techniques are combined in certain sequences, how interventions begin, proceed, and end, and how the constraints of time and location affect the treatment process. In reality, considerable legitimate variation in treatment approach is possible. When presented with the same situation, 10 experienced clinicians will design 10 different interventions, yet there will also be notable similarities! In light of this, this chapter presents an introduction to design basics and includes some advanced considerations toward the end of the chapter.

SUMMARIZE THE CLINICAL FINDINGS AND OUTCOMES OF CARE

As Chapter 2, The Clinical Decision-Making Process, outlines, the starting point for the design of any massage sequence is the summary of clinical findings from the client examination (Fig. 2-2) and a succinct statement of the identified impairment-level and functional outcomes of care (Fig. 2-3). The clinician should prioritize this list of identified outcomes in collaboration with the client before determining which impairments are amenable to treatment.

SELECT TREATMENT TECHNIQUES

Since the selection of treatment techniques is based on their potential impairment-level outcomes of care, the clinician who wishes to use massage techniques within an intervention must be familiar with the impairment-level outcomes and clinical indications for the various massage techniques (see Chapters 5 through 10 and Table 11-1). Clearly, not all massage techniques are useful or indicated for all clinical conditions; consequently, the understanding and application of the impairment-level outcomes of each massage technique are prerequisites for the consistent achievement of the identified outcomes of a treatment regimen.

In developing the plan of care, the clinician must consider which techniques are of potential use in each presenting clinical situation. This goes beyond the matching of techniques to outcomes of care to include broader issues that are related to the client and the context of treatment. For example, the clinician may ask herself some of the following questions. "Has the client indicated an interest in relaxation?" "What is the client's overall energy level and emotional state?" "Is there a problem with the function of a particular tissue or structure?" "Is there any ongoing systemic pathological process?" "Does the client have pain, and if so, should it be treated in and of itself, or can it be treated by addressing the underlying clinical condition?" "Are there restrictions of positioning or draping that would preclude the application of some massage techniques?" and "What are the client's primary treatment goals?" With practice, as answers to questions like these arise during the course of the evaluative phase, the clinician can begin to

determine the need for an emphasis on one or more of the major categories of massage techniques (superficial reflex, superficial fluid, neuromuscular, connective tissue, passive movement, or percussive) and mentally assemble a list of potentially useful massage techniques with which to address the client's needs. She will identify other treatment techniques that are appropriate for the client's clinical condition, impairments, and functional limitations. The clinician will then refine her list of massage and other treatment techniques during the treatment-planning phase as she considers which impairments are amenable to treatment, the contraindications and cautions for each technique, and compensatory strategies that she will use.

Health care professions differ in the extent to which they can use massage techniques, as opposed to other available treatment techniques, within an intervention. This will vary with the clinician's scope of practice, training, knowledge of treatment techniques other than massage techniques, clinical setting, and time available for interventions. Consequently, many clinicians are uncertain how to determine whether to use massage techniques or other appropriate techniques within a given intervention. One approach is to identify which of the client's presenting impairments must be addressed to facilitate the achievement of other impairment-level outcomes of care. In particular, it is valuable for the clinician to identify soft-tissue dysfunction that can impede the remediation of the client's other impairments. Take, for example, the case of a client who presents for physical therapy with a decreased ability to raise his arm that appears to be secondary to muscle weakness. During the client examination, the clinician determines that the client has an abnormal scapulohumeral rhythm and soft-tissue restrictions in the scapular region, in addition to muscle weakness. In this situation, it may be more effective for the clinician to use massage techniques to reduce the soft-tissue restrictions in the client's scapular region and joint mobilization techniques to increase accessory joint motion, prior to initiating therapeutic exercise and as a component of the ongoing treatment regimen. The resolution of the client's soft-tissue dysfunction and decreased accessory joint motion could facilitate his ability to perform the therapeutic exercise that the clinician uses to increase muscular performance and joint mobility. The clinician could also introduce the use of electrotherapeutic modalities, such as neuromuscular electrical stimulation, and physical agents, such as hot packs, to the extent that they facilitate the achievement of the identified outcomes of care. As the client's impairments are remediated, the clinician could progress her use of functional training to address the client's functional limitations. Finally, education in self-care would be an ongoing component of the treatment regimen.

Table 11-1
Summary of Impairment-Level Outcomes of Care for Massage Techniques

The following chart tabulates effects and impairment-level outcomes of care for the categories of techniques discussed in Chapters 5 to 10. ✓ denotes that the impairment-level outcome of care is supported by literature summarized in that chapter, P denotes that the impairment-level outcome of care is probable, and – denotes improbable or nonexistent effects.

Effects/Uses	*Category of Technique (Chapter)*					
	5	**6**	**7**	**8**	**9**	**10**
Decreased capsular restriction	–	–	P	P	P	–
Increased joint mobility	–	P	✓	✓	P	–
Increased joint integrity	–	–	P	P	P	–
Increased muscle extensibility	–	–	✓	✓	P	–
Pain reduction						
Counterirritant analgesia	✓	P	✓	P	P	P
Via sedation	P	P	P	P	P	–
Via treatment of dysfunction	–	P	✓	✓	P	P
Increased venous return (direct)	–	P	P	–	–	–
Increased lymphatic return (direct)	–	✓	P	–	–	–
Decreased joint effusion	–	P	P	–	–	–
Separation/lengthening of fascia	–	–	P	✓	P	–
Promotion of dense connective tissue remodeling (in chronic stage)	–	–	P	P	–	–
Increased connective tissue mobility	–	–	P	P	–	–
Decreased muscle spasm	P	P	P	–	–	–
Decreased resting tension of skeletal muscle	–	P	P	P	P	–
Decreased trigger point activity	–	–	✓	P	–	–
Increased postural awareness	–	–	P	P	P	–
Normalized structural alignment	–	–	P	P	–	–
Normalized sensation/reduction of nerve compression	–	–	P	P	–	–
Enhanced muscle performance (secondary effect)	–	–	✓	✓	P	–
Balanced agonist/antagonist function	–	–	✓	✓	P	P
Increased rib cage mobility	–	–	P	P	P	–
Increased respiration/gaseous exchange	–	–	–	–	–	✓
Increased airway clearance/mobilization of secretions	–	–	–	–	✓	✓
Decreased dyspnea	–	–	P	P	✓	✓
Decreased perceived anxiety	✓	✓	✓	✓	P	–
Increased perceived relaxation	✓	✓	✓	✓	P	–
Decreased level of cortisol	P	P	✓	P	P	–
Systemic sedation	P	P	✓	P	P	–
Normalized neuromuscular tone	P	–	P	–	–	–
Alteration of movement responses	✓	–	✓	✓	✓	P
Stimulated peristalsis	–	–	P	P	P	✓
Stimulated immune function	P	P	✓	P	P	–
Sensory or systemic arousal and enhanced alertness	P	P	✓	P	P	P
Promoted weight gain/development	✓	–	✓	–	P	–

SPECIFY THE SCOPE AND DURATION OF THE MASSAGE

The scope of the massage refers to the amount of the body the intervention will address, and the duration of the massage refers to the amount of time available for that intervention. Although these two considerations are closely related, they are discussed separately.

The scope of massage sequences usually falls into one of two categories: regional sequences or full-body sequences. Conventional anatomical regions that are defined by major bony and muscular landmarks form naturally interrelated body segments that are commonly treated together. In practice, any large contiguous area of the client's body may be the focus of a regional sequence. An exception to this rule is that the hands, feet, and the face and head are often treated as regions in themselves, because of their complexity. Box 11-1 lists body segments that are commonly treated together in massage sequences. Clinicians who are learning how to design massage sequences may find it easier to create sequences for individual regions first and then develop more-extensive sequences as a combination of sequences for regions of similar sizes.

The decision on whether the scope of the massage sequence is to be regional or more-encompassing depends on the client's clinical condition, the techniques being applied, and the amount of time available for the intervention. First, a localized clinical condition such as a tendinopathy, fasciitis, or capsular restriction requires a regional focus. The clinician will also have to perform more-local treatment when orthopedic lesions are severe (in either the acute or chronic stage). Nevertheless, as the section on agonist-antagonist balance discusses, the use of certain massage techniques, such as neuromuscular techniques, will sometimes necessitate that the clinician broaden the scope of the regional massage sequence regardless of the duration of the intervention. When shorter treatment times are the norm within a clinical setting, it is difficult for the clinician to address the entire body within an intervention, except through the use of very general massage techniques. Short, full-body sequences of 20 min or less do not permit time for much local treatment; consequently, this is only advised when the clinician is seeking to achieve general outcomes related to the client's level of arousal, such as sedation or stimulation. When the time available for treatment is short and the outcomes of care are general, the clinician and the client may still prefer to focus on a region of choice, such as the back. Finally, longer treatment times will sometimes permit the integration of a local treatment into a full-body sequence that is being performed as a wellness intervention.

It is essential for the clinician to specify and adhere to a time for the application of a given regional or full-body sequence. Some clinicians object to this approach on the basis that "clock watching" conflicts with the supportive, nurturing nature of a therapeutic intervention or that it inhibits learning. In practice, the contrary is true: Respect for the time boundaries of an intervention reflects a respect for the client and facilitates a respect for the other boundaries that are required for an appropriate client–clinician relationship. Furthermore, the time available for intervention influences all decisions about the number, type, and ordering of the techniques used, even though it may not change the basic emphasis of the intervention. In other words, it is more difficult to design an efficient massage sequence without knowing how much time is available for its execution.

There are some general guidelines for the timing of massage sequences: Regional sequences can take from 5 to 45 min or more to apply, and full-body sequences can require from 15 to 90 min or more. Shorter massage sequences need to address fewer impairment-level outcomes with fewer techniques, to be coherent and effective. The outcomes that a clinician can expect to achieve with treatments of shorter duration will vary with the level of experience of the clinician, the clinical condition being treated, and the massage technique

---

Box 11-1
Areas Commonly Treated Together as Regions

Face and head

Face, head, and neck (all surfaces)

Head and neck (all surfaces)

Posterior shoulders and neck

Arm and hand

Hand

Abdomen

Abdomen and anterior thorax

Anterior thorax

Anterior thorax, shoulders, and neck

Lateral abdomen and thorax (sidelying)

Back and posterior neck

Back

Lumbar and gluteal areas

Posterior thigh, including gluteals, leg, and foot

Posterior thigh, leg, and foot

Posterior leg and foot

Medial thigh, leg, and foot (sidelying)

Lateral thigh, leg, and foot (sidelying)

Foot

Table 11-2
Suggested Times for Massage Sequences That Seek to Achieve Common Impairment-Level Outcomes

The first figure represents a minimum duration of treatment (less time than this would make it difficult to achieve the outcome consistently). The second figure represents a comfortable length of time; more time can often be used to good effect. These figures are based on treatment by an experienced clinician.

Region	Impairment-Level Outcome	Minimum Time (min)
Back	Systemic sedation, decreased anxiety	10–20
Back	Systemic or sensory arousal, enhanced awareness	5–15
Thorax	Increased airway clearance	15–45
Thorax	Increased rib cage mobility	10–30
Limb	Increased lymphatic return	20–60
Limb	Reduced spasticity	10–30
Joint	Increased range (one joint)	5–20
Any	Counterirritant analgesia	15–45
Any	Decreased trigger point activity	3–20
Any	Decreased resting level of tone	5–30
Any	Local fascial lengthening	3–15
Any	Promotion of tendon remodeling	2–15
ALL	Deep systemic sedation	30–60

being used. Table 11-2 provides some suggested minimum times in which experienced clinicians can address discrete tasks within the context of a regional massage sequence. The amount of time that a clinician allocates to the use of massage techniques, in relation to the other treatment techniques, will also be consistent with the relative impact of the soft-tissue dysfunction on the client's functional level and other factors, such as the clinician's scope of practice and clinical setting. All other factors being equal, when soft-tissue dysfunction has a significant impact on the client's functional level, then the clinician can justify a greater emphasis on the use of massage techniques and vice versa.

CHOOSE A PREDOMINANT GENERAL MASSAGE TECHNIQUE

"General" and "specific" are useful, if somewhat imprecise, concepts that summarize several of the defining components for massage techniques. General massage techniques[1] engage and provide information about a large area of the body or a large group of tissues. These techniques have a large amplitude, use a broad contact surface (sometimes repeatedly over contiguous areas), and are inherently not localized to a particular area. Some examples of general massage techniques are superficial effleurage, direct fascial technique performed with a broad contact, palmar compression done in a series, and rocking. By contrast, specific massage techniques have smaller amplitude, use small contact surfaces, and are inherently localized. Examples of these techniques are specific compression and cross-fiber friction. It is a worthwhile exercise to attempt to group massage techniques according to these concepts of general and specific; a suggested organization is provided in Box 11-2.

Massage sequences most often consist of a mix of general and specific massage techniques, although the clinician can use either type of technique by itself. It is unusual to omit a general massage technique in the Western systems of massage. Oriental approaches, however, sometimes consist only of specific compression,[2] an approach that reflects the fact that their rationale for application of massage techniques is very different from that in the Western system (see the discussion of meridian theory in Chapter 7, Neuromuscular Techniques). It is beneficial for the clinician to use one general massage technique to which she can return periodically during the course of the massage sequence. Used in this way, this technique becomes the principal palpation tool and serves to frame and connect the other techniques that are used. A clinician can incorporate a predominant general massage technique into the intervention regardless of the duration of the massage

Box 11-2
General vs. Specific

The following list arranges some massage techniques approximately from the more general (top) to the more specific (bottom):

Rocking

Superficial stroking

Superficial effleurage

Deep effleurage

Broad-contact direct fascial technique

Broad-contact myofascial stretch

Shaking

Wringing

Picking up

Superficial lymph drainage technique

Static contact

Broad compression

Squeezing

Fingertip and thumb kneading

Skin rolling

Friction

Specific compression

Rationalize a different order for the list. Is there a relationship between specificity and depth?

sequence and the relative emphasis on massage within the intervention. The periodic use of this general massage technique can impart a sense of structure to the massage sequence or, as Fritz[1] so aptly puts it, it can act as the "broth" in which the other, more-specific techniques "float." A predominant general massage technique can be used regardless of the duration of the massage sequence and the relative emphasis of massage in the intervention. Consequently, the predominant general massage technique should be chosen with the overall outcomes of the intervention in mind. Furthermore, while the clinician can select more than one general massage technique for use in a given sequence, this practice may result in the loss of coherence of a massage sequence. Table 11-3 lists some of the characteristics of general massage techniques that can influence how the clinician chooses to use them in given situations.

SEQUENCE THE CHOSEN MASSAGE TECHNIQUES ACCORDING TO PRINCIPLES

The next step in designing an effective massage is to sequence the massage techniques. The following is a formal summary of sequencing principles that have been

implicitly introduced throughout the techniques chapters in the sections entitled "Manual Technique," "Context," and "Practice Variations."

APPLY GENERAL MASSAGE TECHNIQUES BEFORE SPECIFIC ONES[3,4]

The clinician should apply general massage techniques before specific ones for two reasons. First, this approach permits an assessment of the broader manifestations of a local problem. Second, general massage techniques can be used to achieve effects on level of arousal. An approach for using general massage techniques and allotting time for their use within an intervention is outlined below.

When the clinician applies general massage techniques prior to performing more-localized treatment, she obtains a full palpatory scan of the tissues that are mechanically connected to the specific area that may be the focus of treatment. This approach to determining the regional context of a set of tissues (the clinical "lay of the land") enables the clinician to identify imbalances in the tissues adjacent to a local lesion that she may have missed during the client examination. For example, antagonist and synergist muscle groups and proximal and distal tissues can be affected by a local lesion, often in predictable patterns that relate to the type of lesion. General treatment over the entire region allows the clinician to investigate and address the broader manifestations of the local problem prior to performing more-specific local treatment.

For example, a clinician who is treating a chronic tendinitis at the common extensor origin (tennis elbow) might use the following progression from general to specific massage techniques. The clinician would first apply the general massage techniques to the client's arm: regional superficial effleurage and broad neuromuscular techniques to reduce the resting level of tone in the agonist, antagonist, and synergist muscles. She would apply specific neuromuscular techniques, such as stripping to the agonist muscle, prior to performing cross-fiber friction on the tendon in question. Toward the end of the time allotted for the sequence, the clinician would reverse the order of massage techniques from specific to general again. The entire sequence leading up to the friction may take as little as 5 min yet can still be beneficial.

General massage techniques are ideal for achieving impairment-level outcomes of care that are related to level of arousal. For example, if reduction of anxiety or sedation are among the desired outcomes of care, then the periodic return to the long flowing strokes of superficial effleurage or the rhythmic undulations of rocking will enhance the sedative effects provided throughout the intervention. The clinician can also use more-specific massage techniques to address local restrictions within the same intervention. If the clinician proceeds too quickly to treatment with specific massage techniques or spends too long on these, it may be more difficult for her to achieve and maintain effective sedation.

The relative amount of time that the clinician will spend using general and specific massage techniques will vary with the impairments that she is addressing, the time available for the intervention, and the mechanical depth to which specific massage techniques must proceed (see the section on the progression from superficial to deeper massage techniques below). For example, a 20-min full-body intervention with reduction of anxiety as the impairment-level outcome of care might consist only of general massage techniques. On the other hand, a 20-min regional intervention for a chronic orthopedic lesion, which is aimed at the promotion of remodeling of deep connective tissue, might include 15 min of very specific massage techniques.

APPLY SUPERFICIAL MASSAGE TECHNIQUES BEFORE DEEPER MASSAGE TECHNIQUES[1-7]

Superficial massage techniques engage structures near the surface of the client's body, whereas deeper massage techniques engage those tissue layers that lie deep to the superficial tissues. The appropriate depth of the massage technique to be applied varies with the client's clinical condition. Deeper massage techniques are not necessarily better, nor is it always necessary to mechanically engage structures far below the surface to produce profound or lasting effects.

There are several reasons to begin with the application of superficial massage techniques. The application of superficial massage techniques enables the client to accommodate to the clinician's touch. In addition, the manner in which superficial massage techniques are applied permits the clinician to palpate the client's body with her hand in the most relaxed and sensitive position.

Consequently, the clinician is able to assess the immediate response of the client's body to her touch. Finally, some clinical conditions can impede the clinician's ability to palpate and appropriately treat the client's underlying tissues. For example, when the edema that accompanies acute inflammation and the fibrosis that is associated with chronic conditions occur at the superficial level, they can limit the clinician's ability to accurately palpate deeper structures. In these situations, the clinician should proceed to the first tissue layer at which she can palpate an abnormality and treat that layer until there is a perceptible (usually palpable) restoration of function. From this point, she may increase her pressure and the depth of the application of the technique to access deeper structures. A useful analogy for this approach to treatment is peeling the layers of an onion.

When the restriction is in multiple layers of muscle or connective tissue, the clinician may not be able to accurately determine where the restriction is located at the outset of the intervention. Nevertheless, the basic procedure remains the same: the clinician proceeds gradually through superficial layers to the first palpable restriction, she normalizes this restriction, and then she treats progressively deeper layers of tissue restriction. Regardless of the massage techniques used, toward the end of the regional sequence, the clinician gradually reduces the pressure she exerts on the client's tissues and briefly reengages each layer that she previously addressed. This allows her to reassess any additional effects that the use of deeper massage techniques may have had on the superficial tissues.

Here are some examples of this progression from superficial to deeper massage techniques. If traumatic edema is present, the clinician will not attempt to engage structures underlying the local edema with massage techniques until the edema has resolved. Usually within

Table 11-3
Characteristics of Some General Massage Techniques

Technique	Requires Oil	Works Through Sheet	Advantages/Disadvantages
Broad-contact compression in a series	No	Yes	Takes more time, but gives information about deeper tissues
Myofascial release	No	±	Slow
Rocking	No	±	Highly sedative, but motion may increase pain
Superficial stroking	No	Yes	Produces only reflex effects
Superficial effleurage	Yes	No	Takes little time

±, the technique may be applied through the fabric, but this may reduce its effectiveness.

a day of initiating treatment, the clinician can perform superficial reflex techniques on the site of trauma and then superficial fluid techniques to the proximal margin of swelling, as tolerated by the client. At the end of this intervention, she would return to superficial reflex techniques. During subsequent interventions, the clinician would apply massage techniques using the same basic pattern of treating from superficial to deep to superficial on the site of the lesion as the edema resolves. With each intervention, the clinician would apply massage techniques in a manner that would enable her to reach progressively deeper tissue layers.

If the client's subcutaneous tissues are normal but a restriction exists in a superficial layer of muscle, the clinician may progress the massage within a minute or two to include the application of neuromuscular techniques that engage this layer. If the difficulty lies in a deeper muscular layer, the clinician would begin as noted in the previous example, then engage progressively deeper layers of muscle before she finally engages the target layer in which the restriction lies.

When designing the progression of the depth of massage techniques in a massage sequence, the clinician must keep in mind that superficial reflex techniques, such as static contact, superficial stroking, and fine vibration, may be used at any time in an intervention and for virtually any length of time. These massage techniques are commonly placed at the beginning and end of full-body or regional sequences. Furthermore, except for a brief application (1 to 2 min) of static contact at the beginning of an intervention, the clinician may omit the use of superficial reflex techniques entirely if the principal focus of an intervention is not pain relief or sedation for an acute or severe clinical condition.

Coordinate and Repeat the Transitions from General to Specific to General and from Superficial to Deep to Superficial

In practice, the clinician executes the transitions from general to specific to general and from superficial to deep to superficial simultaneously. In other words, massage sequences begin with the application of general massage techniques over large areas to engage superficial tissues and then progress to the application of massage techniques that engage deeper tissues to a succession of smaller areas. The clinician returns to the use of a more general and superficial application of massage techniques between her treatment of the smaller areas. When time permits, it is also useful for the clinician to make such transitions in depth and specificity several times during the course of a regional massage sequence. This strategy permits the clinician to continuously assess the tissue responses at different depths throughout the region being treated. Adherence to these guidelines will reduce the occurrence of the agonist/

antagonist imbalances that might otherwise result from the application of deep, specific massage techniques that is required for the treatment of chronic restrictions in muscle and connective tissue (see later in this chapter).

PRINCIPLES RELATED TO ENHANCING FLUID RETURN

The following principles are relevant when the clinician specifically seeks to enhance lymphatic or venous return. While these principles are commonly observed in classical sequences that emphasize effleurage and petrissage, they may in fact be disregarded when the clinician is not attempting to enhance fluid return.

Use Centripetal Pressure and the Assistance of Gravity When Possible

The use of centripetal pressure with minimal pressure on the return stroke ensures that the mechanical flow of fluid receives maximal assistance in the direction of the flow of its normal return.[3–6,8,9]

Begin Proximally, Proceed Distally, Return Proximally, and Repeat [2–4,6,8,9]

When the aim of treatment is to increase lymphatic return from a region, the clinician begins the application of massage techniques as proximally (close to the heart) as time allows and progressively moves in a distal direction until she approaches the region. The direction of pressure of each stroke is, nonetheless, always centripetal. For the limbs, this requires that the clinician begin at least as proximally as the axillary or inguinal lymph nodes. The clinician repeats this sequence of applying massage techniques from proximal to distal as frequently as the time available for the intervention allows. This approach of beginning treatment proximally creates a proximal reservoir into which the fluid that is located in the distal region can be moved.[9] If the client's lymphatics are not intact, the clinician designates a proximal body segment as the reservoir to which the fluid from the distal region will be directed; for example, this may be the client's contralateral trunk or ipsilateral chest.

Maximize the Relaxation of the Proximal Muscle Groups

Earlier this century, Mennell[10] noted that deep veins and deep lymphatics are embedded in skeletal muscle and, consequently, that excessive muscular tone can compress the lumen of the deep veins and lymphatics and thus contribute to a reduction in venous and lymphatic flow. When the clinician ensures that there is maximum pliability of all of the muscles between the heart and the body segment from which drainage is required, she will reduce the internal pressure on the collapsible vessels and passively assist venous and lymphatic return. If possible, then, the clinician will incorporate the application of massage techniques to increase the general mobility and muscular relaxation of the muscles of the thorax. In some cases (e.g., with hand edema secondary to thoracic outlet syndrome), addressing mobility and relaxation in the thorax may be the first priority. In practice, the clinician may sometimes have to shift her focus quickly to the client's affected limb because of time constraints; however, this approach must be judged carefully, since the application of massage techniques to proximal regions may be more effective.

The sequencing of massage techniques is often more flexible when the clinician is applying superficial reflex, connective tissue, specific neuromuscular, and passive movement techniques. Clinicians should note that when circulatory concerns are not the focus of treatment, they may use centrifugal pressure (with the exception of deep centrifugal pressure over incompetent veins or, as some authors suggest, all veins[1,2]), and they may apply massage techniques to distal areas first.

Coordinate All Transitions

Clinicians frequently encounter situations in which the tissues to be engaged in adjacent body segments lie at different depths. For example, with posttraumatic swelling of the wrist, massage on the immediate site of the injury is contraindicated, minimal, or light, depending on the nature and degree of the injury. In this case, the clinician may begin the application of massage techniques to the superficial tissue layers on the proximal portion of the client's arm to enhance his superficial lymphatic return. She would then gradually move her application of massage techniques in a distal direction toward the proximal edge of the swelling. In addition, the clinician might progress to the application of massage techniques to deeper tissue layers of the upper arm to relax the client's muscles and enhance the deep lymphatic return from his proximal arm. To progress the intervention, she might alternate between the proximal application of deeper massage techniques and the distal application of superficial massage techniques, moderating the depth of her application of massage techniques as she moves from one body segment to the other. To complete the intervention, she would apply superficial massage techniques over the entire treated portion of the client's limb.

APPLY MASSAGE TECHNIQUES FROM THE PERIPHERY TO THE CENTER OF THE REGION BEING TREATED[4]

When the clinician is addressing a circumscribed area of local pathology as the focus of an intervention, she begins with the application of regional general massage techniques and gradually moves her application of massage techniques closer to the periphery of the local region. This strategy permits the clinician to palpate related tissue changes that may occur in areas that are remote from the local region being treated. Furthermore, it enables the clinician to gradually introduce the application of massage techniques to an area that may demonstrate tenderness and other altered responses to touch.

The same principle of applying massage techniques from the periphery to the center of the region being treated applies to the treatment of an area of circumscribed swelling. In this case, the clinician applies massage techniques in a centrifugal direction at the periphery of the area of swelling and gradually moves her application of massage techniques toward the center of the area of swelling as the peripheral fluid is absorbed.

ADDRESS AGONIST, ANTAGONIST, AND SYNERGIST MUSCLE GROUPS

When the clinician uses neuromuscular or connective tissue techniques, she must be careful to avoid producing an imbalance in the client's myofascial system. This is particularly important if the clinician is applying these massage techniques in small areas, with a higher force, or for long periods of time. For example, Travell and Simons[11] have noted that releasing trigger points can produce a reactive tightening or cramping in related muscles and may activate other trigger points. Clinicians who use connective tissue techniques routinely note positional shifts in related body segments in response to the local application of massage techniques.

When the clinician applies deep specific massage techniques locally without including the use of other general massage techniques, clients will commonly experience undesirable responses to the treatment within half an hour to 3 days following the intervention. These responses can include reactive tightness and pain in (a) areas that are immediately proximal or distal to the site that was treated, (b) in antagonist or synergist muscle groups that are located on the same side of an adjacent joint, or (c) in antagonist or synergist muscle groups that lie across a joint. Reactive pain and restrictions can be detrimental to the client's clinical condition and may worsen until the imbalance that resulted from treatment resolves or is treated. To avoid this situation, the clinician must also plan to address the related areas where reactive tightening may occur whenever she includes the application of local, deep, specific massage techniques within an intervention. The less-experienced clinician can use the application of nonsuperficial general neuromuscular massage techniques, such as broad-contact compression or petrissage, for this purpose. A very experienced clinician may use a postural assessment to identify relatively shortened areas that must be lengthened to maintain adequate myofascial balance. Regardless of her level of expertise, the clinician should alert the client to the possibility of these sequelae to treatment and ensure that the client understands that it is important to communicate with the clinician if a troublesome shift in pain or symptoms occurs after the intervention. The clinician may also teach the client appropriate stretching exercises to minimize reactive tightening.

In general, the intensity and duration of the application of treatment techniques to balance antagonist and synergist muscle groups will vary in direct proportion to the specificity, depth, and duration of the treatment that is performed on the principal area of treatment. This component of the treatment might require from 10 to 50% of the designated treatment time. The clinician's ability to identify which antagonist and synergist muscle groups are the most prone to reactive tightening and to determine how long to spend on addressing this issue will improve with experience and, one hopes, with a minimum of client distress.

Treatment of the Contralateral Side

The clinician may have to include the treatment of the client's contralateral side or limb within an intervention that addresses a unilateral lesion. For example, the clinician who is treating a client with a unilateral piriformis syndrome may justifiably include petrissage, stripping, and specific compression as the primary massage techniques to lengthen the client's affected piriformis. She must, however, also ensure that she treats the client's unaffected gluteals and lateral rotators, to ensure that the end-result of the intervention is a reasonably balanced bilateral distribution of tension throughout the pelvic musculature. Clinicians vary as to whether they apply massage techniques to the contralateral limb before or after their treatment of the client's affected limb. It may be easier for the clinician to judge the depth and intensity of the treatment that is required to achieve balance with the client's contralateral limb after she has treated the affected limb. When the clinician is treating an acute unilateral orthopedic lesion, she may also treat the client's contralateral side as a means of addressing compensations that may arise from altered patterns of muscular use.

Treatment of the Related Axial Skeleton

If the clinician applies deep specific neuromuscular or connective tissue techniques on one of a client's limbs (even the distal limb), she should also treat the related portion of the axial skeleton, even briefly. For the lower limbs, the clinician applies general petrissage (or a related general technique) to the lumbar musculature bilaterally, and for the upper limbs, she applies general massage techniques to the cervical musculature bilaterally. For example, a clinician who is treating a client with deQuervain's tenosynovitis might apply superficial effleurage to the client's entire arm, broad-contact petrissage to his upper arm and then to his lower arm, additional specific neuromuscular techniques to his lower arm, friction to the tendons in the region of the anatomical snuff box, and broad-contact petrissage and superficial effleurage to his entire arm. Furthermore, she would either precede or follow this massage sequence with the brief application of broad-contact or general petrissage to the client's contralateral arm and cervical musculature (approximately 25% of the treatment time).

SEQUENCE MASSAGE TECHNIQUES WITH OTHER APPROPRIATE TREATMENT TECHNIQUES

The clinician will often apply massage techniques in conjunction with other treatment techniques that are relevant to the client's clinical condition. Examples of how to sequence the use of massage techniques with physical agents and therapeutic exercise are given to illustrate how the clinician may approach this task.

The clinician who is coordinating the application of heat and cold with massage techniques will not alter the sequence of the massage techniques themselves. Instead, she would apply the selected physical agent either before or after the massage techniques. Cryotherapy, such as ice or cold packs, is not routinely applied before massage, since this would result in a decrease in the client's sensation in the region that the clinician is treating. This decrease in sensation would be a concern, since with all massage techniques it is important that the client is able to provide accurate feedback about the tenderness or pain arising from the involved tissues during the massage. The clinician can use cryotherapy after the application of massage techniques to reduce the client's symptoms or the consequences of the overapplication of massage techniques. For example, if the clinician believes that she has overtreated a client with friction, then it would be appropriate for her to ice the treatment area after the application of friction. The clinician may also apply cold packs to another body segment concurrently with the application of massage techniques. This would be the case if the clinician was treating an acute orthopedic injury, such as a sprained ankle, and used cold packs on the site of the lesion (as it was elevated) while she applied massage techniques proximally to reduce edema.

If the clinician is applying massage techniques to healthy tissues or chronic lesions, she can apply heat either before or after the application of the massage techniques. When treating muscle, the clinician can apply heat before the application of massage techniques to relax the muscle, to decrease tissue viscosity, and to allow easier access to deep tissue layers.[12] If, however, the clinician was applying massage techniques to lengthen or stretch dense connective tissue, then it would not be appropriate for her to use heat prior to the application of these massage techniques, since the application of heat prior to any sustained loading of connective tissue can increase the risk of collagenous rupture.[13]

Massage techniques are usually applied before the use of therapeutic exercise. In doing so, the clinician can prepare the client's tissue for active or resisted exercise by increasing tissue extensibility, improving the balance of agonist/antagonist function, and enhancing the client's level of alertness. The clinician can also use massage techniques prior to the application of passive exercise, such as stretching or passive range-of-motion exercises, to enhance the effects of those techniques. A skillful clinician can alternate between the application of massage techniques and passive exercise techniques so that they seamlessly blend together throughout the intervention. Finally, in cases in which the client has abnormal neuromuscular tone, the clinician can use massage techniques as proprioceptive or exteroceptive stimulation techniques to normalize neuromuscular tone and the client's movement responses in preparation for therapeutic exercise or functional activity.[14]

Design of Regional Massage Sequences

The steps involved in designing a massage sequence for a region are summarized in Box 11-3. Using this approach, the clinician can generate a wide variety of sequences that address different outcomes through the use of different massage techniques.

Some simple examples with questions and instructions to guide students and novice clinicians in the art of designing massage sequences follow (see Examples 11-1 to 11-5). These examples are by no means the only possible massage sequences—they are simply illustrations of ways in which the clinician can apply the guidelines discussed in this chapter. Students and novice clinicians are advised not to hurry this portion of their training, since the exploration of a variety of different massage sequences will facilitate their development of a flexible, adaptable approach to treatment. Even the design of seemingly simple regional sequences involves considerable reflection and planning on the part of the clinician. Clinicians who practice in settings where intervention time is short (10 to 20 min) especially need to master the principles of massage design, since there is often no extra time in which to address oversights of planning.

> **Box 11-3**
> ### Steps in the Design of Regional Massage Sequences
>
> Summarize and prioritize impairment-level outcomes of care
>
> Choose relevant massage techniques
>
> Assign the time for regional sequence
>
> Choose the predominant general technique
>
> Order the massage techniques, keeping in mind
>
> - Position of superficial reflex work if included
> - General to specific to general
> - Superficial to deep to superficial
> - Proximal to distal if working to enhance fluid return
> - Periphery to center if working with circumscribed local pathology
> - Agonist/antagonist/synergist balance if including neuromuscular or connective tissue techniques to release local restriction
>
> Do other regions have to be included? If so, design these sequences and revise the time budget for the intervention.

EXAMPLE 11-1
A Regional Sequence for the Back[2,5]

Impairment-level outcomes of care: Decreased resting level of tension throughout the muscles of the back, increased muscle extensibility, increased mobility of spinal joints and rib cage, reduction of pain, reduction of perceived anxiety, sedation

Time: 20-40 min

Predominant general technique(s): Superficial and deep effleurage

Techniques and order of application:

Static contact applied to sacrum and occiput
Superficial palmar stroking down spine
Effleurage progressing from superficial to deep
Wringing, picking up, palmar kneading applied to the whole back
Deep effleurage with forearm; finger and thumb kneading to erector spinae muscles
Stripping along erector spinae muscles with elbow
Bilateral specific compression along erector spinae muscles—10 locations at 20 sec per location
Palmar kneading
Wringing
Superficial palmar stroking, becoming progressively slower
Static contact at sacrum and occiput

Additional: Slow and rhythmic. Apply each massage technique for 1 to 2 min. After you introduce superficial effleurage, return to it for a few strokes before you add each new technique. Switch sides every few minutes. It may exacerbate muscular imbalances to perform all massage techniques on one side of the back before switching. Simply break contact, move around the table and recommence. This type of sequence might be indicated in back pain and/or tightness associated with prolonged bed rest and in the chronic stage of erector spinae strain or lumbar facet derangement.

Further exercises:

1. Why might you have to address the extensors of the hip after this sequence is performed? How would you alter the sequence to include these?

2. For similar aims and techniques, how would you adapt this routine for other regions? Practice several of these in a similar time interval.

3. For similar impairment-level outcomes of care, how would the selected massage techniques differ for a clothed client? Design and practice a regional back sequence with this restriction in mind.

4. How would you alter this sequence if there were only 15 min available for the intervention? If there were 10?

EXAMPLE 11-2

A Regional Sequence for the Abdomen[2,5,15]

Caution: When practicing this sequence, bear in mind that deep abdominal pressure is not advisable immediately preceding or during menstruation because of sensitivity and because local congestion limits the clinician's ability to palpate. Even light abdominal massage during menstruation may alter the flow and duration of the menses. See detailed discussion of contraindications and cautions in Chapter 2, The Clinical Decision-Making Process.

Impairment-level outcomes of care: Stimulated peristalsis, systemic sedation, decreased resting tension throughout the abdominal musculature

Time: 20–30 min

Predominant general technique: Superficial effleurage

Techniques and order of application:

Static contact applied to navel and occiput

Superficial stroking of the abdomen in clockwise circles

Effleurage progressing from superficial to deep in clockwise circles

Wringing, picking up, and palmar kneading applied to the entire abdomen

Specific kneading and stripping to abdominal muscle (moderate pressure can be used as long as there is a high horizontal component—high shear—to localize the force to the skeletal muscle)

Draw knees up to a crook lying position to slacken abdominal wall

Deep specific compression applied in retrograde sequence from the sigmoid colon to the iliocecal valve

Palmar kneading

Wringing

Large-amplitude sedative shaking

Rocking

Static contact at navel and occiput

Additional: Slow and rhythmic. Apply each massage technique for 1 to 2 min. After superficial effleurage is introduced, return to it for a few strokes before each new massage technique is added. Switch sides as required. The application and release of deep specific digital compression must be very slow, and the clinician must pay close attention to the client's comfort level.

The scant literature suggests that abdominal massage may have a reflex or mechanical effect on peristalsis.[16–19] Among the clinicians who use massage extensively, there is a very common perception that abdominal massage will at least promote colonic emptying. Nevertheless, opinion about the mechanisms by which this might occur are varied, since the nervous control of peristalsis itself is vastly complicated. Peristalsis may be promoted by

1. Superficial reflex techniques applied over the abdominal wall
2. Nonspecific neuromuscular techniques that decrease the tone of the skeletal muscle of the abdominal wall and affect intestinal flow via somatovisceral reflexes
3. Deep specific massage techniques that mechanically assist movement in the direction of the colonic flow (Mennell doubted that this was possible[10])

With respect to the three possible mechanisms above, the prevalent practice is for light massage techniques, such as superficial stroking, to be performed in the direction of colonic flow. Neuromuscular techniques, such as wringing, are oriented according to the direction of the muscle fibers being treated. Finally, deep massage techniques, which specifically seek to move intestinal contents, are performed over the colon with pressure in the direction of peristaltic flow in a retrograde sequence from the sigmoid colon to the iliocecal valve.[1,2,5] The last mechanism presupposes that the skeletal muscle that forms the abdominal wall has been sufficiently relaxed to allow the pressure of the technique to physically engage the viscera. It is important to remember that a nonspecific way of promoting peristalsis is to promote a generalized parasympathetic response. This can be done when working on any region.

Further exercises:

1. Design and practice a 20-min abdominal sequence that has the same aims, but is done through a sheet.
2. Design and practice a similar abdominal sequence that is done from one or both sides with the client in sidelying.
3. How might some of the treatment be accomplished with the client prone? Consider, for example, what lumbar wringing might achieve.

EXAMPLE 11-3
A Regional Sequence for the Leg[2,5,9]

Impairment-level outcomes of care: Increased lymphatic return from a leg with an intact lymphatic system, decreased perceived anxiety

Restrictions: Administered directly on skin with talc, cornstarch, or chalk

Time: 20–30 min

Predominant general massage technique: Superficial and deep effleurage

Massage techniques and order of application:

Position client supine with legs elevated 30–45°
Instruct client in deep diaphragmatic breathing
Apply rhythmic palmar compression over the upper ribs for 2–3 min
Superficial effleurage to entire affected leg
Superficial lymphatic technique beginning at proximal thigh and then beginning progressively more distal with each new series of strokes, until the foot is reached (repeat ad lib)
Deep effleurage
Series of centripetally moving palmar compressions applied in a pattern similar to that used in the lymphatic technique above (i.e., beginning proximally and starting progressively more distal with each new series until the foot is reached) (repeat ad lib)
Passive relaxed movements for all joints, beginning at the hip and proceeding to the ankle
Superficial effleurage

Additional: This sequence uses few massage techniques, but they must be repeated. Frequent repetition is required when moving fluid, and it facilitates developing the rhythmic stability that is useful for achieving sedation. Note that there are two general massage techniques used here: superficial effleurage is interspersed with the superficial lymphatic technique, whereas deep effleurage is interspersed with the compressions. This sequence could be used to drain a localized traumatic edema anywhere in the leg, such as an ankle sprain, quadriceps contusion, or hamstring strain, with appropriate modifications to avoid areas of acute tissue damage, to reduce the pressure around these areas, to avoid pushing fluid through areas of congestion, and to perform passive movements only where they can be performed without pain.

Further exercises:

1. How would you address the same impairments with massage techniques that use oil as a lubricant? How would you do this without using lubricant?

2. Design and practice a similar sequence that seeks to drain a designated area on the thorax toward the ipsilateral axilla.

3. How would the sequence change if the application of mechanical techniques was contraindicated in the area of the ankle?

4. How would the sequence change to address swelling in the posterior calf? For example, an acute calf contusion or Achilles tendon rupture.

5. Should the sequence be altered to include other proximal segments or the contralateral leg?

EXAMPLE 11-4

A Regional Sequence for the Shoulders

Impairment-level outcomes of care: Decreased resting tension of skeletal muscle, separation and lengthening of superficial fascial layers, enhanced muscle performance (secondary), increased joint mobility

Restrictions: Minimal lubricant

Time: 30+ min (to do both shoulders)

Predominant general massage technique: Rhythmical mobilization

Massage techniques and order of application:

Rhythmical mobilization

General, broad-contact neuromuscular technique (compression and squeezing) and direct fascial tissue technique, progressing to more-specific neuromuscular and direct fascial technique

Combine direct fascial technique with slow active movements

Rhythmical mobilization

Additional: Split the sequence into the application of techniques with the client in supine, then prone, or perform the entire sequence with the client in sidelying (both sides). Apply all massage techniques from midthorax to occiput and distal to the elbow. Include all muscles that produce motion at the glenohumeral joint and the scapulothoracic articulation. Use minimal lubricant, otherwise there will not be enough drag for the connective tissue work. Return to rhythmical mobilization frequently—ensure that it is not too stimulating. The two shoulders should receive equal time, though in different areas: usually, the dominant shoulder is tighter anteriorly, and the nondominant is tighter posteriorly. It is very instructive to get the client off the table after one side is completed and compare the range and ease of movement of the two shoulders. Once both shoulders are completed, spend at least 5 minutes to address the neck with conventional stretching (or myofascial release) and traction. This would make an acceptable intervention for a capsular restriction. If the client presented with adhesive capsulitis, trigger point work (especially to subscapularis[11]), friction to relevant tendons,[23] and joint play might be added after the specific neuromuscular technique.

EXAMPLE 11-5
A Regional Sequence for the Neck, Head, and Face[2,5]

Impairment-level outcomes of care: Counterirritant analgesia, reduction of trigger point activity, decreased resting tension of skeletal muscle, increased range of motion, systemic sedation

Restrictions: No lubricant

Time: 20–30 min

Predominant general massage technique: Palmar compression

Massage techniques and order of application:

Supine

Palmar superficial stroking

Palmar compression done as a series from the top of the neck to the clavicle, unilaterally, then palmar compression to head; muscle squeezing to neck

Specific compression on either side of spine and to suboccipital muscles, followed by appropriate stretch

Specific compression to sites of upper trapezius and sternocleidomastoid trigger points (use pincer compression for sternocleidomastoid), followed by appropriate stretches; gentle fingertip kneading to face, more vigorous fingertip kneading to scalp

Fingertip fascial technique with short strokes to scalp

Gentle palmar compression from top of neck toward axilla in several series

Superficial stroking throughout with palms, then fingertips

Additional: Spend 3 to 4 min on each item. Turn the client's head frequently and, if necessary, ensure that the client's neck is supported with a small pillow for comfort. Return to the application of palmar compression done as a series from the top of the neck to the axilla between each new massage technique. This sequence with slight adaptations would be valuable in many cases of muscular tension or trigger point headache.

Design of More-Extensive Massage Sequences

The most common example of a more-extensive massage sequence is the "full-body massage." In its simplest form, a full-body massage is simply a series of regional sequences that covers the entire body and is executed in a chosen order. These regional sequences are designed using the guidelines outlined earlier in this chapter, employ similar massage techniques, and are similar in character. The exception to this guideline is that if there is a specific condition in one region that requires a different technical approach, then that sequence will differ from the others and will often be allocated proportionately more time. Specifying an order and time for each regional sequence can help the clinician overcome the problem of being unable to complete treatment in the available amount of time. Furthermore, the clinician must prioritize the outcomes of care for a given intervention, since clinicians are typically faced with more work than they can accomplish in a single intervention. The use of a combination of clear prioritization of outcomes and

adherence to the allocated timing of techniques will minimize the likelihood that the clinician will lose focus or get sidetracked during the intervention.

The practice of including all the regions of the body in an intervention is common for "wellness massage" (general full-body relaxation massage)[1,2,5] and many of the approaches listed in Table 11-5. The regions that the clinician does not treat in an intervention will vary with social norms, the clinician's training, and the preference of the clinician and the client. Within 45 to 60 min, it is often possible for the clinician to address, at least briefly, each region of the client's body. Since many clinical conditions require a more-extended local focus, the time constraints of many clinical settings often require that the clinician omit some regions or treat them in a cursory manner with general massage techniques. Consequently, it is important that the clinician ascertains during the initial interview whether the client expects all regions to be included in a longer massage.

There is no one order in which the clinician must treat the regions addressed during a full-body massage.[1,2,3] An acceptable order is for the clinician to begin regional sequences at the client's head or feet and then proceed region by region to the other end of the client's body in prone, supine, or sidelying. The clinician will then turn the client and repeat or reverse the order of treatment of the regions. If there is a clear emphasis on one category of technique, then there may be some restrictions to the order in which regions can be addressed (see Table 11-4).

APPROACHES TO FULL-BODY WELLNESS MASSAGE

The reader who has systematically practiced the application of individual massage techniques all over the client's body as suggested in the practice sequences of previous chapters has already carried out a number of different approaches to full-body massage that can achieve the impairment-level outcomes of care associated with the technique used. This "one-technique" sequence has limited scope but can be highly effective and rewarding for both client and clinician. More-familiar approaches to full-body massage employ a greater variety of massage techniques and involve the application of these massage techniques at a consistent rate and rhythm to produce a coherent, structured sensory experience for the client.

Classical, or "Swedish" massage, as it is commonly practiced today, uses mostly superficial fluid and neuromuscular techniques. In applying these massage techniques, the clinician uses a broad-contact surface, moderate centripetal pressure, and a rhythmical rate[2,5] (quite slow if the clinician was trained in North America

and faster if she was trained in Europe). When performed in this manner, classical, or Swedish, massage increases the return of lymph (and possibly venous blood), reduces the level of resting muscle tension, reduces anxiety, and enhances the client's awareness (see chapters on superficial fluid and neuromuscular techniques for details of effects). This effective approach to the full-body massage sequence continues to be the cultural archetype for wellness massage in North America.

Increased access to the massage forms of other cultures and the work of modern Western innovators has recently spurred a substantial technical renaissance in the practice of massage. Many of these traditions or approaches use a limited spectrum of massage techniques and refine related client examination and palpation skills to a high degree. Some of these approaches are summarized in Table 11-5.[1-3,5-8,20] Without trivializing the substantial philosophical differences that exist between these approaches, they can each be characterized as the refined application of specialized massage techniques that results in the achievement of particular effects and very different sensory experiences for the client. When appropriate to the clinical situation and executed with skill, any one of these approaches can produce excellent results.

MAXIMIZING RELAXATION IN WELLNESS MASSAGE

A great emphasis is placed on active sympathetic functioning; however, repair and regeneration of the body and mind may occur more effectively when the nervous system is in a parasympathetic state. A central

Table 11-4
Suggestions for Ordering Regions When Emphasis Is Placed on Particular Massage Techniques

Emphasized Technique	*Suggestions for Ordering Regions*
Connective tissue	If there is extensive connective tissue work, start and/or end with work around the sacrum and iliac crest
Connective tissue, passive movement	Include the axial skeleton (i.e., neck, back, pelvis, sacrum); if there is deep, specific, or extensive work around the lumbar/pelvic region, include at least briefly the lower legs and feet
Neuromuscular	If there is deep, specific work on limbs, conclude with the related axial skeleton, i.e., cervical or lumbar area
Percussive	Rarely if ever emphasized throughout the body; if concentrated in the thorax for an extended period, finish with sedative reflex technique
Superficial fluid	Start on upper thorax and proceed distally to region of focus; work distally from next major proximal set of lymph nodes
Superficial reflex	Start and finish with sacrum, occiput, face hands, or feet

Note: The basis for most of these suggestions is discussed in the individual techniques chapters.

Table 11-5
Characteristic Massage Techniques of Some Popular Massage-Related Approaches

Approach, System, or School	*Characteristic Massage Techniques*
Lomilomi	Fast, superficial and deep effleurage and fast, broad neuromuscular technique
Manual lymph drainage	Superficial effleurage and superficial lymphatic technique
Myofascial release	Myofascial release, craniosacral techniques
Neuromuscular technique	Specific kneading, stripping, specific direct fascial technique
Polarity	Static contact and compression
Rolfing,® Bindegewebsmassage	Direct fascial technique
Shiatsu	Compression, specific (ischemic) compression, stretching
Therapeutic Touch, Reiki	Static contact
Trager®	Rocking, and sedative rhythmical mobilization and shaking

Data from references 1–3, 5–8, 20.

premise of wellness massage is that systemic sedation (a "relaxation response") is a desirable impairment-level outcome of care in most situations. This fact is also true for the application of massage techniques to clinical conditions, although other goals related to presenting impairments may be a higher priority for both the client and the clinician.

An important axiom of practice is that to produce relaxation in a client, the clinician must be relaxed. The corollary is equally true: clients will not relax in the hands of an agitated clinician. It is as if the physical state of relaxation or tension is transmitted from person to person. This axiom is worthy of consideration and is very easy to forget in a busy practice. Suggesting that a clinician work from a place of deep calm does not in any way imply that she will exhibit a lack of attention, inquiry, or intention, nor that she will suspend her capacity for critical thinking. A good clinician is highly adept at achieving a relaxed, attentive state in herself while maintaining her focus on the objectives of treatment and using precise technique. As discussed in the chapter on the process of clinical care, the clinician is advised to practice gentle stretching, conscious breathing, and some ritual of calming the mind throughout the workday, especially in the few minutes preceding a massage intervention. The use of conscious diaphragmatic breathing and controlled repetitive movement using correct mechanics can also deepen a clinician's relaxation during the application of massage techniques.

Students and novice clinicians often learn how to perform a general full-body massage for relaxation in an environment that is relatively free of pressure. When they are later faced with the pressures of completing client examinations, handling complex clinical situations, and managing the time constraints of practice, they commonly fail to maintain and refine the skill of being relaxed when performing a massage intervention. The resulting massage intervention may be technically competent but may feel somewhat disjointed or ineffective to both clinician and client because it lacks the critical element of relaxation that contributes so much to the experience of both parties.

Box 11-4 summarizes some hints to help clinicians achieve and maintain effective sedation in their clients. These suggestions must be tempered with the observation that what produces deep relaxation will differ from client to client and from intervention to intervention. In light of this, the clinician must continually monitor the client's subtle body cues and make judicious inquiries about the client's response to treatment to determine the effectiveness of an intervention with the goal of producing deep relaxation.

ADDRESSING THE EFFECTS OF STRESS

While there is no direct link from the autonomic nervous system to skeletal muscle, research suggests that a generalized elevation of muscle resting tension is one of the effects of stress and the activation of the sympathetic nervous system.[21,22] As a result, massage techniques that reduce muscle resting tension are among the most valuable for treating the short-term and long-term effects of stress. Since neuromuscular techniques, connective tissue techniques, and movement techniques can all affect the level of resting tension in skeletal muscle and the quality and quantity of movement, they are obvious choices for returning a client's body to homeostasis after periods of stress.

Nevertheless, addressing the effects of stress by altering the level of resting muscle tension and improving the quality and quantity of movement is not the same as reducing anxiety or producing sedation, although they may all be addressed with the same massage techniques. If a principal outcome of treatment is the amelioration of ongoing stress in otherwise healthy individuals, the clinician usually seeks to achieve (at least) three outcomes: to produce and maintain sedation throughout the massage, to decrease the level of resting tension of skeletal muscle, and to improve the quality and quantity of movement, since movement is often restricted by stress-related muscular tension. If the clinician only achieves sedation with her intervention, the client may soon feel not much different than before the massage intervention. If the level of resting muscle tension and the movement patterns of skeletal muscle are also altered,

---

Box 11-4
To Maximize a Client's Relaxation During Massage

Prior to touch, ensure that the

Client

- needs/desires sedation
- has expressed expectations and preferences
- is comfortable!
- is breathing fully but without forcing, using the diaphragm

Clinician

- is breathing fully using the diaphragm
- has a clear logistical plan for the intervention
- has a calm mind, free of distracting self-talk
- is relaxed, free of stress or pain

Environment is quiet and as private as possible

While in contact, ensure that

- The rate and rhythm of similar strokes is constant
- Pressure transitions within each stroke are smooth
- Transitions from one type of stroke to another are smooth
- Contact is made and broken gently and carefully
- Communication is minimal
- The client is comfortable after each change of position
- YOU DO NOT EVER RUSH OR HURRY

After contact Allow a rest period of 10 to 60 min

Box 11-5
An Unpleasant Experiment: The Incoherent Massage

Allow about 20 min

Prepare for prone or supine

Choose massage techniques with conflicting intentions

Randomly and rapidly vary rate, rhythm, and pressure

Arbitrarily switch back and forth from region to region

Ignore your posture: slump, lean in an uncontrolled fashion

Talk to the client about whatever crosses your mind

It usually takes less than 5 min to make an unforgettable point to the person on the table. Once the clinician terminates the exercise, help the client return to homeostasis with some sedative massage.

---

the combination of aims will be synergistic. A good clinician can seamlessly incorporate massage techniques that alternately or simultaneously address all of these outcomes during the massage sequence and may also be able to address other impairment-level outcomes.

THE ART OF COHERENCE

In the context of outcome-based massage, coherence is defined as the consistent order or structure of an intervention. Coherence is the result of clear and consistent intention(s) on the part of the clinician. Maintaining coherence is relevant in all massage interventions, but it is of particular importance in massage sequences that last longer than 15 min and that address multiple impairment-level outcomes of care with a wide variety of massage techniques. Coherent massage interventions produce in the client a overall feeling of being in harmony and balanced throughout the massage sequence and afterward. It is fairly easy to imagine an incoherent full-body sequence: vigorous fast shaking on one leg, smooth slow superficial effleurage on the other, similarly mismatched massage techniques on the arms, myofascial release on the back, and light percussion on the face. Other examples of strategies that result in lack of coherence are in Box 11-5.

Several strategies that can help the clinician produce coherent massage interventions have been previously introduced. The most important of these is unwavering relaxation of the clinician around the treatment table. Constant relaxation throughout the intervention conveys a consistency of manner and approach to the client, regardless of the technical content of the intervention.

Another strategy for making an intervention coherent is to achieve and maintain a generalized nervous response in the client throughout the intervention: this would usually be sedation, or the "relaxation response." A third way of increasing the coherence of a massage sequence is to use the same type of general stroke (palpatory stroke, connecting stroke) to touch all regions of the client's body throughout the intervention. Returning periodically to the same technique imparts a sense of sensory regularity to the sequence, which can put the client at ease. Touching all regions of the body—even if only briefly with general strokes—can strongly reinforce a client's sense of being addressed as a whole person, not merely as an instance of an illness or disorder. This is often a crucial and unstated concern when the client has experienced long-standing pain or physical disability. Nevertheless, it is not how much of the body is touched, but the manner in which it is touched that is critical. Coherence can be unwittingly reduced when the clinician uses too many massage techniques with a large variation in rate, pressure, and palpatory focus. Strategies to enhance coherence of full body massage sequences are summarized in Box 11-6.

Practitioners of massage would also be wise to experience and/or observe the work of practitioners of the various massage-related approaches listed in Table 11-5. Their methods of practice often artfully demonstrate many of these strategies for enhancing coherence.

DESIGN OF MORE-EXTENSIVE SEQUENCES THAT DO NOT HAVE A LOCAL FOCUS

It is quite common for beginning students of massage to be taught one well-choreographed, coherent, generic routine that incorporates a variety of massage techniques (predominantly neuromuscular) according to general principles.[5–8] This approach has both good and bad points. In learning the routine, students unconsciously absorb sound principles; however, students almost always develop a certain rigidity of technical approach that can be detrimental in later clinical practice and that is very hard to retrain. It is generally preferable to have beginning students design and practice a variety of coherent full-body sequences of 15-, 30-, 45-, and 60-min duration that address different outcomes. This practice teaches students mental flexibility and physical adroitness; it prepares students to later deal with time-consuming clinical problems without having to sacrifice the emphasis on treating the whole person that is the hallmark of good wellness massage.

A thorough training will allow students to both give and receive a large number of varied massage sequences

that are performed with a strict observance of the character and duration of each sequence. Students are cautioned against the early development of a particular "style," since this is often technical limitation in disguise or a projection of personal preference. The student is better served by attempting to master many massage styles and to understand how the impairment-level outcomes of care largely define the style of any given outcome-based massage intervention.

Box 11-7 expands on the steps required for the design of regional sequences so that they can be applied to more-extensive sequences. Note that in the examples that follow (Examples 11-6 to 11-9), the same general impairment-level outcomes of care are addressed in all regions, with an approximately equal allocation of time between regions.

DESIGN OF MORE-EXTENSIVE SEQUENCES THAT HAVE A LOCAL FOCUS

The clinician who practices in a setting where longer interventions (30 to 60 min) are possible may wish to integrate the specific treatment for a local condition with a more-extensive sequence for the entire body. In this situation, the clinician will give the region of focus more time within the intervention than it might be given in a full-body sequence that has no regional focus. The clinician has two options for allocating treatment time: including all of the remaining regions and shortening

---

Box 11-6
Strategies to Enhance Coherence of More-Extensive Sequences

Let yourself relax thoroughly and continuously while giving the massage

Choose a small number of impairment-level outcomes and stick to them

Aim for a generalized nervous response in the client (i.e., sedation or arousal)

Use the same predominant general stroke in all regions

Maintain consistent rhythm in all regions

As far as possible, maintain a comparable rhythm in all massage techniques

Use similar (not necessarily identical) massage techniques in all regions

Be cautious of overloading a sequence with many different sensations

> **Box 11-7**
> ***Steps in the Design of More-Extensive Massage Sequences***
>
> Summarize findings from the client examination
>
> Identify appropriate functional outcomes of care
>
> Summarize and prioritize impairment-level outcomes of care
>
> Choose relevant massage techniques to address the impairments
>
> Assign time for the entire intervention
>
> Choose regions to be included/excluded
>
> Specify initial times and order for regions
>
> Choose the predominant general technique(s)
>
> Sequence the massage techniques for regional sequences, keeping in mind
>
> > Position of superficial reflex work if included
> >
> > General to specific to general
> >
> > Superficial to deep to superficial
> >
> > Proximal to distal if working to enhance fluid return
> >
> > Periphery to center if working with circumscribed local pathology
> >
> > Agonist/antagonist/synergist balance if including neuromuscular or connective tissue techniques to release local restriction
>
> If you are including a regional sequence(s) to address a particular condition, does the initial time budget need to be readjusted?

the treatment time proportionally or eliminating some regions so that the final sequence addresses less than the full body (e.g., just the upper body). This approach to the design of massage sequences may seem reasonable for clinicians who have first practiced full-body wellness massage. However, outcome-based interventions that address specified impairments should not be conceptualized as full-body wellness massage with slight alterations; often, the alterations to the basic full-body massage must be so radical that the result bears scant resemblance to the massage sequences that are commonly performed for relaxation.

EXAMPLE 11-6

A Full-Body Sequence for Stress When Clothing Cannot Be Removed

Impairment-level outcomes of care: Sedation, decreased perceived anxiety (and cortisol levels), increased perceived relaxation, improved immune function, decreased resting level of muscle tension

Restrictions: Client is clothed

Time: 20, 40, or 60 min for all regions

Predominant general massage technique: Rocking, broad-contact compression

Massage techniques and order of application in each region:

Begin prone

Static contact

Rocking

Once reflex and movement techniques are performed in each region, introduce broad-contact compression all over the region (you may synchronize its application on the thorax with the client's exhalations); then alternate between broad-contact compression, and specific compression in areas where muscular tension is higher

Intersperse these with rocking ad lib

Finish each region by returning to rocking and static contact again

Additional: The more the clinician uses compression (especially if it is specific), the greater the decreases in muscle resting tension. It is both possible and extremely useful to learn to cover all regions in as short an interval as 20 min, although the amount of specific compression that can be included will be very limited. In doing so, ensure that the general character of the sequence remains the same regardless of the time in which it is performed. The clinician is advised not to increase the speed with which she applies the individual techniques when she is faced with less time for the intervention; it is preferable to use fewer repetitions of a technique and more-general massage techniques. This sequence would be suitable for reducing the effects of stress. It might also be incorporated, with the use of additional techniques, into longer interventions when anxiety and stress are playing a secondary role in the exacerbation of primary symptoms in clinical conditions such as asthma (between attacks), fibromyalgia, or chronic whiplash injuries.

Further exercises:

1. Where would you incorporate superficial stroking and muscle squeezing into this sequence?
2. Design and perform a sequence that accomplishes the same aims using lubricant.
3. Design and perform a version of this exercise with the client in sidelying position (i.e., left sidelying, then right sidelying).

EXAMPLE 11-7

A Full-Body Sequence to Increase Range of Motion

Impairment-level outcomes of care: Generalized increased joint mobility, decreased perceived anxiety, systemic sedation

Restrictions: No lubricant

Time: 30, 45, or 60 min for all regions

Order of regions: Various orders are possible, finish with at least 15 min on the back, neck, and pelvis

Predominant general massage technique: All massage techniques are general

Massage techniques and order of application in each region:

Perform one or two strokes of direct fascial technique with a broad contact, then perform one myofascial stretch with wide hand placement
Stretch associated joints (stretch hands and feet as a unit)

Additional: This sequence might be used for a basically healthy individual who complains of generalized stiffness a day after vigorous physical activity. Sixty minutes permits treatment in about 15 to 20 localized areas that should be distributed evenly throughout the body unless an obvious deficit in range exists in one joint. Because the chosen massage techniques require time for a viscoelastic response to occur in the client's tissues, the tempo must be slow and the pressure of application moderate. The depth of release and the resulting increase of range of motion in any one area will be very small compared with what would be possible if the procedure was concentrated on one or two regions of the body for the entire treatment time. Students are initially advised not to concentrate connective tissue technique around one joint, because compensations can arise quickly.

Further exercises:

1. Perform a version of this exercise with the client in sidelying. Try to foresee and deal with difficulties regarding positioning before you start.

EXAMPLE 11-8

A Stimulating Full-Body Sequence

Impairment-level outcomes of care: Systemic arousal, enhanced awareness, marginal decrease in resting level of muscle tension, increased perceived relaxation

Restrictions: No lubricant

Time: 20 or 40 min for all regions

Order of regions: Supine and prone, head to feet

Predominant general massage technique: Coarse running vibration

Massage techniques and order of application in each region:

Coarse running vibration
Shaking
Fast rhythmic palmar compression and muscle squeezing (1–2 techniques/sec)
Light hacking
Superficial fingertip stroking (limit the time spent on this last massage technique or the effect may be too stimulating for the client)

Additional: This sequence has a character similar to that of some precompetition sports massage sequences and might also be used to temporarily alleviate lethargy and fatigue. Because of the brisk tempo and relatively short time, the neuromuscular techniques cannot penetrate much below the superficial layers of muscle.

Further exercises:

1. Outline and provide a rationale for the selection of massage techniques and tempo for a precompetition sports situation.
2. For the same outcomes and duration of treatment, how would you alter the sequence if a lubricant were used?
3. How short can you make the duration and still have the massage feel coherent to the client?

EXAMPLE 11-9
A Gentle Full-Body Sequence to Relieve Pain and Maintain Joint Range

Impairment-level outcomes of care: Maintained joint mobility and integrity, prevention of capsuloligamentous restrictions, increased lymphatic return, analgesia, decreased perceived anxiety, sensory arousal

Restrictions: None

Time: 30 to 40 min for all regions (full body)

Order of regions: Supine then prone, head/thorax toward limbs (i.e., proximal to distal)

Predominant general massage technique: Superficial effleurage

Massage techniques and order of application in each region:

At the outset of the intervention encourage full breathing using both diaphragmatic and costal segments
Superficial effleurage progressing deeper to engage superficial muscle layers

Gentle wringing and nonspecific kneading
Gentle rhythmical mobilization and rocking
Passive relaxed movements (no overpressure)
Return frequently to, and end with, superficial effleurage

Additional: This sequence is similar to that recommended to treat rheumatoid arthritis in the noninflammatory phase;[23] it is relatively short, to prevent fatiguing the client. As with Example 11-7, because of time constraints, the depth of massage techniques is limited.

Further exercises:

1. How might you modify this sequence to specifically address reduced range and complaints of stiffness in the hands?
2. How could you integrate the use of a hot pack into this sequence?
3. If a client fell asleep during this sequence, what massage techniques—gently applied—could be used to awaken him?

Treatment Regimens

Until the last 40 years, the use of massage was elaborated on as a standard part of treatment regimens for a wide variety of orthopedic, medical, and surgical conditions.[23] Following a period in which massage was deemphasized or discarded as a primary intervention,[24] empirical research is again suggesting the merits of massage for a growing variety of conditions.[25] In the modern treatment paradigm, effective treatment regimens that include massage are developed through an iterative process of examination, evaluation, and treatment planning that has been described in Chapter 2, The Clinical Decision-Making Process.

PROGRESSION OF MASSAGE REGIMENS

The treatment of a client's clinical condition progresses through stages that reflect the clinical course and prognosis for that condition as well as client-specific

factors that are discussed in Chapter 2, The Clinical Decision-Making Process. The clinician monitors the client's progression from stage to stage by assessing changes in the client's impairments and functional limitations rather than by calculating the amount of time that has elapsed from the time of onset of the clinical condition. At each stage, the clinician modifies or redirects her plan of care so that it remains consistent with the client's current impairments and functional limitations.

Broad guidelines for the duration of the regimen and number of visits for various conditions can provide the clinician with a general framework for treatment planning. An example of these guidelines for physical therapy interventions for selected musculoskeletal and neurological disorders is provided in Table 11-6.[26] The number of massage interventions within an episode of care will often be lower than the overall number of visits noted in guidelines for general treatment. This occurs because the overall treatment will address a broader range of impairments and functional limitations than those that are specific to the use of massage. The appropriate number of massage interventions will vary with many factors, including the cause, severity, acuity, and complexity of the client's clinical condition; the use of complementary modalities; the overall health status of the client; and the age of client. Clinicians are referred to the numerous condition-specific practice guidelines and those that exist for professions, such as the American Physical Therapy Association's[26] "Guide to Physical Therapist Practice," that provide a general guide to prognoses, expected numbers of visits per episode of care, outcome measures, and relevant types of intervention for a range of clinical conditions.

Notwithstanding the existence of general practice guidelines, the clinician is encouraged to avoid using a standard progression of massage techniques for all clients with a given clinical condition. Instead, she should remain outcome-based in her practice and tailor the progression of massage techniques within a given episode of care to the client's presenting impairments and functional limitations. The ability to progress treatment regimens effectively can improve with appropriate clinical experience. Consequently, novice clinicians are encouraged to develop their strategies for progressing massage regimens through the consistent application of the principles of outcome-based massage, preferably in collaboration with an experienced clinician. Examples of the possible progression of massage regimens for clients with acute orthopedic injuries and chronic tissue restrictions are presented below to provide an illustration of how treatment progressions can be formulated.

PROGRESSION WHEN THE CLIENT PRESENTS WITH AN ACUTE ORTHOPEDIC INJURY

Clinicians whose clients present for treatment in the early stages after an orthopedic injury can apply a predictable and orderly succession of massage techniques on the site of injury. Early intervention on or near the site of injury is often geared toward the reduction of pain through counterirritant analgesia and to the reduction of edema. When lesions are less severe, the clinician can apply superficial reflex techniques on the site of the lesion, provided this does not exacerbate the client's pain. When the client's lesion is more severe and touch is locally contraindicated, the clinician can achieve counterirritant analgesia through the application of superficial techniques proximally in the related dermatome, to antagonist muscle groups, or even to the contralateral side (see the impairment-level outcomes of care for fine vibration in Chapter 5, Superficial Reflex Techniques). The clinician can also apply superficial fluid techniques at the proximal edge of swelling and more proximally to reduce edema. As local sensitivity at the site of the injury declines and the edema lessens, the clinician can apply superficial fluid techniques beginning at the periphery of the location of the swelling and moving closer to the center of the site of the injury. Once the local edema has resolved, the clinician can increase the pressure of the massage technique through the superficial tissues to engage the investing layer of the deep fascia and then the superficial muscular layers. Light neuromuscular and connective tissue techniques and movement techniques of small amplitude are appropriately introduced to apply a stress to the newly deposited connective tissue elements. Finally, in the chronic stages of rehabilitation (consolidation and maturation), the clinician can apply

Table 11-6
Duration of Physical Therapy Regimens and Expected Number of Visits for Selected Orthopedic and Neurological Conditions[26]

Condition	Duration of Expected Physical Therapy Regimen	Number of Visits
Tendinitis, bursitis, fasciitis	8–16 weeks	6–24
Postural conditions	12 months	6–20
Sprain/strain/dislocation	2–16 weeks	3–21
Uncomplicated joint arthroplasty	6 months	12–60
Disk herniation	1–6 months	8–24
Cerebrovascular accident (stroke)	Until maximal independence is achieved	10–60
Peripheral nerve injury	4–8 months	12–56

Data from American Physical Therapy Association. Guide to physical therapist practice. Phys Ther 1997;77(11):1155–1674.

more-aggressive neuromuscular and connective tissue techniques to address shortness or poor modeling of connective tissue. This is often unnecessary, since the appropriate application of massage techniques in the earlier stages of healing promotes adequate tissue modeling. To summarize, the progression of massage techniques on the site of injury involves the application of massage techniques that are directed to layers of increasing depth in a regimen that can take from 1 to 4 weeks or longer.

Off the site of injury, the clinician can use a broader variety of massage techniques from the outset of treatment, provided that she heeds the appropriate contraindications and cautions and does not attempt to force fluid through a congested area or place an excessive mechanical stress on remote sections of structures that may pass through the injury site.

PROGRESSION WHEN THE CLIENT PRESENTS WITH CHRONIC TISSUE RESTRICTIONS

Chronic soft-tissue restrictions can be the result of a number of clinical conditions, such as orthopedic injuries, postural malalignment, long-standing immobility, general deconditioning, and arthritic conditions. When clients present with chronic tissue restrictions, several patterns of progression through the tissue layers are available to the clinician. If the client's condition is relatively recent, the clinician can use a less-complicated progression with a local focus similar to the one described above. This would involve first freeing the more superficial muscular and connective tissue layers and then proceeding to deeper ones. The clinician will have to spend relatively more time on these tasks if the client has received no prior treatment.

On sites of old injury that were inadequately treated or not treated at all and with long-standing pain of musculoskeletal origin, the clinician may have to use some force and persistence over several interventions to progress through the restrictions in the different layers of muscle and connective tissue. The progression of treatment in these conditions is further complicated by the factors outlined below.

Compensatory Changes

Chronic injuries are complicated by the fact that compensatory changes in the musculoskeletal system, such as restrictions in mobility, movement, and coordination, can arise in response to local damage. The severity and extent of these compensatory changes are typically in proportion to the severity of the original damage and the amount of time that has elapsed since the injury. While the clinician may productively begin treatment by addressing the layers of restriction at the original site of injury, she must also periodically address the compensatory changes to achieve a satisfactory resolution of the client's impairments and associated functional limitations. Chronic complaints of insidious onset may be related to these compensatory changes; furthermore, the client may be unaware of the causal relationship between a forgotten injury and his current complaints. In this situation, the clinician will need to find and treat the restrictions in the different tissue layers at the original site(s) of injury.

Multiple Sources of Pain

Since long-standing chronic conditions can result in the development of widespread restrictions in multiple layers of soft tissue, the client may present with multiple sources of local and referred pain in her muscles, fascia, and joints. As a result, the clinician may find it impossible to identify any one tissue or structure as the primary focus of treatment. In this situation, at the outset of treatment the clinician may be justified in applying several interventions of progressively deeper neuromuscular and connective tissue techniques to reduce the tension in the superficial layers of muscle and connective tissue throughout the body, in the hope of reducing both compensatory changes and multiple sources of pain. As the clinician progressively reduces the tension in the superficial, and then deeper, tissue layers, the client may experience a succession of both familiar and unfamiliar symptoms that may endure for days or weeks, finally arriving at a point where one tissue or structure can be identified as the primary focus of treatment.

A Strategy to Achieve Adequate Depth in the Treatment of Chronic Lesions

Inexperienced clinicians who are treating chronic lesions commonly attempt to cover too wide an area with too general a focus; therefore, their massage never proceeds to therapeutic depth in any one area and fails for that reason. The application of specific deep massage techniques is indispensable but time consuming; a single area, such as the shoulder, gluteal, or hand, can take anywhere from 20 to 60 min. When the clinician needs to use extensive, deep, specific massage techniques, she must subdivide the client's body into smaller manageable areas and schedule the treatment of the various areas on two or more consecutive interventions. The clinician must also take great care to include the application of general techniques and to address the client's antagonist and synergist muscle groups, to minimize the potential for imbalances in the client.

Discharge

If the clinician follows the principles of progression of interventions and treatment regimens outlined in this and other chapters, then the transition from the treatment phase to the discharge phase will be gradual and imperceptible. Chapter 2, The Clinical Decision-Making Process, outlines the steps that the clinician follows for the physical and psychological preparation of the client for discharge. Some additional clinical issues are worthy of mention. As the clinician identifies the resolution of

the client's impairments through the ongoing reexaminations, she can progress her use of techniques, such as functional training, for the remediation of the client's functional limitations as her scope of practice permits. Finally, as discharge approaches, the clinician will ensure that she addresses the client's needs for education in self-care, equipment, and the coordination of ongoing services that are appropriate given the clinician's scope of practice.

References

1. Fritz S. Fundamentals of therapeutic massage. St Louis: Mosby-Lifeline, 1995.
2. Tappan FM, Benjamin P. Tappan's handbook of healing massage techniques. 3rd ed. Stamford, CT: Appleton & Lange, 1998.
3. Salvo SG. Massage therapy. Philadelphia: WB Saunders, 1999.
4. Quality Assurance Committee of the College of Massage Therapists of Ontario. Code of ethics and standards of practice. Toronto: College of Massage Therapists of Ontario, 1999.
5. de Domenico G, Wood EC. Beard's massage. 4th ed. Philadelphia: WB Saunders, 1997.
6. Holey E, Cook E. Therapeutic massage. London: WB Saunders, 1997.
7. Beck M. The theory and practice of therapeutic massage. Albany, NY: Milady, 1988.
8. Wood EC, Becker PD. Beard's massage. 3rd ed. Philadelphia: WB Saunders, 1981.
9. Lederman E. Fundamentals of manual therapy. New York: Churchill Livingstone, 1997.
10. Mennell JB. Physical treatment by movement, manipulation and massage. 5th ed. Philadelphia: Blakiston, 1945.
11. Travell JG, Simons DG. Myofascial pain and dysfunction. The trigger point manual, vol 1. Baltimore: Williams & Wilkins, 1983.
12. Michlovitz S. Thermal agents in rehabilitation. 3rd ed. Philadelphia: FA Davis, 1996.
13. Cummings GS, Tillman LJ. Remodeling of dense connective tissue in normal adult tissues. In: Currier DP, Nelson RM, eds. Dynamics of human biologic tissues. Philadelphia: FA Davis, 1992:45–73.
14. O'Sullivan SB. Strategies to improve motor control. In: O'Sullivan SB, Schmitz J. Physical rehabilitation, assessment and treatment. 2nd ed. Philadelphia: FA Davis, 1988.
15. Hollis M. Massage for therapists. Oxford: Blackwell, 1987.
16. Ernst E. Abdominal massage therapy for chronic constipation: a systematic review of controlled clinical trials. Forsch Komplementarmed 1999;6(3):149–151.
17. Emly M. Abdominal massage. Nurs Times 1993;89(3):34–36.
18. Resende TL, Brocklehurst JC, O'Neill PA. A pilot study on the effect of exercise and abdominal massage on bowel habit in continuing care patients. Clin Rehabil 1993;7:204–209.
19. Klauser AG, Flaschentrager J, Gehrke A, Muller-Lissner SA. Abdominal wall massage; effect on colonic function in healthy volunteers and in patients with chronic constipation. Z Gastroenterol 1992;30:246–251.
20. Stillerman E. The encyclopedia of bodywork. New York: Facts on File, 1996.
21. Hoehn-Saric R. Psychic and somatic anxiety: worries, somatic symptoms and physiological changes. Acta Psychiatr Scand Suppl 1998;393:32–38.
22. Millensen JR. Mind matters: psychological medicine in holistic practice. Seattle: Eastland Press, 1995.
23. Wale JO. Tidy's massage and remedial exercises in medical and surgical conditions. 11th ed. Bristol: John Wright & Sons, 1968.
24. Thomson A, Skinner A, Piercy J. Tidy's physiotherapy. 12th ed. Oxford: Butterworth-Heinemann, 1991.
25. Field TM. Massage therapy effects. Am Psychol 1998;53(12):1270–1281.
26. American Physical Therapy Association. Guide to physical therapist practice. Phys Ther 1997;77(11).

Suggested Readings

Arvedson J. Medical gymnastics and massage in general practice. London: JA Churchill, 1930.

Baumgartner AJ. Massage in athletics. Minneapolis: Burgess, 1947.

Beard G. History of massage technique. Phys Ther Rev 1952;32:613–624.

Bohm M. Massage: its principles and techniques. Gould E, trans. Philadelphia: JB Lippincott, 1913.

Claire T. Bodywork: what type of massage to get and how to get the most out of it. New York: William Morrow, 1995.

Collinge W. The American Holistic Health Association complete guide to alternative medicine. New York: Warner Books, 1996.

Cyriax J. Theory and practice of massage. In: Textbook of orthopedic medicine, vol 2. Treatment by manipulation, massage and injection. 11th ed. London: Bailliere Tindall, 1984.

Cyriax JH, Cyriax PJ. Cyriax' illustrated manual of orthopaedic medicine. 2nd ed. Oxford: Butterworth-Heinemann, 1993.

Hoffa A. Technik der massage. Stuttgart: Verlag von Ferdinand Ernke, 1897.

Jahnke R. The body therapies. J Holistic Nurs 1985;Spring:7–14.

Joachim G. Step by step massage techniques. Cancer Nurs 1983;4:32–35.

Kellogg JH. The art of massage. Battle Creek, MI: Modern Medicine Publishing, 1923.

Kellogg JH. The art of massage: a practical manual for the nurse, the student and the practitioner. Battle Creek, MI: Modern Medicine Publishing, 1929.

King RK. Performance massage. Champaign, IL: Human Kinetics, 1993.

Licht S, ed. Massage, manipulation and traction. Baltimore: Waverly Press, 1960.

Loving J. Massage therapy. Stamford, CT: Appleton & Lange, 1999.

Macias Merlo ML. [Abdominal massage: therapy for the control of chronic constipation]. Rev Enferm (Spanish) 1985;8(79–80):16–19.

McMillan M. Massage and therapeutic exercise. 2nd ed. Philadelphia: WB Saunders, 1925.

Meagher J. Sports massage. Barrytown, NY: Station Hill Press, 1990.

Prosser EM. A manual of massage and movement. 2nd ed. London: Faber & Faber, 1941.

Rattray FS. Massage therapy: An approach to treatments. Toronto, Ontario: Massage Therapy Texts and MA Verick Consultants, 1994.

Seyle H. History and present status of the stress concept. In: Goldberger L, Breznitz S, eds. Handbook of stress: theoretical and clinical aspects. New York: Macmillan, 1982.

Seyle H. The physiology and pathology of exposure to stress. Montreal: Acta, 1950.

Tappan FM. Healing massage techniques. Norwalk, CT: Appleton & Lange, 1988.

Tidy NM. Massage and remedial exercises. London: John Wright, 1932.

Westland G. Massage as a therapeutic tool, parts 1 and 2. Br J Occup Ther 1993;56(4):129–134; 56(5):177–180.

Yates J. A physicians' guide to massage therapy; its physiological effects and their application to treatment. British Columbia, Canada: The Massage Therapists Association, 1990.

Ylinen J, Cash M. Sports massage. London: Stanley Paul, 1980.

Zhang Y, Zhang YL, Cheng YQ. [Clinical observation of constipation due to deficiency of vital energy treated by massage and finger pressure methods]. Chung Hua Hu Li Tsa Chih (Chinese) 1996;31(2):97–98.

Appendix A: Glossary

Abnormal connective tissue density: Irregular connective tissue remodeling that occurs during the consolidation and maturation stages of connective tissue healing.

Accessory joint motion: The range of motion within synovial and secondary cartilaginous joints that is not under voluntary control and can therefore only be obtained passively by the clinician. These motions, also known as joint play movements, are essential for full and painfree active range of motion.

Active range of motion: The amount of joint motion that can be achieved by the client during the performance of unassisted voluntary joint motion.

Active trigger point: A trigger point which refers pain in a characteristic pattern whether the muscle in which it is located is working or at rest.

Acupoint: In Traditional Chinese Medicine and related systems, a point on a meridian which can be stimulated by various methods to achieve complex effects on physiological function that are usually manifested in areas that are remote to the point of application.

Acupressure: A type of massage which uses specific compression to stimulate acupoints and meridians to achieve complex effects on physiological function that are usually manifested in areas that are remote to the point of application.

Acute pain: Pain provoked by noxious stimulation produced by injury and/or disease with unpleasant sensory and emotional experiences (see Pain).

Adhesions: A binding together with dense connective tissue of tissues that normally glide or move in relation to each other, with resultant loss of mobility. Like scars, adhesions may result from the replacement of normal tissue that has been destroyed by burn, wound, surgery, radiation, or disease with connective tissue.

Airway clearance: Ability to move pulmonary secretions effectively through the use of normal mechanisms of cough and the mucociliary escalator.

Amplitude of technique: An indication of the size of the area that is covered by a technique.

Anatomic barrier in soft tissue: The final resistance to normal tissue range of motion that is provided by bone, ligament or soft tissue. Motion beyond the anatomic barrier results in tissue damage.

Armoring: Myofascial hardness associated with chronically elevated resting level of tone.

Arousal: The process of awaking or stimulating.

Attention: The clinician's capacity to focus on the sensory information that she receives primarily, but not exclusively, through her hands.

Barrier-release phenomenon: The clinician engages the tissue barrier at the point at which the clinician palpates a resistance to tissue motion. If the clinician sustains the pressure on the tissue barrier, a "release" may occur after a latency period that will vary with the nature and state of health of the tissue. This release results in a reduction of the resistance that will enable the clinician to move the tissue beyond the location of the original barrier without increasing the pressure of palpation.

Bodywork: A contemporary term which embraces massage and related approaches which contact or move the client's tissues to achieve educational or therapeutic effects.

Broad-contact compression: A non-gliding neuromuscular technique, delivered with a broad contact surface, which engages the client's muscle with the pressure and release of the stroke administered perpendicular to the surface of the client's body.

Broad-contact kneading: A gliding petrissage technique performed in circles or ellipses with a large contact surface such as the palm.

Capsular laxity: Anatomical or pathological lengthening of the joint capsule.

Capsular restrictions: Anatomical or pathological shortening of the joint capsule.

Capsulitis and synovitis: Inflammation of the joint capsule and associated internal ligaments, and of the synovium.

Caution: A sign, symptom, evaluation, or diagnosis which directs the clinician to be prepared to modify a given procedure in order to reduce the risks associated with its application.

Centrifugal: (1) Directed away from the heart or distally; (2) directed away from an area of local pathology.

Centripetal: Directed towards the heart or proximally.

Chronic obstructive pulmonary disease: Pulmonary disorders that are characterized by the presence of increased airway resistance.

Chronic pain: Pain that persists beyond the usual course of healing of an acute disease or beyond the reasonable time in which the injury is expected to heal. Some authors define chronic pain in terms of duration of pain, with a lower limit of duration ranging from six weeks to six months; others define chronic pain in terms of an increasing dissociation from the physical etiology and increasing affective and cognitive dimensions of pain.

Chronic pain syndrome: A clinical syndrome in which clients present with high levels of pain that is chronic in duration, functional impairment, and depression.

Chronic restrictive pulmonary disease: Pulmonary disorders that are characterized by the restriction of lung expansion, such as interstitial fibrosis.

Chronic stress: A prolonged and heightened state of arousal that has negative physiological and psychological consequences.

Clapping: A form of percussion which is used to mechanically loosen secretions in the lungs and to facilitate airway clearance.

Classic massage or classical massage: See Swedish massage.

Clinical decision-making: The process by which clinicians synthesize and analyze information on their clients' conditions and use the results of their analysis to formulate and progress a therapeutic regimen for their clients. Also known as clinical reasoning and clinical problem-solving.

Clinical hypothesis: The clinician's hypothesis about the client's key clinical problems.

Clinical indication: A sign, symptom, evaluation, or diagnosis which directs the clinician to apply a certain procedure.

Clonus: A cyclical, spasmodic hyperactivity of antagonistic muscles that occurs at a regular frequency in response to a quick stretch stimulus.

Cognitive Transactional Model of Stress: Lazarus and Folkman's model of stress as the condition that results when a person's interactions with his environment leads him to perceive a discrepancy between the demands of the situation and the resources of the person's biological, psychological, or social systems.

Cogwheel rigidity: A ratchet-like response to passive movement, alternating between giving way and resistance.

Coherence: Consistent order and structure of a massage sequence or intervention that results from clear and consistent intention(s) on the part of the clinician.

Combines with: When one technique is said to "combine" with another, it means that the two techniques may be executed simultaneously.

Complex decongestive therapy (also known as complex or complete decongestive physiotherapy, CDT, CDT, or CDP): A treatment regimen for lymphedema which includes massage, bandaging or compression garments, specific exercises, and education on hygiene.

Compression: Any force that is oriented in a manner so that its effect is to shorten or compact a tissue or structure.

Conceptual framework: A set of empirical generalizations that provides a means of organizing and integrating observations about a specific set of behaviors that one observes in a particular setting.

Conceptual model: A diagram that shows the proposed causal linkages among a set of concepts that the individual believes to be related to a particular health problem.

Connective tissue: Tissues that consist of several different types of cells, such as fibroblasts and fat cells, and elastin and collagen fibers embedded in a matrix of gelatinous material, the consistency of which varies in response to many factors. Nerves, blood vessels, lymph vessels, myofibrils, and organs are found within connective tissue.

Connective Tissue Massage: A system of massage developed by Elizabeth Dicke and popular in Europe in which connective tissue techniques are applied in precise sequences to the skin and superficial fascial layers to elicit specific physiological reflex effects.

Connective tissue techniques: Massage techniques that palpate, lengthen, and promote remodeling of connective tissue.

Contact surface: The portion of the clinician's hand or arm that is used to execute the stroke.

Context: A brief description of how a massage technique is conventionally sequenced in relation to other techniques.

Contractile tissue: Muscle, with its enveloping fascial layers, associated tendon(s), and periosteal attachments.

Contracture: A permanent muscular shortening due to a variety of physiological changes in muscle, such as fibrosis or loss of muscular balance.

Contraindication: A sign, symptom, evaluation, or diagnosis which directs the clinican to avoid applying a certain procedure.

Controlled lean posture: An inclined, aligned posture used to efficiently transfer the clinician's body weight to the client in a controlled manner.

Creep: Visco-elastic stretch of connective tissue that occurs when it is subjected to sustained tension, and which is palpable.

Crepitus: A vibration of variable fineness that is associated with roughened gliding surfaces of a tendon or its sheath, or of the articulating surfaces of a joint. Crepitus can sometimes be heard, as well as palpated.

Decerebrate rigidity: Rigidity that occurs as a result of brainstem lesions. It presents clinically as sustained contraction and posturing of the trunk and lower limbs in extension.

Decorticate rigidity: Rigidity that occurs as a result of brainstem lesions. It presents clinically as sustained contraction and posturing of the trunk and lower limbs in extension and the upper limbs in flexion.

Deep effleurage: A general gliding manipulation performed with moderate-to-heavy centripetal pressure that deforms superficial or deep layers of muscle.

Deep fascia: Connective tissue layer that lies immediately superficial to, or between, muscle fibers. The primary functions of the deep fascia are to allow muscles to move freely, to carry nerve and blood vessels, to fill the space between muscles, and to provide an origin for muscles.

Deformation: The change in shape of a tissue or structure when it is subjected to pressure.

Dependent edema: An increase in extracellular fluid volume that is localized in a dependent area, such as a limb.

Dermatomal pain: Pain in the pattern of a dermatome. A dermatome is an area of skin supplied by one dorsal nerve root. Injury of a dorsal root may result in sensory loss in the skin or may be felt as a burning or electric pain.

Dermis: The first layer of connective tissue.

Diagnosis: The process and result of analyzing and organizing the findings from the client examination into clusters or syndromes.

Direct fascial technique: A slow, gliding connective tissue technique that applies a moderate, sustained tensional force to the superficial fascia or to the deep fascia and associated muscle. It results in palpable visco-elastic lengthening and plastic deformation of the fascia.

Direct inhibitory pressure: Specific compression applied to a tendon as a means of inhibiting the tone of the related muscle for a short period of time.

Direction of technique: The direction of the applied force. The direction given in the description of techniques is the direction in which the greatest force is applied during the pressure phase of the stroke.

Disability: When an individual is unable to perform his socially defined tasks, activities, or roles to the expected level.

Discrimination: The clinician's ability to distinguish fine gradations of sensory information.

Drag: (1)Tensile force, stretching force, or tractional force exerted along a single tissue layer; (2)inherent tissue resistance to such force.

Draping: The process by which the clinician covers and uncovers portions of the client's body during treatment, while maintaining modesty and respecting appropriate client-clinician boundaries.

Duration of technique: An estimate of a reasonable length of time for which a single technique may have to be applied by a competent clinician to begin to achieve the specified impairment-level outcomes of care.

Dyspnea: Shortness of breath, labored or difficult breathing, or uncomfortable awareness of one's breathing.

Edema: An accumulation of fluid in cells, tissues, or serous cavities. Edema has four main causes: increased permeability of capillaries, decreased plasma protein osmotic pressure, increased pressure in capillaries and venules, and lymphatic flow obstruction.

Effleurage: A group of general gliding manipulations performed with centripetal pressure and varying pressures.

Effusion: Excessive fluid in the joint capsule, indicating irritation or inflammation of the synovium.

Elastic barrier in soft tissue: The resistance that the clinician feels at the end of the passive range of motion of the tissue when she is taking the "slack" out of the tissue.

Elastic deformation: Deformation in response to applied force that disappears after the force is removed; spring-like behavior.

End feel: The qualities of motion or resistance to motion that the clinician palpates in the joint at the end of passive range of motion.

Endangerment sites: Areas of the human body over which the use of direct or sustained pressure is contraindicated.

Engage: To enter into contact with. In this text, a tissue is said to be "engaged" during a technique, if it is significantly deformed during the technique's application.

Entrapment neuropathy: Nerve compression that can result from muscle and connective tissue shortening and inflammation associated with trigger point activity, fascial restrictions, overuse syndromes, and other clinical conditions.

Episode of care: A single period of treatment—initial visit to discharge—that a client receives for a specific condition.

Epithelium: A layer of closely packed columnar or squamous cells that have little intercellular material between them.

Evaluation: The synthesis of the information from the client examination.

Examination: The collection of information on the client's health status and clinical condition through history-taking, a general systems review, and tests and measures.

Fascial restrictions: The loss of mobility of one fascial layer with respect to another because of the loss of fluid consistency of ground substance and development of collagenous cross-links. Fascial restrictions can result from repair of tissue damage and from prolonged immobility.

Fasciculations: Localized, subconscious muscle contractions that result from the contraction of the muscle cells innervated by a single motor axon and thus do not involve the entire muscle.

Fine vibration: A superficial reflex technique in which a fast, oscillating or trembling movement is produced on the client's skin that results in minimal deformation of subcutaneous tissues.

Fremitus: A pulmonary vibration that a clinician can palpate over the rib cage as the client speaks or vocalizes.

Friction: A repetitive, specific, non-gliding, connective tissue technique that produces movement between the fibers of dense connective tissue, increasing tissue extensibility.

Functional limitation: A restriction of the individual's ability to perform actions or activities within the range considered normal for the organ or organ system.

Functional outcome of care: The outcome of care that is related to the client's functional limitation.

General technique: A technique that is applied to an entire region or a larger portion of the body, or applied using a broad surface such as the palm, or both.

Glide: Movement of the clinician's hand across the client's skin.

Health-related quality of life: The objective and subjective dimensions of an individual's ability to function in, and derive satisfaction from, a variety of social roles in the presence of impaired health status.

Hypertonia: A general term used to refer to muscle tone that is above normal resting levels, regardless of the mechanism for the increase in tone.

Hypotonia: A general term used to refer to muscle tone that is below normal resting levels, regardless of the mechanism for the decrease in tone.

Identification: The clinician's ability to distinguish between healthy and dysfunctional tissue states, and to identify tissues and structures and their responses to applied force.

Impairment: A loss or abnormality of the affected individual's physiological, anatomical, cognitive, or emotional structure or function that occurs as a result of the initial or subsequent pathophysiology.

Impairment-level outcome of care: The outcome of care that is related to the client's impairment.

Indication: A sign, symptom, evaluation, or diagnosis that directs the clinican to apply a certain procedure.

Inquiring touch: Intelligent Touch is inquiring touch. A good clinician is constantly asking questions, and the use of massage is no exception to this requirement. The use of inquiring touch does not imply that the clinician's touch feels tentative to the client or that it lack firmness when required.

Intelligent touch: The learned skills essential for successful clinical use of massage: attention and concentration, discrimination, identification, inquiry, and intention.

Intergrades with: To merge gradually one into another. When one technique is said to "intergrade" with another, the two techniques can be performed consecutively and will merge gradually one into another since there are intermediate hybrid forms of the technique that lie between and resemble both techniques.

Intervention: A single purposeful and skilled interaction between the clinician and the client.

Investing layer of the deep fascia: Dense connective tissue that lies between the superficial fascia and muscle.

Ischemic compression: *See* Trigger point pressure release.

Joint integrity: The extent to which a joint conforms to the expected anatomical and biomechanical norms.

Joint range of motion: The capacity of the joint to move within the anatomic or physiological range of motion that is available at that joint based upon its arthrokinematics and the ability of the periarticular connective tissue to deform. Range of motion reflects the function of the contractile, nervous, inert, and bony tissues and the client's willingness to perform a movement.

Kneading: A gliding neuromuscular technique, performed in circles or ellipses, which repeatedly compresses and releases muscle. *See also* Petrissage.

Latent trigger points: Trigger points which are not painful in and of themselves unless they are being palpated.

Lead-pipe rigidity: Constant resistance to passive movement.

Life Events Model of Stress: Holmes and Rahe's model of stress that examined the nature and consequences of negative life events and proposed that interpersonal stressors are predictive of increases in disease activity.

Ligament insufficiency: Anatomical or pathological shortening of the capsular ligament.

Ligament laxity: Anatomical or pathological lengthening of the capsular ligament.

Lymphedema: Accumulation of abnormal amounts of lymph fluid and associated swelling of subcutaneous tissues that results from the obstruction, destruction, or hypoplasia of lymph vessels.

Manual lymph drainage: Comprehensive massage systems designed to enhance lymphatic return (e.g., Vodder, Leduc). These systems may incorporate various massage techniques, but often rely extensively on what is termed in this text superficial lymph drainage technique.

Meridian: In Traditional Chinese Medicine, a conduit or channel through which energy (qi, chi, ch'i) circulates through the body in well-defined cycles.

Muscle endurance: A muscle's ability to contract, or maintain torque, over a number of contractions or a period of time. Conversely, fatigue is inability to maintain torque, or the loss of power, over time.

Muscle extensibility: The ability of a muscle and its associated fascia to undergo lengthening deformation during the movement of a joint through its anatomic range.

Muscle integrity: The extent to which a muscle conforms to the expected anatomical and biomechanical norms.

Muscle performance: A muscle's capacity to do work, based on its length, tension, and velocity. Neurological stimulus, fuel storage, fuel delivery, and balance, timing and sequencing of muscle contraction influence integrated muscle performance.

Muscle power: Work produced by a muscle per unit of time (strength × speed).

Muscle resting tension: The firmness to palpation at rest observed in muscles with normal innervation.

Traditionally, resting muscle tension has been described as resulting from the physiological properties of muscle, such as viscosity, elasticity, and plasticity rather than from motor unit firing.

Muscle spasm: Involuntary contraction of a muscle that results in increased muscular tension and shortness that cannot be released voluntarily.

Muscle squeezing: A petrissage technique in which one or both hands are used to grasp, lift, and squeeze a muscle, muscle group, or body segment without glide.

Muscle strain or tear: Lesion or inflammation of muscle fibers that can occur in response to trauma.

Muscle strength: The force or torque produced by a muscle or group of muscles to overcome a resistance during a maximum voluntary contraction.

Myofascial trigger point: A hyperirritable spot in skeletal muscle that is associated with a hypersensitive palpable nodule in a taut band. The area is painful on compression and can give rise to a variety of symptoms, such as referred pain, referred tenderness, motor dysfunction, and autonomic phenomena.

Myofascial pain syndrome: The sensory, motor, and autonomic symptoms caused by myofascial trigger points.

Myofascial release: (1)A connective tissue technique that combines nongliding fascial traction with varying amounts of orthopedic stretch and that results in palpable visco-elastic lengthening and plastic deformation of the fascia. (2) A system of treatment that uses the myofascial release technique, in conjunction with cranial sacral, osteopathic, and other soft-tissue techniques.

Myotomal pain: Pain in a myotome, or a group of muscles that are supplied by one nerve root.

Neurogenic pain: Pain that results from noninflammatory dysfunction of the peripheral or central nervous system that does not involve nociceptor stimulation or trauma.

Neuromuscular or muscle tone: Muscle resting tension and responsiveness of muscles to passive elongation or stretch.

Neuromuscular technique: As defined by Chaitow and others, a complex massage system that includes specific finger and thumb techniques that resemble stripping and direct fascial technique.

Neuromuscular techniques: Massage techniques that palpate muscle, affect the level of resting tension of muscles, and have additional psychoneuroimmunological effects.

Nociceptive pain: Sensitization of peripheral nociceptors as a result of injury to a muscle or a joint that causes increased release of neurotransmitters in the dorsal horn of the spinal cord. The sensitized dorsal horn neurons demonstrate increased background activity, increased receptive field size, and increased responses to peripherally applied stimuli.

Nonmyofascial trigger points: A hyperirritable spot in scar tissue, fascia, periosteum, ligament, or joint capsule that is associated with a hypersensitive palpable nodule in a taut band.

Object being palpated: The chosen portion of the sensory field on which the clinician focuses attention during palpation. The object being palpated is not necessarily a physical object; instead, it may be a characteristic, such as temperature, or a phenomenon, such as resistance to movement.

Outcome of care: The results of an intervention or the treatment regimen as a whole.

Pain: An unpleasant sensation associated with actual or potential tissue damage that is mediated by specific nerve fibers to the brain where its conscious appreciation may be modified by various factors.

Parkinsonian rigidity: Rigidity that occurs as a result of basal ganglia lesions. It presents clinically as a tight contraction of both agonist and antagonist muscles throughout the movement (lead-pipe rigidity).

Passive movement techniques: Massage techniques that primarily palpate the movement of tissues and structures, and result in the repetitive movement of soft tissue masses over the underlying structure(s) with varying degrees of joint motion.

Passive range of motion: The amount of joint motion available when an examiner moves a joint through its anatomic or physiological range, without assistance from the client, while the client is relaxed.

Percussion, or percussive techniques: Massage techniques that deform and release tissues quickly through controlled, repeated, rhythmical, light striking.

Petrissage: A group of related neuromuscular techniques that repetitively compress, shear, and release muscle tissue with varying amounts of drag, lift, and glide.

Physiological barrier in soft tissue: The resistance that determines the range of motion of soft tissue that is available under normal conditions. In other words, the range of motion of the tissue lies between the two physiological barriers, with the least amount of resistance being apparent at the midrange.

Physiological Model of Stress: Hans Selye's model of stress that is based on the interaction of the adrenal cortex and the neuroendocrine and immune systems during stress. Stress in this model is defined as the body's automatic response ("fight or flight") to a demand that is placed on it.

Picking up: A one-handed or two-handed gliding petrissage technique in which muscle is lifted and squeezed between the fingers and the abducted thumb.

Pitting edema: Edema that retains the indentation produced by the pressure of palpation.

Plastic deformation: Deformation in response to applied force which remains after the force is removed; putty-like behavior.

Pliability: The inherent quality of tissue that refers to the ease with which it is bent, twisted, sheared, elongated, or compressed.

Positional release: A group of related osteopathic techniques which relieve tension and pain in muscles through positioning and gentle sustained pressure.

Positioning: The alignment and support of the client's body by the clinician in preparation for the application of massage.

Postural drainage: The use of positioning to promote the movement of bronchial secretions through the lungs; conventionally used in conjunction with percussion.

Postural malalignment: Abnormal joint alignment caused by soft-tissue imbalance or deformity within a bone.

Postural tone: The development of muscular tension in skeletal muscles that participate in maintaining the positions of different parts of the skeleton. The cerebellum regulates postural tone. Unlike muscle resting tension, constant muscle activation is required for the maintenance of postural tone, and the self-sustained firing of motoneurons may reduce the need for prolonged synaptic input in this situation.

Posture: The positioning and alignment of the skeleton and associated soft tissues in relation to gravity, the center of mass, and the base of support of the body.

Pressure of technique: The amount of force per unit area of contact surface that the clinician applies.

Process of care: The manner in which care is delivered—the activities that take place within and between the clinician and the client. This encompasses the interpersonal aspects of the client-clinician interaction and the technical aspects of how the clinician provides care.

Prognosis: The process of predicting the client's level and timing of improvement.

Proprioceptive palpation: A form of palption in which the clinician uses priopriceptive sense to gauge how the client's compressed tissues are deforming under the application of the clinician's body weight.

Radicular pain: Pain that is felt in a dermatome, myotome, or sclerotome because of direct involvement of a spinal nerve or nerve root. Also known as nerve root pain.

Rate of technique: An indication of how fast the force is applied. The rate may describe the speed of the movement of the clinician's hand over the client's skin (distance per second), or the frequency of repetitions of a described technique (repetitions per second), or both.

Referred pain: Pain that is felt at another part of the body that is at a distance from the tissues that have caused it because the referred site is supplied by the same or adjacent neural segments.

Reflexology: A system of manual treatment which applies specific compression to reflex points in the foot or hand to normalize function in distant body segments or organs.

Resilience: The inherent quality of tissue which restores original form after deformation by applied force.

Resistance: That inherent quality of tissue which counteracts the tendency of applied force to produce movement of the tissue.

Resting tension of muscle: *See* Muscle resting tension.

Restrictive or pathological barriers in soft tissue: Barriers that are observed when soft tissue dysfunction is present. They can be located anywhere between the normal physiological barriers, can limit the available range of motion within the tissues, and can alter the position of the midrange. A restrictive barrier will change the quality of the movement and the "feel" at the end of the tissue range of motion. This is analogous to the abnormal end feels observed in joints.

Rhythmical mobilization: A technique in which entire structures are repetitively moved, resulting in the movement of soft tissue over bone and the movement of related joints and internal organs

Rib cage mobility: The capacity of the rib cage to move within the available anatomic range of motion during respiration, based on the arthrokinematics of the joints of the rib cage and the thoracic spine, and the ability of the periarticular connective tissue to deform.

Rigidity: Increased muscular tone that results from brainstem or basal ganglia lesions. Rigidity involves a uniformly increased resistance in both agonist and antagonist muscles, resulting in stiff, immovable body parts, independent of the velocity of the stretch stimulus.

Rocking: A technique in which gentle, repetitive oscillation of the body is produced by repeatedly pushing the pelvis or torso from a midline resting position into lateral deviation and then allowing it to return.

Scar: The fibrous tissue that replaces normal tissues that have been destroyed by a burn, wound, surgery, radiation or disease.

Sclerotomal pain: Pain in a sclerotome, an area of bone or fascia innervated by one segmental nerve root.

Sedation: The process of calming or allaying nervous excitement.

Sequence: A structured, outcome-based series or succession of massage techniques that comprise an intervention or a part of an intervention.

Shaking: A passive movement technique in which soft tissue—primarily muscle—is repetitively moved back and forth over the underlying bone, with minimal joint movement.

Shiatsu: A complex Japanese system of massage, based on the meridian system, which makes extensive use of specific compression.

Skin: A layer of epithelium, the epidermis, and the dermis.

Skin rolling: A gliding connective tissue technique in which tissue superficial to the investing layer of deep fascia is grasped, continuously lifted, and rolled over underlying tissues in a wave-like motion.

Societal limitations: Those limitations to an individual's level of function that can be attributed to physical or attitudinal barriers in society.

Soft tissue range of motion: Available range of motion of soft tissue that is analogous to the range of motion available in joints. Within this range of motion, normal soft tissue has three barriers or resistances that can limit movement.

Spasticity: Increased muscular tone results from an upper motor neuron lesion that may or may not be associated with reflex hyperexcitability. Spastic muscle exhibits velocity-dependent increase in tonic stretch reflexes. The quicker the stretch, the more pronounced the resistance of the spastic muscle.

Specific compression: A nongliding neuromuscular technique in which pressure is applied to the target tissue with a specific contact surface in a direction that is perpendicular to the target tissue.

Specific kneading: A gliding petrissage technique performed in circles or ellipses and delivered with a small contact surface such as the thumb.

Specific technique: A technique that is applied to a localized area or applied with a small contact surface, or both.

Sports massage: Massage performed on athletes for the purpose of preparation, recovery, maintainance, or rehabilitation.

Static contact: A superficial reflex technique in which the clinician's hands contact the client's body without motion and with minimal force.

Stress response: The individual's cognitive, physiological, affective, or behavioral response to the stressor, or stress causing agent.

Stripping: A slow, specific, gliding, neuromuscular technique that is applied from the origin of a muscle to its insertion for the purpose of reducing the activity of trigger points.

Structural integration: A generic term for the massage systems descended from the work of Ida Rolf, whose practitioners use connective tissue techniques and education to realign clients' bodies in a series of 10 interventions.

Structure of care: The human, physical and financial resources that are available for the delivery of care.

Superficial effleurage: A gliding manipulation performed with light centripetal pressure that deforms subcutaneous tissue down to the investing layer of the deep fascia.

Superficial fascia: Connective tissue layer that is deep to the skin that houses fat and water; provides a path for nerves and vessels; and which may contain, in certain areas of the body, striated muscle that controls the movement of the skin, such as the platysma muscle.

Superficial fluid techniques: Massage techniques that are applied to tissues superficial to muscle that increase the return flow of lymph and possibly venous blood.

Superficial lymph drainage technique: A nongliding technique performed in the direction of lymphatic flow using short, rhythmical strokes with light pressure, which deforms subcutaneous tissue without engaging muscle.

Superficial reflex techniques: Massage techniques that palpate the skin and primarily affect level of arousal, autonomic balance, or the perception of pain.

Superficial stroking: A superficial reflex technique that involves unidirectional pressureless gliding over the client's skin with minimal deformation of subcutaneous tissues; usually applied over large areas.

Supports: Objects such as pillows and bolsters that are used to make the client more comfortable, stable, or accessible during massage.

Swedish Massage: A system of massage, consolidated by Per Henrik Ling (1776-1839), which includes effleurage, petrissage, friction, tapotement, and shaking (or vibration) and which constitutes one of the technical foundations for *Outcome-Based Massage.*

Swelling: An abnormal enlargement of a segment of the body.

Tapotement: *See* Percussion.

Tendinitis: Inflammation of the peritendinous tissues, which can occur in response to repetitive mechanical trauma.

Tendinosis: Unlike tendinitis, which is an inflammatory condition, tendinosis refers to common overuse conditions of tendon that have a histopathology that is consistent with a noninflammatory, degenerative process of unclear etiology.

Tension, or tensile force: Any force that is so oriented that its effect is to lengthen a tissue or structure.

Theory: An organized set of facts that explains the relationships between a group of observed phenomenon.

Thixotropy: The property of some colloids by which they become more fluid when subjected to movement or heat, and less fluid when subjected to stasis or cold.

Tissues engaged by technique: The target tissues or layers of tissue to which the clinician directs the pressure of the stroke and that are mechanically deformed by application of the technique.

Treatment: A series of interventions that make up an episode of care.

Tremors: Rhythmic movements of a joint that result from involuntary contractions of antagonist and agonist muscle groups.

Trigger point: *See* Myofascial trigger point.

Trigger point pain: Referred pain that arises in a trigger point, but is felt at a distance, often entirely remote from its source. The pattern of referred pain is diagnostic of the site of origin. The distribution of referred trigger point pain rarely coincides entirely with the distribution of a peripheral nerve or dermatomal segment.

Trigger point pressure release: Sustained specific compression applied to a trigger point to reduce its activity.

Visceral pain: Pain in areas of the viscera that are supplied by a nerve root.

Viscosity, or fluid viscosity: The property of fluids and semifluids that offers resistance to flow, i.e., stickiness.

Visco-elastic deformation: Deformation in response to applied force, which partially remains after the force is removed; visco-elastic deformation combines spring-like and putty-like behavior.

Wellness massage: General massage in which the main outcomes of care are the reduction of anxiety, stress response, and muscle resting tension.

Wringing: A petrissage technique in which muscle is lifted and sheared between contact surfaces that are moving in opposite directions.

Appendix B: Selected Soft-Tissue Examination Techniques

Assessment of Pain

Visual Analog scales, pain drawings, pain interviews, palpation and pressure algometry can be used to assess pain.

VISUAL ANALOG SCALE

The Visual Analog Scale (Fig. B-1) is a written rating scale of pain intensity that is widely used both clinically and in research because of the ease with which it can be administered.[1–3] The Visual Analog Scale (VAS) consists of a straight line measuring 10 cm in length. "No pain" is written at the left end of the line and 'the worst pain I have ever experienced' is written at the right end. Test-retest reliability for the VAS has been reported by Scott[4] as $r = 0.99$. Concurrent validity between the VAS and the Numeric Pain Rating Scale ranged between $r = 0.77$ to 0.91.[5]

STEPS IN ADMINISTERING THE VISUAL ANALOG SCALE

1. Explain the pain rating levels at either extreme of the scale to the client.
2. Ask the client to mark the line at the point that corresponds to the intensity of pain that she is experiencing at the time at which she is completing the VAS.
3. Measure the distance from the beginning of the line to the client's mark; this value represents the intensity of the client's pain.
4. On re-examination present the client with a new diagram rather than her previous pain rating.

THE PAIN DRAWING

The pain drawing is often used as a means of systematically guiding the client through a description of her pain and related symptoms. The pain drawing that a client produces on a body diagram can serve several purposes (Fig. B-2). First, it can also be used as an adjunct to the pain interview as a means of facilitating the client's discussion of her symptoms. It is a simple and reliable method of identifying the location of a client's pain and associated symptoms, such as paresthesia and tightness.[2] In addition, it can be used to guide treatment planning and to document the client's response to treatment.

STEPS IN USING THE PAIN DRAWING

1. Provide the client with a diagram of the human body (see Fig. B-2) and colored pens.
2. Explain the purpose of the pain drawing and any pre-defined symbols, such as dotted lines, that are used to represent pain and associated symptoms.
3. Inform the client what time period the pain drawing is intended to represent. For example, this may be pain and symptoms experienced over the previous 24 hours. This time period will vary with the nature of the client's clinical condition.
4. Ask the client to indicate on the diagram the location of any pain and associated symptoms that the client has experienced during the specified time period, using colors and predefined symbols. If the client is unable to complete this task independently, the clinician may provide the appropriate level of assistance.
5. When the client has completed the pain drawing, discuss the drawing to clarify and expand on the information that the client has provided. This may be done as part of the pain interview discussed below. Document this supplemental information on the pain drawing or elsewhere in the client's record. The section on general pain behavior in the pain interview notes some issues that may be worthy of additional attention, depending on the client's clinical condition. The clinician may wish to identify asymptomatic areas that are immediately adjacent to the symptomatic area on the pain drawing.

No pain   The worst pain I have ever experienced

Figure B-1. Visual Analog Scale for Pain Measurement

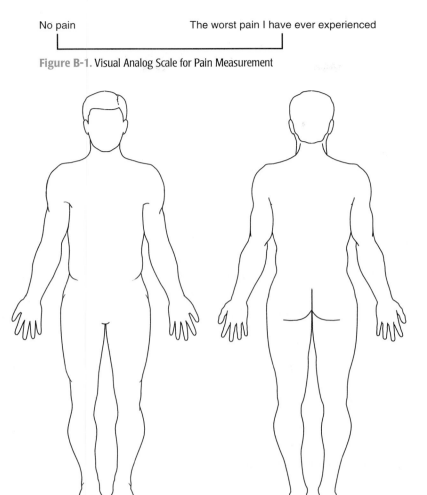

Figure B-2. Body diagram for the pain drawing.

THE PAIN INTERVIEW

Pain is a subjective experience; consequently, the pain interview is an important means of eliciting information on the different components of the client's experience of pain: pain intensity, pain location, pain behavior, and the client's response to pain.[2,6] Through the pain interview, the clinician can determine the nature of the client's symptoms and the behavior of the client's symptoms over a 24-hour period. General guidelines for a pain interview are outlined below; the clinician should modify the number of issues covered in the pain interview to be consistent with the clinical setting and the client's clinical condition. For example, a more-detailed pain interview may be more appropriate for a client with chronic back pain in an occupational medicine clinic than it would be for a client with an acute episode of shoulder pain. Readers are also referred to the texts on client examination for their health care profession for guidelines on

issues related to pain assessment for specific clinical conditions. The clinician can use the information from the pain interview during the Evaluative Phase to confirm or refute his hypothesis about the client's clinical condition. The pain interview findings can also be used to clarify the impact of the client's pain on her functional level and thus guide the identification of functional outcomes of care.

STEPS IN PERFORMING THE PAIN INTERVIEW
Location of Pain and 24-Hour Pain Behavior
Discuss the following issues with the client as a means of outlining the behavior of the client's pain over a 24-hour period. Bear in mind that the relevance of these issues will vary with the client's clinical condition.

1. Location of symptoms: The client clarifies any locations marked on the pain drawing that are unclear.

2. Priority of symptoms: The client distinguishes between primary and secondary symptoms that are noted on the pain drawing.

3. Nature of pain: The client selects a pain identifier, such stabbing or burning, that best describes the pain in a particular location.

4. Intensity of pain: The client defines the intensity of pain that has occurred during a specified time period. The clinician may use a numeric rating scale of 0 to 10, in which 0 represents the absence of pain and 10 represents the most pain the client has ever experienced, for this purpose.[2]

5. Additional symptoms: The client describes associated symptoms, such as paresthesia, that are noted on the diagram.

6. Frequency and duration of symptoms: The client indicates if pain is constant or intermittent. The client also indicates how frequently and for how long the symptoms occur. A distinction between the duration of symptoms that occur during the day and those at night may be relevant to the client's clinical condition. The frequency of the symptoms may be stated as a percentage, such as "50% of waking hours," or in relation to a time of day or an activity, such as "pain starts after 11:00 am and persists until bedtime," or "burning sensation occurs after 30 minutes of keyboarding."

Positions That Aggravate Pain

1. Ask the client to list the positions, such as sitting or standing, in which she notices an increase in her pain and associated symptoms.

2. For each position, elicit the following information:
   a. What is the time period for which the client can maintain the position before noticing that the symptoms start (or increase if there is a constant baseline level of pain)?
   b. What is the time period for which the client can maintain the position before the symptoms reach a level of intensity that causes her to move out of the position?
   c. When the symptoms are changed as a result of being in the position, what is the change in level of intensity of the symptoms (use the scale of 0 to 10 discussed above to show the difference)?
   d. Once the client's pain and other symptoms have been aggravated by the use of the position, what does the client do to ease these symptoms? For example, note the positions, modalities, exercises, and medication the client uses to ease pain.
   e. Once the client has moved out of the position and used some means of pain relief, how much time elapses before the client notices that the symptoms have returned to the original level?

Activities That Aggravate Pain

1. Ask the client to list the activities during which she notices an increase in her pain and associated symptoms. These activities can include:
   a. Self-care activities, such as grooming, feeding, and functional mobility.
   b. Community management activities (instrumental activities of daily living), such as driving, taking the bus, and grocery shopping.
   c. Work-related activities, such as lifting, keyboarding, and telephone use.
   d. Leisure activities, such as sexual activity, walking, watching television, and playing sports.
   e. Sleeping. Since clients' symptoms are frequently aggravated during sleep, this activity usually warrants additional discussion of issues, such as sleep position, bed type, and sleeping behavior.

2. For each activity, elicit the following information:
   a. What is the time period for which the client can perform the activity before noticing that the symptoms start (or increase if there is a constant baseline level of pain)?
   b. What is the time period for which the client can perform the activity before the symptoms reach a level of intensity that causes her to cease the activity?
   c. When the symptoms are changed as a result of performing the activity, what is the change in level of intensity of the symptoms (use the scale of 0 to 10 discussed above to show the difference)?
   d. Once the client's pain and other symptoms have been aggravated by the performance of the activity, what does the client do to ease these symptoms? For example, note the activities, modalities, exercises, and medication the client uses to ease the pain.
   e. Once the client has ceased the activity and used some means of pain relief, how much time elapses before the client notices that the symptoms have returned to the original level?

Self-Management

1. Ask the client to describe the strategies she uses to manage her symptoms. Include details of the frequency, duration, and effects of these activities.

2. Ask the client if she has received a self-care program in the past. Determine whether this is still being carried out. If so, discuss the frequency, duration, and effects of this self-care program.

Ergonomics

1. Ask the client to describe and demonstrate the following:
   a. Usual positions in which she performs her work

b. Any repetitive activities that are associated with performance of her job.

c. Positions that she uses at work that she feels are safe and comfortable.

d. Positions that she uses at work that she feels cause her pain.

e. Positions that she uses at work that she feels are adaptations to her pain or that she uses to minimize her pain.

2. Ask the client if the placement of the furniture and equipment in her work area appears to be contributing to her pain.

3. Ask if the client has had an ergonomic evaluation of her workplace by a qualified professional. If so, what were the results?

PALPATION FOR PAIN

Palpation can be used as a means of obtaining further information on the location of the client's pain and the sensitivity of the client's tissues.

STEPS IN PERFORMING PALPATION FOR PAIN

1. Ensure that your hands are warm and dry.

2. Position the client in a comfortable position in which the area to be palpated is readily accessible to you.

3. Drape the client appropriately (see Chapter 4, Preparation and Positioning for Treatment).

4. Explain the purpose of palpation and the procedures to be followed to the client.

5. Ask the client to inform you when she experiences tenderness, a referral of pain, tingling, or any other symptoms as a result of your palpation.

6. Select the location where you will begin palpation based on the client's reports of the locations of pain, patterns of referred pain, or areas of tissue tightness that may be contributing to a postural dysfunction.

7. Begin palpation using a light pressure. Gradually increase the depth of palpation since a rapid change of depth may elicit a guarding response.

8. As you palpate each location, ask the client if pressure on a given area causes any tenderness, localized pain, or referred pain. Move between locations slowly to avoid eliciting a painful spasm.

9. Observe the client for twitching, vasomotor responses, and changes in breathing.

10. As you progress with palpation, identify and palpate areas in which there are abnormalities of tissue texture, such as bogginess or taut tissue bands (see the section on palpation in Chapter 3, Review of Client Examination Concepts for Massage).

11. If palpation with light pressure does not reproduce the client's symptoms or the results of this palpation

are inconclusive, then increase the depth of palpation and repeat the process.

12. In addition to palpating the locations of pain the client has reported, you may also wish to palpate the following:

a. Trigger points that may refer to the painful areas

b. Related dermatomes

c. Related sclerotomes

13. Document all locations in which the client's symptoms are reproduced by palpation, and note the patterns of referred pain that result from palpation.

Note: Tenderness on palpation of a given area may be referred from another area and may not be a reliable finding. The clinician is advised to corroborate the findings of palpation for pain with other clinical tests and measures.

MEASURING TISSUE SENSITIVITY USING A PRESSURE ALGOMETER OR PAIN THRESHOLD METER

Tissue sensitivity to pressure can be measured using a pain threshold meter or pressure algometer. There are a variety of types of pressure algometers available. Typically, these devices consist of a component that is used to apply pressure, such as a hard rubber tip, that is attached to a pressure (force) gauge. The dial of the gauge shows pressure readings, often in kg/cm^2 or lb/cm^2. Pressure sensitivity readings are obtained by applying a gradually increasing force on the client's tissues with the algometer and noting the pressure reading at the point at which the client reports experiencing pain or discomfort. Reeves et al. [7] found that interrater reliability for pressure algometer scores had values for intraclass correlations of greater than $r = 0.78$, while Delaney and McKee[8] reported Pearson correlation coefficients of $r > 0.82$. The pressure algometer is valuable for documenting and re-assessing the effects of trigger point therapy and other interventions that change tissue sensitivity, since it provides a means of quantifying the client's subjective complaints.

STEPS IN PERFORMING TISSUE SENSITIVITY TESTING

1. Stand in a position that will enable you to apply an even pressure to the client's tissues when the pressure algometer is positioned perpendicular to the client's skin.

2. Position the client in a relaxed and well-supported position.

3. Explain the overall procedure to the client, and demonstrate the application of the pressure algometer on an unaffected area of the client's body. In particular, instruct the client to say "yes" when she first feels discomfort, and explain that you will cease

the application of pressure as soon as she does so, so that she does not experience undue discomfort. Explain that rubor and capillary breakage can occur following tissue sensitivity testing with a pressure algometer, and provide basic instructions for the application of ice to the areas that were tested if this occurs.[9]

4. Identify the location where you want to test tissue sensitivity. For example, in the case of a trigger point, palpate for a taut band and an area of tenderness in the location specified for that trigger point. Once you have located the area to be tested, you may wish to mark it.

5. Ensure that the pressure gauge is at zero. Place the contact surface of the pressure algometer on the location to be tested.

6. Hold the pressure algometer so that the shaft of the instrument is at a 90° angle to the surface of the client's skin.

7. Using your free hand, gradually apply pressure on the client's tissues with the pressure algometer. Continue to increase the pressure gradually until the client reports feeling discomfort.

8. Cease applying pressure as soon as the client reports discomfort, and note the pressure algometer reading that was recorded at that point.

9. Reset the gauge to zero prior to the next episode of testing.

Assessment of Scarring

Palpation, photography, and linear measurements can be used to assess scarring.

STEPS IN PERFORMING PALPATION OF SCARRING

1. Position the client so that the scar is not in a stretched position and is readily accessible to you.

2. Explain the purpose of palpation and the procedures to be followed to the client. In particular, instruct the client to indicate when she feels any discomfort, and explain that you will cease the application of pressure as soon as she does so, so that she does not experience undue discomfort. This is especially important if the client has reported that the scar is painful.

3. Begin palpation using a light pressure. Gradually increase the depth of palpation.

4. As you palpate the scar, identify differences in the mobility of the scar tissue and areas in which the scar appears to be adherent to tissues that are adjacent to

or deep to it. The scar should move as freely as the surrounding tissues. Document this information using the positions of a clock, (e.g., 3:00 versus 6:00) to describe the relative positions of sections of the scar.

5. Ask the client to report when she experiences pain at the site of the scar or elsewhere during palpation. Movement of the scar should be pain free.

6. Identify areas of the scar that are puckered, and document this information.

7. Adjuncts to palpation as means of assessing changes in the dimensions of scars include the measurement of the depth of the scar using a ruler and photography. The clinician is advised to follow his facility's guidelines for obtaining the client's written permission for photographs.

Assessment of Posture

Soft tissues exert a stress on bony structures; consequently, pathological changes in the tension of muscles and connective tissue can affect bony alignment. The purpose of the postural analysis is, therefore, to document both soft tissue and bony structure and alignment. This information provides objective data that can be used to corroborate or refute findings from other examination techniques and the client's functional limitations and to assist in the identification of appropriate outcomes of care (Box B-1). Visual analysis and accompanying palpation are the commonly used approaches to postural analysis. Photographs and videotapes, which facilitate documentation of posture, are also useful adjuncts to this approach.

CLINICIAN'S POSITION FOR THE POSTURAL ANALYSIS

ANTERIOR VIEW

The clinician is positioned directly in front of the client at a distance of approximately 8 to 15 ft for the examination of the anterior view with the client in standing or sitting. If the client is in supine, the clinician is positioned at the foot of the treatment table (standing upon a stool may offer a clearer view).

POSTERIOR VIEW

The clinician is positioned directly behind the client at a distance of approximately 8 to 15 ft for the examination of the posterior view with the client in standing or sitting. If the client is in prone, the clinician is positioned at the foot of the treatment table (standing upon a stool may offer a clearer view).

LATERAL VIEW

The clinician is positioned to the side of the client in alignment with the client's external auditory meatus for the examination of the lateral view with the client in standing or sitting. If the client is in sidelying, the clinician is positioned at the side of the treatment table (standing upon a stool may offer a clearer view). Standing at the side of the treatment table may provide a less-obstructed view of the client's upper body than the anterior view, if the client has a large abdomen or considerable amounts of pectoral or breast tissue.

CLIENT'S POSITION FOR THE POSTURAL ANALYSIS

Observation of the client from different views and in different positions can provide the clinician with a greater understanding of the client's postural alignment. For example, a client whose postural alignment differs in standing versus supine may have a pelvic malalignment, a leg-length discrepancy, muscular weakness, or an impaired postural awareness. In addition, the clinician can also determine whether the client has a pelvic malalignment or a leg-length discrepancy by comparing the client's postural alignment in sitting and standing. If the client is nonambulatory, the clinician may use sitting and supine for this purpose.

STEPS IN PERFORMING A POSTURAL ANALYSIS

1. Ask the client to remove her shoes and to don clothing or a gown that will permit viewing of landmarks while ensuring appropriate draping.
2. Select a view to be assessed, for example the anterior view, and identify the appropriate position for doing so.
3. Position the posture grid or plumb line.
4. Position the client in relation to the posture grid or plumb line so that the selected view of the client is unobstructed and the posture grid or plumb line provides an appropriate frame of reference.
5. Ask the client to assume a relaxed posture, rather than what she thinks is "good" posture. Allow the client to settle into that position for a minute to get a more accurate representation of her usual posture. If this is painful, then decrease the amount of time the client spends in this position.
6. Assume the appropriate position from which to observe the landmarks for the selected view.
7. Perform the visual inspection of the selected view, identifying the positions of the landmarks for the selected view noted below and noting the symmetry of body contours and muscle bulk throughout the client's body. Perform a bilateral comparison wherever this is appropriate.

8. Confirm or refute the findings of visual analysis with palpation.
9. Document the findings of visual analysis.
10. Note findings are an indication for further client examination using other tests and measures.
11. Reposition the client for the next view to be assessed.

LANDMARKS FOR POSTURAL ANALYSIS[6,10–16]

Note the positions of the following landmarks, and assess the symmetry of body contours and muscle bulk throughout the body. Landmarks that occur bilaterally should be symmetrical. These landmarks can be viewed with the client in standing or lying. When the client is in sitting, assess the landmarks listed for all areas that are readily visible. In addition, note the degree of hip abduction in sitting.

ANTERIOR VIEW

Head and Neck
1. Orientation of the end of the nose with the manubrium, xiphoid process, and umbilicus (the umbilicus is often not in vertical alignment with these other landmarks)
2. Vertical alignment of the head; for example, excessive lateral flexion or rotation
3. Level of the eyes
4. Vertical alignment of the jaw
5. Contours of the trapezius muscle

Upper Extremities
1. Carrying angle of elbows (5 to 15° is the normal range of the carrying angle for an elbow)
2. Levels of hands (used in identifying asymmetrical shoulder levels)
3. Direction of palms (used in identifying asymmetrical shoulder rotation)

Trunk
1. Trunk in vertical alignment: Note asymmetry of skin folds or the distances of the client's arms to her trunk
2. Level of acromioclavicular joints
3. Level and length of clavicles
4. Sternum and costicartilage aligned: Note superior, inferior, or lateral deviations of these landmarks
5. Ribs aligned and symmetrical bilaterally
6. Differences in weight bearing on the lower extremities as reflected by the position of the trunk over the extremities

Lower Extremities and Pelvis
1. Levels of the anterior superior iliac spines
2. Torsion of the tibia or femurs

3. Orientation of the knees; for example, varus or valgus
4. Orientation of the patellae
5. Levels of the fibular heads
6. Levels of lateral malleoli
7. Levels of the medial malleoli
8. Foot angle (10° of external rotation or toeing out is normal)
9. Orientation of the arches of the feet (e.g., neutral, pronated, supinated, pes cavus, or pes planus) with the feet in their usual posture and then with the great toes aligned. If the client wears orthotics, it may be appropriate to observe foot position with the client wearing shoes.

LATERAL VIEW

1. Deviation from an imaginary vertical line running through the following landmarks: earlobe, through the bodies of the cervical vertebrae, through the acromion process, through the lumbar vertebrae, through the highest point of the iliac crest, through the hip joint, anterior to the knee joint, anterior to the ankle joint
2. Position of the glenohumeral joint
3. Position of the sternum: Note if it is overly prominent or depressed
4. Tilt of the pelvis
5. Alignment of the knees: Note recurvatum, or excessive flexion

POSTERIOR VIEW

Head and Neck
Vertical alignment of the head

Upper Extremities
Level of the shoulders

Trunk

1. Levels and alignment of the spines and inferior angles of the scapulae (the scapulae should rest on the thorax between the levels of T2 and T8. Note if the scapulae are abducted, adducted, elevated, or depressed.
2. Position of the scapulae against the thorax: Note if they are winging.
3. Distance of the vertebral borders of the scapulae from the thoracic vertebrae.
4. Vertical alignment of the spine: Note any lateral curvature.
5. Distance between the 12th rib and the iliac crest.

Lower Extremities and Pelvis

1. Level of the iliac crests
2. Level of the posterior superior iliac spines

> ### Box B-1
> ### *Incorporating Postural Data into Outcomes of Care*
>
> ***Subjective findings:*** Client reports pain after performing keyboarding tasks for 5 min
>
> ***Objective findings:*** Client has an anterior head posture—earlobe is 2.5 cm anterior to the acromion
>
> ***Evaluation:*** Client's anterior head position is biomechanically inefficient, decreases her endurance in performing keyboarding tasks, and contributes to her pain as a result of excessive loading of the posterior cervical and shoulder musculature. Correction of the soft-tissue restrictions that contribute to this posture may reduce the client's complaints of pain and facilitate enhanced alignment of head and cervical spine, biomechanical efficiency, and work tolerance.
>
> ***Functional outcome of care:*** Client will be able to perform keyboarding tasks for 30 continuous minutes without complaints of pain with the earlobe in vertical alignment over the acromion.

3. Levels of the gluteal folds
4. Levels of the knee joints
5. Angle of Achilles tendons (should be vertical)
6. Position of hind foot with the feet in their usual posture and then with the great toes aligned. If the client wears orthotics, it may be appropriate to observe foot position with the client wearing shoes. Note if the hindfoot is in varus or valgus.

Note

Pelvic malalignment or a small hemipelvis can present as changes in thoracic alignment in sitting. In addition, a more-detailed examination of pelvic misalignment may be warranted if the client's anterior superior iliac spines or posterior superior iliac spines are asymmetrical. Clinicians are referred to sources on the detailed examination of pelvic alignment.[10–15]

Assessment of Trigger Points

Trigger points are commonly implicated in a wide variety of musculoskeletal conditions and myofascial pain syndromes (see Chapter 7, Neuromuscular Techniques).[15,16]

STEPS IN PERFORMING PALPATION FOR TRIGGER POINTS [15,16]

1. Explain the purpose of palpation and the procedures to be followed to the client.
2. Ask the client to inform you when she experiences tenderness, a referral of pain, tingling, or any other symptoms as a result of your palpation.
3. Determine the muscle to be palpated for the presence of trigger points. This may include a review of the client's reported pain behavior in the subjective examination for references to possible trigger-point referral zones. In addition, muscles in which the range of motion was limited on examination are other potential locations of trigger points.
4. Ensure that your hands are warm and dry.
5. Position the client with the muscle to be examined in a position that is approximately two-thirds of its normal stretch position. Refer to *Myofascial Pain and Dysfunction*[15,16] for the positions in which specific trigger points are tested.
6. Drape the client appropriately (see Chapter 4, Preparation and Positioning for Treatment).
7. Ensure that the client is warm and the muscle to be palpated is relaxed.
8. Identify the possible location of the trigger point.
9. Palpate the location of the trigger point using one of the following approaches:
   a. Flat palpation: Slide your finger or thumb along the taut band in the client's muscle until the client reports that you have reached the location of maximum tenderness that represents the trigger point.
   b. Pincer palpation: This is used for muscles that can be lifted easily. Grasp the belly of the muscle between your finger and thumb. Squeeze and roll the muscle tissue between your fingers to locate the taut band in the muscle. This maneuver can be repeated along the muscle belly until the trigger point is located.
   c. Snapping palpation: Once you locate the taut band using pincer palpation, roll the taut band quickly under your fingers to produce a local twitch response.
10. During palpation, determine if the following are present:
    a. Taut bands. The fiber direction (as well as the pain referral pattern) will permit identification of the involved muscle.
    b. Local hardness. The trigger point itself may present as a very small area of focal hardness (palpable nodule) in the taut band. Compress this area against the underlying tissues, and determine whether the characteristic pain referral pattern for the trigger point in question is reproduced.
    c. Twitch responses. Twitch responses may be palpated in superficial muscles.
    d. Jump sign. A client may produce a large involuntary contraction and other gross affective signs of pain if the trigger point is palpated too forcefully.
    e. Generalized hardness. If there are adjacent trigger points in overlapping layers as, for example, what commonly occurs between the scapulae, the clinician may find it difficult to palpate anything other than a generalized hardness.
11. During palpation, have the client compare the pain produced by palpating the trigger point with her presenting symptoms. The client should be able to recognize the pattern of pain referral if the trigger point is in fact the contributing cause of her pain.

References

1. Cole B, Finch E, Gowland C, Mayo N. Physical rehabilitation outcome measures. Ontario, Canada: Canadian Physiotherapy Association, 1994:80–81.
2. Ross RG, LaStayo PC. Clinical assessment of pain. In: Van Deusen J, Brunt D, eds. Assessment in occupational therapy and physical therapy. Philadelphia: WB Saunders, 1997.
3. Cohen H, Pertes R. Diagnosis and management of fascial pain. In: Rachlin ES, ed. Myofascial pain and fibromyalgia: trigger point management. St. Louis: Mosby–Year Book 1994:361–382.
4. Scott J, Huskisson E. Vertical or horizontal visual analogue scales. Ann Rheum Dis 1979;10:38–56.
5. Downie W, Leatham P, Rhind V, et al. Studies with pain rating scales. Ann Rheum Dis 1978;37:378–381.
6. Magee DJ. Orthopedic physical assessment. Philadelphia: WB Saunders, 1997.
7. Reeves J, Jaeger B, Graff-Radford S. Reliability of the pressure algometer as a measure of myofascial trigger point sensitivity. Pain 1986;24:313–321.
8. Delaney G, McKee A. Inter- and intra-rater reliability of the pressure threshold meter in measurement of myofascial trigger point sensitivity. Am J Phys Med Rehabil 1993;72: 136–139.
9. Swift T, Brescia N. Intra and inter-rater reliability of pressure algometer measurements taken by student physical therapists. Unpublished masters research paper. Oakland, CA: Samuel Merritt College, 1997.
10. Kisner C, Colby LA. Therapeutic exercise: foundations and techniques. 3rd ed. Philadelphia: FA Davis, 1996.
11. Greenman PE. Principles of manual medicine. 2nd ed. Baltimore: Williams and Wilkins, 1996:43.

12. Rolf IP. Rolfing®: the integration of human structure. New York: Harper and Row, 1977.
13. Hertling D, Kessler RM. Management of common musculoskeletal disorders. 3rd ed. Philadelphia: Lippincott-Raven, 1996.
14. DiGiovanna EL, Schiowitz S. An osteopathic approach to diagnosis and treatment. 2nd ed. Philadelphia: Lippincott-Raven, 1997.
15. Simons DG, Travell JG, Simons LS. Travell and Simons' myofascial pain and dysfunction: the trigger point manual vol. 2: lower half of body. 2nd ed. Baltimore: Williams and Wilkins, 1999.
16. Simons DG, Travell JG, Simons LS. Travell and Simons' myofascial pain and dysfunction: the trigger point manual vol. 1: upper half of body. 2nd ed. Baltimore: Williams and Wilkins, 1999.

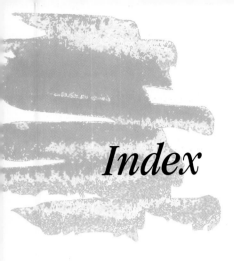

Index

Page numbers in *italics* denote figures; Those followed by a "t" denote tables; Those followed by a "b" denote boxes.